Human Biology and Health: An Evolutionary Approach

Edited by Basiro Davey, Tim Halliday and Mark Hirst

Published by Open University Press

Written and produced by The Open University

Health and Disease Series, Book 4

OPEN UNIVERSITY PRESS

Buckingham • Philadelphia

The U205 *Health and Disease* Course Team

The following members of the Open University teaching staff and external colleagues have collaborated with the authors in writing this book, or have commented extensively on it during its production. We accept collective responsibility for its overall academic and teaching content.

Basiro Davey (Course Team Chair, Senior Lecturer in Health Studies, Department of Biological Sciences)

Helen Dolk (Professor of Epidemiology and Health Services Research, School of Health Sciences, University of Ulster)

Tim Halliday (Professor of Biology)

Mark Hirst (Lecturer in Human Genetics, Department of Biological Sciences)

Heather McLannahan (Senior Counsellor, Science Faculty)

Kevin McConway (Senior Lecturer in Statistics)

Judith Metcalfe (Senior Lecturer and Staff Tutor, Department of Biological Sciences)

Caroline Pond (Reader in Biology, Department of Biological Sciences)

The following people have contributed to the development of particular parts or aspects of this book.

Gail Block (BBC producer)

Heather Davies (electronmicroscopist)

Sheila Dunleavy (editor)

Rebecca Graham (editor)

Alastair Gray (critical reader), Director, Health Economics Research Centre, Institute of Health Sciences, Oxford University

Celia Hart (picture researcher)

Pam Higgins (designer)

Jean Macqueen (indexer)

Jennifer Nockles (designer)

Philip Payne (critical reader), Visiting Professor of Nutrition, Department of Nutrition and Food Science, School of Biological and Molecular Sciences, Oxford Brookes University

Rissa de la Paz (BBC producer)

Denise Rowe (course secretary)

John Taylor (graphic artist)

Joy Wilson (course manager)

Authors

The following people have acted as principal or co-authors for the chapters listed below.

Chapters 1, 3, 5 and 6

Basiro Davey, Senior Lecturer in Health Studies, Department of Biological Sciences, The Open University.

Chapters 2 and 7

Caroline Pond, Reader in Biology, Department of Biological Sciences, The Open University.

Chapters 3 and 5

Tim Halliday, Professor of Biology, Department of Biological Sciences, The Open University.

Chapters 4 and 9

Mark Hirst, Lecturer in Human Genetics, and Judith Metcalfe, Senior Lecturer and Staff Tutor, both in Department of Biological Sciences, The Open University.

Chapter 8

Heather McLannahan (Senior Counsellor, Science Faculty)

Chapters 10 and 11

Helen Dolk, Professor of Epidemiology and Health Services Research, School of Health Sciences, University of Ulster.

External assessors

Course assessors

Professor James McEwen, Henry Mechan Chair of Public Health and Head of Department of Public Health, University of Glasgow.

Professor John Gabbay, Professor of Public Health Medicine, University of Southampton, and Director of the Wessex Institute for Health Research and Development.

Book 4 assessor

Professor Lewis Wolpert, Professor of Biology as Applied to Medicine, Department of Anatomy and Developmental Biology, University College and Middlesex School of Medicine, London.

Acknowledgements

The Course Team and the authors wish to thank the following people who, as contributors to previous editions of this book, made a lasting impact on the structure and philosophy of the present volume.

Steve Best, Nick Black, Geoff Einon, Gerald Elliott, John Greenwood, Richard Holmes, Rosemary Lennard, Perry Morley, Jennie Popay, Rob Ransom, Steven Rose, Phil Strong.

Cover images

Background: Nebulae in the Rho Ophiuchi region (Source: Anglo-Australian Observatory/Royal Observatory Edinburgh). *Middleground*: Globe (Source: Mountain High Map™, Digital Wisdom, Inc). *Foreground*: Chromosomes from a human male which have been chemically treated and coloured using chromosome-specific 'paints' to reveal their banding patterns. (Source: L. Willatt, East Anglian Genetics Service/Science Photo Library)

Open University Press, Celtic Court, 22 Ballmoor,
Buckingham, MK18 1XW.

e-mail: enquiries@openup.co.uk

website: www.openup.co.uk

and

325 Chestnut Street, Philadelphia, PA 19106, USA.

First published 1985. Completely revised second edition
published 1994.

This revised full-colour third edition published 2001.

A catalogue record of the book is available from the
British Library.

Library of Congress Cataloging-in-Publication Data is
available

Edited, designed and typeset by the Open University.

Printed and bound in the United Kingdom by the Alden
Group, Oxford.

ISBN 0335 20839 8

This publication forms part of an Open University level 2
course, U205 *Health and Disease*. The complete list of
texts which make up this course can be found on the
back cover. Details of this and other Open University
courses can be obtained from the Call Centre,
PO Box 724, The Open University, Milton Keynes
MK7 6ZS, United Kingdom: tel. +44 (0)1908 653231,
e-mail ces-gen@open.ac.uk

Alternatively, you may visit the Open University website
at http://www.open.ac.uk where you can learn more
about the wide range of courses and packs offered at all
levels by the Open University.

3.1

Contents

A note for the general reader

Human Biology and Health: An Evolutionary Approach presents an evolutionary history of human health and disease, starting from the premise that patterns of resistance and susceptibility to illness and disability in modern human populations have been influenced by the biological and cultural evolution of the human species over the last five million years. The book focuses on the evolution of infectious, genetic and degenerative diseases and emphasises the degree of variation in susceptibility between individuals and between human populations. The authors are biologists who have written an introduction to human biology that is accessible to a general readership, but which aims to teach some fundamental aspects of the subject, from the structure of DNA and the nature of genes to the physiology of the whole organism and its interaction with the surrounding cultural and physical environment. However, this is not a book aimed exclusively at biology students, but at anyone with an interest in human social organisation and cultural development who wishes to add a biological dimension to their studies.

After an introductory chapter, Chapter 2 describes early human evolution and considers the impact of human cultural developments, such as the farming of grains and domestic animals, on human health. Chapter 3 is a speculative account of the origins of life on Earth, interwoven with a basic introduction to the structure and activity of human cells and the genetic code, and the theory of evolution by natural selection. Chapter 4 extends the discussion of normal genetic variation between individuals and populations and focuses on the inheritance of characteristics that affect health. In Chapter 5, we consider the long evolutionary history of close human contact with other organisms such as bacteria and larger parasites, and in Chapter 6 we describe the defence mechanisms which have evolved in response to the threat of infection. Chapter 7 describes human digestion and the absorption of nutrients and examines the interaction between cultural changes in the composition of the diet and the biological evolution of the digestive system. In Chapter 8, we investigate the mechanisms that underlie the ageing process and ask 'Why do we die?'.

In the final chapters of the book, the authors turn their attention towards the future. Biomedical technology promises to offer partial solutions to a few major health problems and Chapter 9 discusses the implications of transplanting cells and organs from person to person, and of the newest techniques aimed at manipulating human genes. Chapter 10 focuses on the chemical industrial environment and its possible impact on the global environment and on human health. The book ends in Chapter 11 with the suggestion that the pace of cultural change is now seriously challenging human capacity to evolve genetic and cultural adaptations to maintain and improve health.

The book is fully indexed and referenced and contains a list of abbreviations and an annotated guide to further reading and to selected websites on the Internet. The list of further sources also includes details of how to access a regularly updated collection of Internet resources relevant to the *Health and Disease* series on a searchable database called ROUTES, which is maintained by the Open University. This resource is open to all readers of this book.

Human Biology and Health: An Evolutionary Approach is the fourth in a series of eight books on the subject of health and disease. The book is designed so that it can be read on its own, like any other textbook, or studied as part of U205 *Health and Disease*, a level 2 course for Open University students. General readers do not need to make use of the Study notes, learning objectives and other material inserted for

OU students, although they may find these helpful. The text also contains references to a collection of previously published material and specially commissioned articles (*Health and Disease: A Reader*, Open University Press, second edition 1994; third edition 2001) prepared for the OU course: it is quite possible to follow the text without reading the articles referred to, although doing so will enhance your understanding of the contents of *Human Biology and Health: An Evolutionary Approach*.

Abbreviations used in this book

ADD	adenosine deaminase deficiency
AIDS	acquired immunodeficiency syndrome
ALARA principle	as low as is reasonably achievable
ATP	adenosine triphosphate
B cell	bone-marrow derived lymphocyte
BATNEEC principle	best available technology not entailing excessive cost
BSE	bovine spongiform encephalopathy
CF	cystic fibrosis
CFCs	chlorofluorocarbons
CHD	coronary heart disease
CVS	chorionic villi sampling
DNA	deoxyribonucleic acid
GM	genetically modified
HFEA	Human Fertilisation and Embryology Authority
HGAC	Human Genetics Advisory Commission
HGC	Human Genetics Commission
HGP	Human Genome Project
HIV	human immunodeficiency virus
HRT	hormone replacement therapy
IVF	*in vitro* fertilisation
MDR	multi-drug resistant (strains of bacteria)
mRNA	messenger RNA
NHS	National Health Service
NIH	National Institute of Health
NK cell	natural killer cell
OPCS	Office of Population Censuses and Surveys
PCBs	polychlorinated biphenyls
PKU	phenylketonuria
RNA	ribonucleic acid
STD	sexually transmitted disease
T cell	thymus-derived lymphocyte
TB	tuberculosis
TCP	trichlorophenol
UV	ultraviolet (radiation)
UV-B	a particular band of UV radiation
vCJD	variant Creutzfeldt–Jakob disease
WHO	World Health Organisation

Study guide for OU students

(total around 64 hours, including time for the TMA, spread over 4 weeks)

Chapters 1 and 11 are very short, but the other chapters vary considerably in length; Chapters 8 and 10 are the shortest of the central chapters and Chapters 3, 4 and 9 are the longest. The earlier chapters introduce the largest number of new terms and concepts; the later chapters extend and reinforce material taught earlier in the book. You should pace your study accordingly.

1st week

Chapter 1	**Why 'an evolutionary approach'?**
Chapter 2	**The human biological heritage** Reader article by Bogin (1993); revise Reader article by Diamond (1992)
Chapter 3	**The story of life in a few pages** TV programme 'Bloodlines: A family legacy' is relevant to Chapters 3, 4 and 9

2nd week

Chapter 4	**Inheritance and variation** TV programme 'Bloodlines: A family legacy'
Chapter 5	**Living with other species**
Chapter 6	**Surviving infectious disease** revise Reader article by Strassburg (1982)

3rd week

Chapter 7	**Digestion and dietary change**
Chapter 8	**On living longer**
Chapter 9	**Tinkering with nature** Reader articles by McGowan (1999), Müller-Hill (1993), Watson (2000); audiotape 'Tinkering with nature'; TV programme 'Bloodlines: A family legacy'

4th week

Chapter 10	**Living with the chemical industrial environment** Reader article by Epstein (1999)
Chapter 11	**The impact of modern culture** Reader article by Jones (1993)
TMA completion	

Human Biology and Health: An Evolutionary Approach presents the study of human biology as a dynamic evolutionary process which cannot be understood except in the context of human cultural evolution. It builds on knowledge of biomedical research methods discussed in *Studying Health and Disease*, and of human epidemiology described in *World Health and Disease*; in turn, it informs the development of biological themes in two later books in this series, *Birth to Old Age: Health in Transition* and *Experiencing and Explaining Disease.* The structure of the book is outlined in the 'Note for the general reader' (p. 6), and is described further in Chapter 1.

Study notes are given at the start of every chapter. These primarily direct you to important links to other components of the course, such as the other books in the course series, the Reader, and audiovisual components. Major learning objectives are listed at the end of each chapter, along with questions that will enable you to check that you have achieved these objectives. The index includes key terms in orange type (also printed in bold in the text), which can be easily looked up as an aid to revision as the course proceeds. There is also a list of further sources for those who wish to pursue certain aspects of study beyond the scope of this book, either by consulting other books and articles or by logging on to specialist websites on the Internet.

The time allowed for studying *Human Biology and Health: An Evolutionary Approach* is around 64 hours spread over 4 weeks. The schedule (left) gives a more detailed breakdown to help you to pace your study. You need not follow it rigidly, but try not to let yourself fall behind. Depending on your background and experience, you may well find some parts of this book much more familiar and straightforward than others. If you find a section of the work difficult, do what you can at this stage, and then return to reconsider the material when you reach the end of the book.

There is a tutor-marked assignment (TMA) associated with this book; about 5 hours have been allowed for writing it up, *in addition to* the time spent studying the material it assesses.

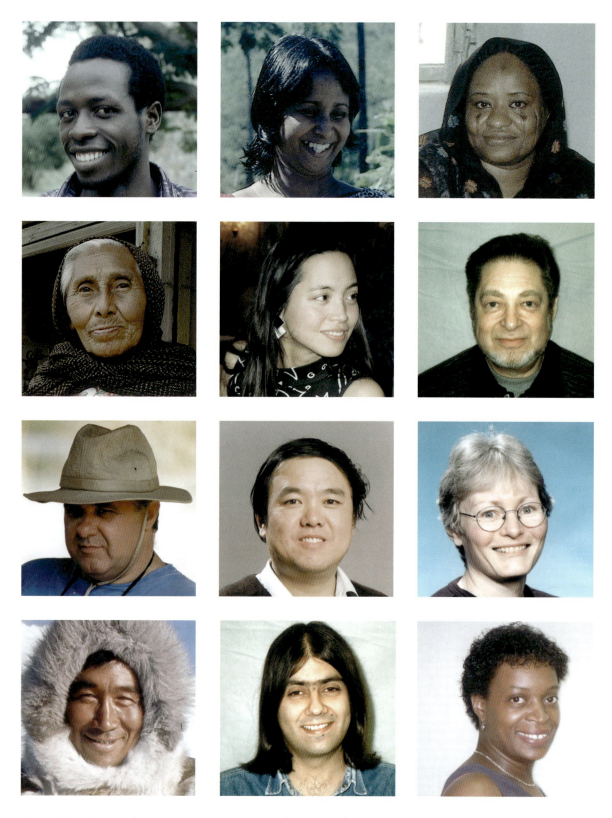

Figure 1.1 *Humans display exceptional variation in their outward appearance, which is matched by invisible variations between individuals in the activity of the molecules, cells and organs of which their bodies are composed. Yet these varied individuals are members of a single species,* Homo sapiens. *(Photos: (bottom left-hand image) Camera Press; (other images) Marion Hall, Mike Levers, Caroline Pond, Jonathan Silvertown, Tina Wardhaugh, Mike Wibberley)*

CHAPTER 1

Why 'an evolutionary approach'?

1.1   An unusual approach to human biology

1.1.1   Why study biology?

This book about human biology is rather unusual for several reasons. First, the authors have assumed that the readers don't know any biology beyond the most rudimentary general knowledge that organisms come in many different shapes and sizes and all are composed of cells made from lots of different chemicals. Anything else you need to know is taught within the pages of this book. We are aware that some readers will already know a lot of biology, but we confidently expect that the unconventional structure of this book will shed a novel and interesting light on the presentation even of familiar terms and concepts.

Second, we have kept in the forefront of our minds the question 'Why does a non-biologist interested in human health need to know this bit of biology?'. With so much to choose from in the vast field of biological knowledge, what has guided our selection of certain aspects for attention here? To some extent our selection reflects the interests and expertise of the contributors, but our guiding principle has been to focus on the unique contribution that a study of biology can bring to a modern understanding of human health and disease. For example, it gives an important insight into the susceptibility and resistance to illness of individuals and populations, and why they vary between people and places. Biological explanations are among the most compelling for fluctuations in the patterns of disease that human populations display across long time periods and between geographical locations, and during the span of each life from birth to old age.

For many people, biology is a daunting and impenetrable subject, principally because conventional teaching texts are crammed with new terms and detailed explanations of complex mechanisms. We have attempted to side-step that approach by 'telling stories' wherever possible and keeping the terminology to an essential minimum. As a result, there are plenty of gaps in the details, but we hope this sacrifice ensures that you reach the end of the book with an understanding of the 'big picture' of human health and disease from a biological vantage-point.

Biological phenomena intrude into people's lives constantly and in many diverse ways. When we catch a cold or suffer heart disease we are experiencing biological changes, which are shared by at least some other animals. Understanding such events from a biological standpoint gives us insights that are not provided by a purely medical approach. There is a more general point here, too. The authors of this book believe that there is a need for greater 'scientific literacy' in our society. We find it odd that an 'educated' person is expected to know who wrote *Romeo and Juliet*, for example, but is not generally expected to understand the essential properties of DNA, the chemical that influences every aspect of our biology, and hence our lives, and about which you will learn a great deal in this book.

1.1.2 Biological and cultural evolution

The third unusual aspect of this book is that we have taken *evolution*, of humans and of other living things, as the 'backbone' of the story. It is a constant theme running through every chapter and the ultimate purpose of all the descriptions of mechanisms and molecules is to illuminate this theme. We are interested in discovering how and why the human species has arrived at the highly successful body structure and internal activity that it presently enjoys, and how and why that same body is prey to certain characteristic illnesses and disabilities. These are questions that biologists can only partially answer and about which there is much dispute, so you can expect to be challenged by uncertainty in this book as much as in all the others in this series. But there is one basic certainty: the conviction among the authors that the humans we see today are the consequence of several million years of evolution from ancestral species. In adhering to this central dogma of modern biology, we mean no offence to readers who reject evolution in favour of divine creation, but we have to disagree.

However, we have broken with traditional biology by using a very broad definition of **human evolution**. We take it to mean 'gradual changes over successive generations in the biological *and* the cultural development of the human species'. Though biological and cultural evolution have both been very important in shaping modern humans, they are very different processes, as we discuss in later chapters of this book. Cultural evolution does not usually figure at all in conventional biological texts. Note that our definition of human evolution does not imply a linear progression from simple to complex, either in the form and function of human biology nor of human culture. Change does not march forward on a united front: as some aspects become more complex, so others simplify; the gains of one age can be reversed by the next. But, like the Spanish-American philosopher and poet, George Santayana, we believe that:

> The tide of evolution carries everything before it, thoughts no less than bodies, and persons no less than nations. (Santayana, Little Essays, number 44, quoted in Daintith and Isaacs, 1989, p. 68)

1.1.3 Ethical considerations

A further unusual feature of this book is its emphasis on questions of ethics. As the pace of acquisition of new biological knowledge hots up and new techniques for manipulating human biology are developed, individual members of society are faced with the ethical implications of such developments. Moreover, cultural change continues to have profound effects on the environment and on human health which have provoked discussion of the ethics of industrialisation, deforestation, pollution and population growth. In this book, we join the ethical debate by identifying major causes of concern about the development of biological science — particularly genetics — and certain aspects of human culture (such as industrialisation) and their possible impact on the future health of the human species. We do not claim any special expertise in ethics, nor have we attempted to reach a judgement about the rights and wrongs of any issue. We have written simply from the viewpoint of biologists who are personally concerned to disseminate relevant information and encourage non-biologists to become engaged in the debate.

1.2 Distant origins and future prospects

With the overview of the general approach taken in this book in mind, we can look briefly at the individual chapters in the sequence in which you will study them. Broadly speaking, the book begins in the distant past, considers the present situation of humans and, finally, looks forward to the future.

Chapter 2, 'The human biological heritage', starts 60 million years ago and identifies some special features of the ancestors of present-day humans. It traces the evolution of some uniquely human characteristics, including upright posture and the ability to walk on two legs, the body changes we call puberty, and the practice of cooking food. These features of human biology and culture have had major consequences for our health. For example, the backache that afflicts millions today may have had its origins in the move from a forested to a grassland environment made by early humans about 3 million years ago.

1.2.1 Elements, atoms and molecules

In Chapter 3 we go further back in time to tell 'The story of life in a few pages'. We start with the coalescence of *atoms* of certain *chemical elements* into *molecules* of *DNA* in the 'primeval soup' cooling on the surface of the newly formed planet Earth. Then we sketch in the evolution of large creatures such as ourselves, composed of billions of cells organised into recognisable structural features such as the major organs, muscles and bones. For readers who are new to this series and new to science, the italicised terms earlier in this paragraph are likely to be familiar, but may not be understood in their scientific sense. Before moving on, we need to ensure that you know their scientific meaning.

All matter, whether it is in a living organism like a tree or a person, or in non-living material such as the rocks and the atmosphere, is composed of **chemical elements**. There are about 100 different elements in nature and among the most familiar are the most abundant constituents of living things: oxygen, carbon and hydrogen, which together form over 90 per cent of the mass of every organism. Under natural conditions on the surface of the Earth, one element cannot be turned into another, so you can think of them as the basic building blocks of the material world. (In the Earth's core and in the upper atmosphere, elements *are* transformed one into another, but this does not concern us here.) Each element exists in the form of extremely small 'particles' known as **atoms**, which can be joined together by energy fields known as chemical *bonds*. An assembly of two or more atoms is called a **molecule** (a common representation of a water molecule is shown in Figure 1.2).

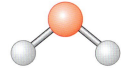

Figure 1.2 *A ball-and-stick representation of a water molecule, consisting of two atoms of the element hydrogen attached to one atom of the element oxygen. Each water molecule is so small (about 0.000 000 000 2 m across), that there are about 10^{20} (or 1 followed by 20 zeros) in a single raindrop.*

Molecules often contain atoms of more than one element, so for example *water* molecules are formed from two atoms of hydrogen and one atom of oxygen, written in the familiar chemical notation of H_2O. Water is an extremely small molecule because it has only three atoms, but molecules can be millions of times larger than those of water and contain the atoms of several different elements. One of the largest is the 'thread of life', deoxyribonucleic acid or DNA. In an era in which medical science is influenced more and more by the breakthroughs and applications of new genetic technology, we will spend time explaining the structure and functions of DNA in Chapter 3.

1.2.2 Individuals interact with environments

In line with our evolutionary theme, and because it acts as the universal canvas upon which biological evolution is painted, DNA runs as a thread through subsequent chapters.

In Chapter 4, 'Inheritance and variation', we describe the contribution of DNA to the variation between individuals and its role in passing on characteristics, such as height and susceptibility to a particular disease, from one generation to the next. Chapter 4 takes us into the realm of genetic disease and genetic resistance to disease, but it also emphasises the *interaction* of a person's genetic makeup with the environment in which he or she develops, in producing the normal variation between individuals we see all around us. The frontispiece to this book (Figure 1.1) illustrates the exceptional external variation seen in members of the human species.

Chapter 5, 'Living with other species', considers the interaction between human populations and the organisms that have a major impact on our health. Most obvious among them are the *pathogenic* (disease-causing) species, which include some types of bacteria, viruses, fungal infections, single-celled parasites and larger parasitic animals like the tapeworms and liver flukes. This interaction has had a major impact on the evolution of large multicellular organisms, including humans, and has played a role in fundamental aspects of our lives; even the fact that we reproduce sexually may be an adaptation against infection! But human survival also crucially depends on bacteria and other minute creatures such as the plankton in the sea, as Chapter 5 will reveal.

In Chapter 6, 'Surviving infectious disease', we examine the dynamic balancing act that goes on whenever a pathogenic organism invades the human body. Over the long time-scale of life on Earth, pathogens have evolved numerous adaptations to evade the defensive strategies evolved by their 'hosts'. As a consequence of this evolutionary history, the human immune system is a network of mind-boggling complexity, which has solved the problem of attacking infection without destroying the body itself. Chapter 6 gives a glimpse into this inner world of threat and counter-attack.

But there is more to survival than resisting infection. According to the English clergyman, W. R. Inge, 'the whole of nature is a conjugation of the verb to eat, in the active and in the passive' (from his *Outspoken Essays,* quoted in Daintith and Isaacs, 1989, p. 145). Chapter 7, 'Digestion and dietary change', is about the mechanisms of digestion and absorption and how they cope with the modern human diet. The chapter ends with a case study on variation in the ability to digest milk among different human populations.

1.2.3 Changing the future: for better or for worse?

In Chapter 8 we move more firmly into the present to examine the biological consequences of increased longevity. 'On living longer' describes the biological changes underlying the familiar signs of ageing and asks: Why, in evolutionary terms, do we grow old and die? Are we genetically programmed to grow old? The increased prevalence of degenerative diseases is one of the driving forces behind biological research aimed at improving human health in the future. Another is the desire to alleviate the hitherto intractable consequences of certain degenerative or genetic diseases.

In Chapter 9, 'Tinkering with nature', we examine some of the most controversial methods that medical science in the new millennium is in the process of developing to increase the quantity and the quality of human life. These include organ transplant surgery, gene therapy and genetic screening. Some of these procedures have the potential not only to reduce human suffering but may also change the nature of human evolution. These topics are the subject of far-reaching ethical debates.[1]

As it nears its conclusion, the book progresses steadily deeper into the vexed territory of modern life. In Chapter 10, 'Living with the chemical industrial environment', we turn from the intentional manipulation of human biology to the consequences of a prevalent feature of industrial development, the *unintentional* dissemination of chemicals. What evidence do we have that this activity is damaging human health in any general sense, or is human biology able to adapt sufficiently to defend the species from chemical pollution? What responsibility must we take for protecting other life-forms from the 'fallout' of human cultural evolution?

The book closes in Chapter 11 by looking back over the sweep of human evolution and putting 'The impact of modern culture' in the context of this extensive time frame. We consider the interaction of biological and cultural evolution and speculate about the future. We conclude by posing the question 'Is the pace of change too fast for human evolution to keep up?'.

OBJECTIVE FOR CHAPTER 1

When you have studied this chapter, you should be able to:

1.1 Define and use, or recognise definitions and applications of, each of the terms printed in **bold** in the text.

[1] The ethical dimensions of advances in genetics are also explored further for Open University students in a TV programme 'Bloodlines: A family legacy' and an audiotape 'Tinkering with nature'.

C H A P T E R   2

The human biological heritage

Study notes for OU students

This chapter is written in the style of an essay and is intended to give you the 'big picture' rather than to teach biological details. It synthesises information and points of view from a variety of different sources, so in most cases, it is not possible to attribute any particular fact or conclusion to a single author, but the Further sources list at the end of the book includes several sources that enlarge upon topics mentioned here.

The origins and incidence of many of the diseases discussed in *World Health and Disease* (Open University Press, second edition 1993; third edition 2001) can be partly explained in terms of human evolutionary history and our interactions with other organisms. Chapter 5 of that book introduced the theory of evolution by natural selection and gave the general meaning of the terms 'adaptation' and 'fitness'. We discuss the biological significance of these terms in greater detail later in the present book (Chapters 3 and 5).

There is one Reader article associated with Section 2.4.1 of this chapter, entitled 'Why must I be a teenager at all?' by Barry Bogin. It appears in *Health and Disease: A Reader* (Open University Press, second edition 1995; third edition 2001). A reader article you have already studied during *World Health and Disease* is also relevant to Section 2.6.4 and you could usefully read it again if you have time; it is 'Agriculture's two-edged sword' by Jared Diamond.

2.1 Introduction

In many ways, humans are unique; some of our uniqueness arises from our evolutionary origin, some from our habits and culture. Many of our unique features and habits predispose us to certain diseases. Like all other animals, humans interact with many other organisms to obtain food and shelter. Although some modern city-dwellers appear to live largely isolated from their biological environment, the parasites and pathogens with which we came into contact when our distant ancestors lived as 'wild' creatures are still with us, and can be important causes of disease.

Parasites are organisms that spend part or all of their lives *on* (ectoparasites) or *in* (endoparasites) the body of another **species** called a **host**.[1] Many parasites do little harm to their hosts beyond minor irritation or taking small quantities of their food, but some may cause disease, either directly or indirectly by provoking damaging responses in their host, or by harbouring a third kind of organism that in turn causes disease. **Pathogen** is the term used in this book to refer to organisms that cause disease. The term refers not only to harmful **micro-organisms**, which consist of a single cell and are only visible through a microscope, such as *bacteria* and single-celled organisms like *Amoeba* (biologists call this group of organisms *protoctists*), but also to **multicellular parasites** such as tapeworms, which consist of many cells and can be very large, and to viruses and prions, which are not true cells at all. (All these terms come up again many times in later chapters, where they are explained in greater biological detail. In particular, the meaning of a *cell* is given in Chapter 3.)

In this book, we are concerned mainly with the pathogens that cause disease in *mammals*. All mammals are physiologically similar in a great many ways (for example, they all give birth to live young and feed them on milk), so experiments and observations on rats, guinea-pigs and other laboratory mammals can help scientists to understand the mechanisms of both normal and pathological processes in humans.[2] However, such studies tell us little about the origins or incidence of disease, or why people suffer frequently from disorders that are very rare in other kinds of animals. In this chapter, we look back into the distant past for clues about the origin of our anatomy, sensory and intellectual abilities, dietary requirements and diseases.

The evidence for human evolution is fragmentary, often consisting of only a few bones or stone tools. In spite of an intensive, worldwide search, we have very few human remains older than about 50 000 years, and those from earlier than 10 000 years ago are rare. Consequently, there are several contrasting theories, some of them mutually exclusive, about such crucial events as the evolution of sparse body hair, the origin of speech and conscious thought, and when and by what route people colonised the world's major continents. A thorough review of all the evidence is beyond the scope of this book, so we present a simplified picture, highlighting aspects of the story that clearly pertain to health and disease. But you may find alternative accounts in other texts, and theories may be revised as new fossils and artefacts are discovered and existing remains are re-interpreted.

---

[1] The definition of a 'species' is a population of organisms that usually interbreed in their natural habitat and produce fertile offspring (*Studying Health and Disease*, Open University Press, 2nd edn 1994; colour-enhanced 2nd edn 2001, Chapter 9). The Latinised names for organisms given in this book uniquely and unambiguously identify each species.

[2] *Studying Health and Disease* (Open University Press, 2nd edn 1994; colour-enhanced 2nd edn 2001), Chapter 9, discusses the practical and ethical issues raised by using laboratory animals as substitutes for humans in experiments to investigate human health problems and to evaluate medical treatments.

2.2 Humans as primates

2.2.1 Primate characteristics

Humans are **primates**, a distinctive group of mammals that first appeared more than 60 million years ago and which includes monkeys, apes, lemurs, lorises and many less familiar species. Most primates live in tropical forests, where they eat leaves, flowers, fruit, soft seeds and small animals such as insects. They have unspecialised teeth and guts and relatively long, flexible limbs that enable them to alternate between several different postures and modes of locomotion, including climbing and leaping. The five toes and fingers on each limb are relatively long and flexible, and are tipped with blunt, flat 'fingernails' in place of claws. Primates grip branches and grasp food between the fingers or toes rather than use sharp claws for climbing and manipulating things.

The brain is relatively large in all primates (compared to that of similar-sized mammals) and the eyes are prominent, forward pointing and, with the possible exception of some nocturnal species, capable of excellent colour vision and pattern discrimination. Hearing is also acute but, particularly in larger primates, the snout is relatively short and olfaction (the sense of smell) is not as sensitive as it is in most other mammals (e.g. dogs).

Nearly all monkeys and apes are social and most live in extended family groups led by a dominant adult, which in most species, but not all, is a male. Most species have frequent and elaborate social interactions between adults of both sexes as well as between infants and adults, and communicate by means of sounds (grunts, whistles, screams and more complex noises), facial expressions and gestures.

Compared to other mammals of similar size, primates grow slowly, live a long time, and breed slowly, having only 1–4 babies at a time with many months or, in large species, several years between pregnancies. In contrast to most other mammals, the young are not born in a permanent nest or den, and they cannot walk efficiently at birth. Instead, they are carried continually by one or both parents, giving the juveniles a 'front-seat' view of what their parents are eating, how they handle their food and how they detect and respond to danger and to other members of the group. Experiments in which infant monkeys are reared in isolation or by other species show that such experience is very important for successful foraging and for establishing normal social and sexual relations when adult.

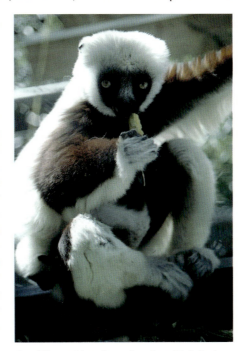

A ruff lemur Varecia variegata *with infant (whose head is visible at the lower left). Lemurs are primitive primates but they have most of the typical primate characters, including large, forward-pointing eyes, short nose and a large, rounded braincase. The limbs are long and mobile, with long flexible fingers and toes adapted to grasping. (Photo: Caroline Pond)*

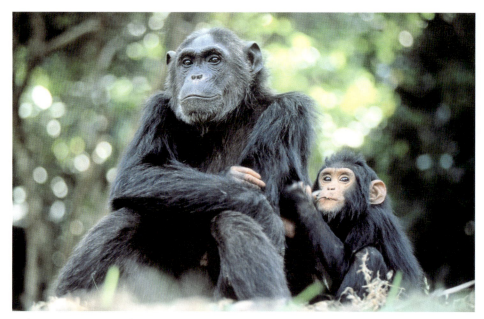

*A chimpanzee (*Pan troglodytes*) mother and child (Mahale Mountains, Tanzania). Early hominids probably lived in family groups, as do most living species of apes. During their long juvenile period, infants associate closely with and learn from adult males and other adult and subadult females, as well as their own mother on whom they are dependent for milk. They learn where to find food, how to detect and evade predators and how to deal with social and sexual interactions with other chimps. (Photo: Karl Amman/BBC Natural History Unit Picture Library)*

2.2.2 Humans and apes

The largest kinds of primates are the humans and the **apes**, which consist of two kinds of gibbons, orang-utans, gorillas, two kinds of chimpanzee (the common chimp and the bonobo) and several extinct species. Apes differ from other primates (e.g. lemurs and monkeys) in that the tail is greatly reduced, the chest is flattened from front to back instead of side to side, the lumbar region of the back (between the ribs and the pelvis) is shorter and stiffer and the shoulders and forelimbs are long and flexible. The apes are among the last major groups of primates to appear, the oldest fossils being about 30 million years old. As well as their fundamental anatomical differences, apes also differ from monkeys in intellectual and perceptual abilities. Apes can monitor, and hence anticipate, each other's activities and are much better than monkeys at learning by observing the actions and experiences of other members of their species, as well as from their own experience. Gibbons and orang-utans live almost entirely in the crowns of tall trees, but the other modern apes, although primarily forest-dwellers, can walk on the ground as well as climb trees.

All the basic features of apes are present, and in many cases enhanced, in humans, but we live longer, grow more slowly and have still more elaborate forms of communication. Human ancestors probably lived in more open grasslands and savannah than other apes, and were almost certainly itinerant, walking from food source to food source over a large home range, carrying their infants with them. The prolonged contact between adults and children became increasingly important as foraging skills, social behaviour and communication became more elaborate, and so took longer to learn.

2.2.3 Evolution of hominids

The direct ancestors of humans and their close relatives are collectively called **hominids**. Their remains can be recognised among fossils in central and east Africa from about 5 million years ago. Hominids are all primates belonging to several extinct species as well as the sole living species, *Homo sapiens*, which are the only hominids correctly referred to as 'people'. Hominid fossils are distinct from those of other ape lineages, and the last common ancestor of humans and modern apes lived well over 5 million years ago.

Between about 3 and 1.8 million years ago, the climate became drier and possibly more variable, and in south-east Africa, dense rainforests gave way to grasslands and savannah. Fossil remains of hominids became more abundant (but still very rare compared to those of animals such as antelopes) and are found in south as well as east Africa. All known fossil hominids from 2 to 4 million years ago are found in sediments that contain animal remains and pollen typical of unforested areas, mostly grasslands, marshes and riversides, and many of the unique and fundamental features of our species may have evolved during this period.

- Compared to primates in general and to other apes, how recently have hominids appeared in evolutionary time?

- Very recently. The time since hominids took to living on grasslands is only about 5 per cent (3/60 million years) of the time since primates first appeared, and only 10 per cent (3/30 million years) of the age of the oldest fossils of apes.

The evolution of hominids involved many anatomical changes that probably accompanied major changes in diet and foraging habits; hominids became more carnivorous than their tree-dwelling ancestors, eating carrion as well as animals that they killed for themselves. They probably lived and hunted in bands, cooperating to kill animals much larger than themselves (as do some carnivores, such as wolves and hyenas), and sharing or exchanging food with others. However, plant food almost certainly never disappeared completely from the diet and may have been the main source of nourishment at certain seasons.

2.3   Erect posture and bipedality

Upright posture is one of the most obvious and fundamental features of hominids. Although chimps and gorillas can stand erect and walk *bipedally* (on two legs) for a few metres, we are the only mammals that stand on our hind legs with straight knees and fully extended hips. Erect posture is among the first uniquely human characteristics to have evolved; analysis of skeletal remains and footprints indicate that, by 2 to 4 million years ago, hominids probably walked bipedally and stood erect, or nearly so.

The evolutionary shift to an upright posture and **bipedality** involved several profound changes in the structure of the leg, foot, pelvis, spine and neck, which have had major consequences for human health and disease. Figure 2.1 is a summary of the main adaptations to erect posture. The leg became longer, the knee and hip joint are almost fully extended and the ankle is flexed (Figure 2.1a), so that the human foot is directly under the body.

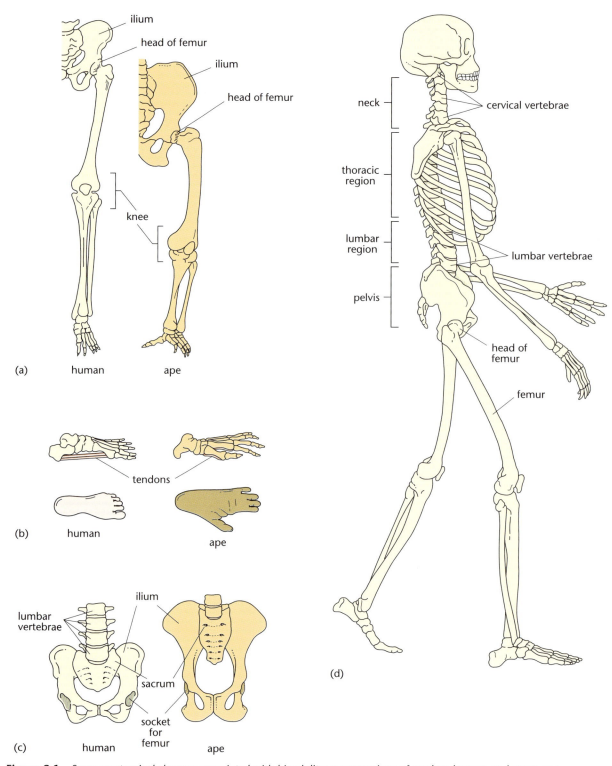

Figure 2.1   *Some anatomical changes associated with bipedality: a comparison of modern human and great ape.*
(a) The pelvis, leg and foot bones, (b) the foot bones and footprint, (c) the pelvis and lower spinal column, and
(d) the human skeleton. (Based on Martin, R. D., 1992, Primate locomotion and posture, Chapter 2.8, p. 78, in Jones, S.,
Martin, R., Pilbeam, D. and Bunney, S. (eds) The Cambridge Encyclopedia of Human Evolution, *Cambridge University*
Press, Cambridge.)

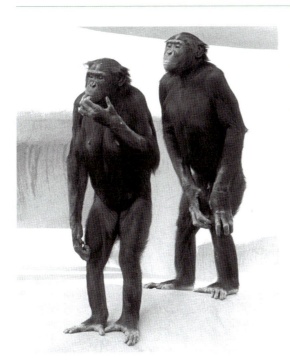

Chimpanzees and other apes can stand upright, but like all non-human primates, they cannot completely straighten their knees or extend the hip fully, so they stand with a pronounced forward stoop. They do not go far in this posture: a four-legged gallop is faster and seems to be more comfortable, even for these bonobo chimps (Pan paniscus) whose erect posture is closest to that of humans. (Photo: Dr Franz B. M. de Waal, Living Links Center, Emory University)

The foot (Figure 2.1b) became specialised for walking, almost completely losing the other functions it had in hominid ancestors and still has in living apes, such as the capacity to grasp objects using opposable digits, in the same way as the hand does. Hominid toes are relatively shorter and more or less parallel, and the bones of the first ('big') toe are stout and strong because most of the weight of the body is carried on this toe when the foot is flexed in stepping or running. The foot becomes arched rather than flat as it is in apes; the tendons strung between the bones of the middle of the foot (see Figure 2.1b) absorb impact energy, cushioning the impact with the ground, and releasing the energy thus absorbed during the following stride. The hominid pelvis became shorter and more rounded, mainly due to the curving of the ilium and widening of the sacrum (Figure 2.1c), and there is greater curvature of the spine (Figure 2.1d) than is seen in ape skeletons.

2.3.1 Effects on locomotion

The changes that took place as the hominid skeleton evolved are also related to the enlargement of muscles that stabilise the hip on one side, while the other leg swings forward in a stride. Although they do not actually swing the legs, the contribution of these muscles is essential to long strides, and powerful, rhythmic walking and running. Chimpanzees, severely emaciated people (in whom the hip muscles are wasted and weakened), those with paralysed hip muscles and people recovering from 'hip replacement' operations, walk upright by shuffling rather than by striding and cannot run at all. The head of the human femur (the thigh bone) is proportionately longer but less massive than in the tree-living apes, and has less efficient internal buttressing (Figure 2.1a).

● Can you suggest why this change in the head of the femur evolved in association with walking upright, and what consequence this might have for human health?

■ The head of the human femur has evolved a less robust structure because it is stressed only in the fairly uniform forces of walking, rather than by the more variable forces generated by leaping and climbing, as in other primates. This contributes to the tendency of the neck of the femur to break in older people. The increased porosity of bone in old age, especially in women, is also a contributory factor, to which we return in Chapter 8.

Walking requires correct coordination of the activity of the hip muscles, which may become weak or inefficient in old age, thus increasing the risk of falling. Fractures of the head of femur often occur almost spontaneously, or following a very minor fall and, although much more effective treatment has been developed in recent years, they are still fatal in roughly a quarter of cases.

The pelvis of modern humans is deeper from front to back than that of other primates, so the pelvic canal is more nearly round than that of early bipedal hominids (Figure 2.1c). Some anthropologists believe that these changes actually reduced slightly the efficiency of walking and running, and since they are especially pronounced in adult women, this may explain why even elite female athletes have a lower average maximum running speed than equivalently trained men.

2.3.2 Effects on childbirth

The changes in the shape and size of the pelvis described above also had important implications for the organisation of the soft tissues, and particularly for the process of *birth*. Although the anterior (upper) end of the pelvis is wider in hominids than in apes, the posterior (lower) end is narrower (Figure 2.1c) and the baby's head has to rotate in the birth canal as it is born. The problems of birth were probably much exacerbated by the increase in brain size among later hominids. The nervous system is among the first tissues to develop in the fetus, and the brain (and with it, the skull) is large relative to the rest of the body throughout development. Hominids that had larger brains as adults almost certainly had bigger heads at birth. The size and shape of the pelvis evolved to accommodate the passage of the baby's head down the birth canal — always the most difficult stage of birth. For these reasons, difficulties with childbirth are relatively common in humans, especially in very young women whose pelvis is not yet fully grown.

Since mammalian births usually take place at night and in secluded nests or dens, there is very little detailed information about them, but so far as we can tell, the stress of giving birth is less severe, and perinatal and maternal mortality much less frequent in other mammals than they are in humans. Although labour is sometimes prolonged and apparently painful, maternal death is almost unknown among the few other primates in which many births have been observed.

2.3.3 Effects on the head and neck

In quadrupedal (four-footed) mammals, the head points forward and is attached to the neck by a stout ligament and strong muscles, which can be massive in animals such as wolves, pigs and bears. By comparison, the human neck is positively flimsy, and has so little muscle that large blood vessels and lymph nodes (sometimes called lymph 'glands') can be felt through the skin. Feel the crests of your own cervical (neck) vertebrae at the back of your neck (Figure 2.1d). You may be able to locate all seven, although the first and last are often difficult to distinguish. In most other mammals, including dogs, horses and large apes such as chimps and gorillas, most of the cervical vertebrae are deeply buried in massive, powerful muscles so you could not feel them through the skin as you can your own.

Human heads are somewhat lighter than those of apes because, although the brain is proportionately much heavier, the skull contains less bone and the jaw muscles are proportionately smaller and less powerful. However, the reduction in the neck muscles cannot be explained solely by the lighter head; it arises mainly from a fundamental change in posture made possible by bipedality. The human neck is almost vertical in all natural postures except lying down, and the skull is balanced on the cervical vertebrae, rather than braced against them (Figure 2.1d). The occiput, the junction between the first cervical vertebra and the skull, is in the middle of the base of the skull and supports it from underneath, with the much smaller muscles just acting like 'guy ropes' around a flag pole. Areas of bone to which muscles were attached are easily identified on fossilised bones, so this integral feature of bipedality can often be identified even in small fragments of the skull.

2.3.4 Advantages of walking upright

● What cultural change could have promoted the evolution of upright posture and walking bipedally in early hominids?

■ The change from living in dense forest to open grassland may have promoted the shift from climber to walker. The erect posture is appropriate for walking and running on open ground, but much less suited to climbing or leaping in trees.

Although modern people, and presumably their anatomically similar hominid ancestors, can walk and run bipedally further and faster on flat ground than any other ape-like primate, humans still run slowly compared to quadrupedal mammals of similar size. Olympic races are won at average speeds of 6–11 metres per second (depending upon the distance), compared to 15–17 metres per second for racehorses and greyhounds. Bipedality also does not significantly improve the efficiency of locomotion; a person *walking* on two legs uses slightly *less* energy than a quadrupedal mammal covering the same distance at the same speed, but *running* requires proportionately *more* energy. So speed and efficiency of locomotion are unlikely to be explanations for why hominids adopted the upright posture.

Anthropologists have discussed several other suggestions for the circumstances that promoted the evolution of bipedality, for example: it enabled early humans to carry large items (tools, food, children, etc.), thereby promoting food sharing and improvements in hunting technology; erect hominids could feed in bushes and/or could see prey and enemies more efficiently, particularly on open savannah; upright hominids have a smaller proportion of the body exposed to direct sunlight, and so heat up less rapidly under the tropical midday Sun than quadrupedal animals of similar size, enabling them to run faster for longer without overheating.

Whatever the cause, a consequence of bipedality was to release the forelimb from direct involvement in locomotion. In other species

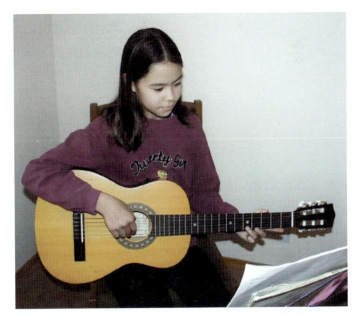

The evolution of an upright posture released the forelimbs from involvement in locomotion; modern humans have become extremely skilled in finely controlled movements of the arms, hands and fingers. (Photo: Yvonne Ashmore)

in which comparable changes have taken place (e.g. kangaroos), the forelimbs became reduced, but in hominids the opposite happened. Tactile sensation and fine control of finger movement improved (though the length and maximum power output decreased compared to those of tree-climbing apes), making possible delicate manipulations of small objects, probably at first mostly food items such as seeds, and later tools.

The prevalence among modern people of lower back pain, arthritis of the hip and knee, and other skeletal disorders of the lower limb and pelvis is often attributed to incomplete or ineffective adaptation to the erect posture. However, when viewed on an evolutionary time-scale, this explanation is not convincing. Relative to traits such as large brains, bipedality is ancient. Almost all the anatomical features that distinguish modern humans, *Homo sapiens*, from their probable direct ancestor, *Homo erectus*, relate to the skull, teeth and jaws; the rest of the skeleton has hardly changed for at least 2 to 2.5 million years, suggesting that an upright posture and bipedality were satisfactory for humans' habits over a very long period of time. Any possible disadvantages arising in old age seem to be outweighed by advantages earlier in life, a subject to which we return in Chapters 5 and 8.

2.4   Human growth and life history

The development of humans, from a fertilised egg to a fully mature adult, is described elsewhere in this series.[3] Here we take an overview of human growth, maturation and ageing across the lifespan. Humans live longer, take longer to reach sexual maturity and, in proportion to their size, grow more slowly than any other mammal.

To understand how atypical the pattern of human growth is, we must compare it with that of a non-primate mammal such as the mouse and with another primate. In most mammals (Figure 2.2a), there is a steady weight gain between birth and puberty and little difference in the pattern of growth between the sexes. In chimpanzees (Figure 2.2b), juveniles of both sexes gain weight at a rate of 4–6 kilograms per year for about the first six years of life. Females continue to put on weight at approximately this rate until they reach **menarche** — the first menstrual cycle — when their growth rate declines; whereas male weight gain accelerates from about the age of 5–8 years before stabilising at the adult weight at somewhere between 10–14 years.

●   Compare Figure 2.2c with 2.2b, and list two features of the pattern of weight gain over time that are peculiar to humans.

■   The first difference is the very slow weight gain in childhood; human children grow at only 2–3 kilograms per year during years 1–6, which is about half the growth rate of young chimps. Second, there is an acceleration of weight gain in humans in both sexes beginning about age 9–10, but proceeding at a faster rate and peaking at an earlier age in females. Much of this later period of female weight gain *precedes* the menarche; (indeed, menarche is delayed in girls who are significantly underweight for their height, particularly so in cases of anorexia nervosa).

[3] *Birth to Old Age: Health in Transition* (Open University Press, 2nd edn 1995; colour-enhanced 2nd edn 2001).

2.4.1 Adolescence

The acceleration in human growth rate shown in Figure 2.2c is called the **adolescent growth spurt**. The fact that it peaks about two years earlier in girls results in a brief period when girls on average are slightly taller than boys of the same age. **Secondary sexual characteristics** (i.e. sex differences other than those of the reproductive organs) such as the growth of pubic hair, development of breasts or enlargement of the penis, onset of menstruation, and adult voice appear during the adolescent growth spurt. But, whereas boys' sperm is fully fertile as soon as the testes and penis assume their adult form, girls cannot normally bear children until several years after acquiring other secondary sexual characteristics. The adolescent growth spurt and this period of adolescent sterility in girls has no parallels in other mammals, which always become fertile and capable of adult sexual and parental behaviour in the next breeding season after they reach sexual maturity.

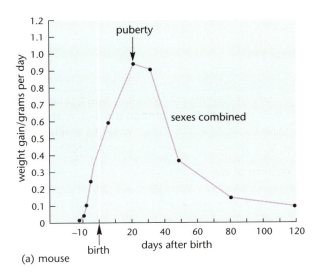

(a) mouse

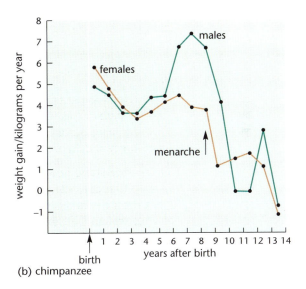

(b) chimpanzee

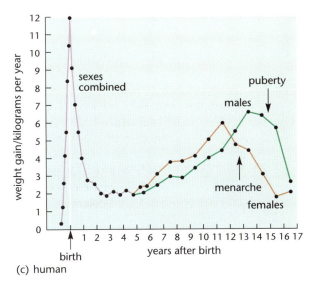

(c) human

Figure 2.2 *The average rates of growth in weight of (a) laboratory mice, (b) chimpanzees, (c) boys (green line) and girls (orange line) in the United Kingdom in the mid-twentieth century. (Based on Tanner, J. M., 1992, Human growth and development, Chapter 2.13, p. 100, in Jones, S., Martin, R., Pilbeam, D. and Bunney, S. (eds)* The Cambridge Encyclopedia of Human Evolution, *Cambridge University Press, Cambridge)*

Adolescence is associated with major changes in habits and desires as well as in appearance and physical strength, some of which can lead to medical and social problems.[4] As Shakespeare put it:

> I would there were no age between ten and three-and-twenty…for there is nothing in the between but getting wenches with child, wronging the ancientry, stealing, fighting. (Shakespeare, 1610, *The Winter's Tale,* Act III, Scene 3)

Some recent scientific theories about the evolutionary origin and biological functions of human adolescence are discussed in an article, 'Why must I be a teenager at all?', first published in 1993 by Barry Bogin, an American professor of anthropology. Bogin's account puts forward just one of several theories and is unlikely to be the last word on the topic; active research into human growth and sexual and social maturation is still in progress. (Open University students should read the article now.[5])

● Summarise the differences between the ages at which adolescent girls and boys begin to display secondary sexual characteristics, reach adult stature and achieve full reproductive capacity.

■ Girls develop secondary sexual characteristics first (around 11 years), then go on to reach adult stature (around 17 years), but only achieve full reproductive capacity at around 18 to 19 years of age. By contrast, boys develop secondary sexual characteristics and achieve full reproductive capacity at around the same age (roughly 14 years), but they don't reach adult stature until several years later.

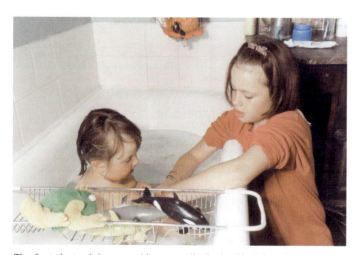

The fact that adolescent girls generally 'look older' than boys of the same age may reflect differences in the evolution of male and female characteristics, and play a part in behavioural differences between the sexes, e.g. in their involvement in rearing younger siblings. (Photo: John Birdsall Photography)

● What does Bogin suggest are the advantages for human survival of these sex differences in the timing of growth and maturation?

■ Adolescent girls start to look like 'women' long before they are reproductively mature, so they are *invited into* adult female society, where they help with child rearing and learn essential skills which later enhance their own children's chances of survival. Conversely, adolescent boys are *excluded* from many aspects of adult male society, even though they are reproductively mature, because they don't look like 'grown men'. This situation may enable boys to practise adult male behaviours, without running the risk of injury in competition with mature men,

[4] The physical and psychological health of adolescents in the UK is discussed in *Birth to Old Age: Health in Transition* (Open University Press, 2nd edn 1995; colour-enhanced 2nd edn 2001), Chapter 6; legal issues to do with sexual maturity and the age of consent are covered in Chapter 7.

[5] Bogin's article is reproduced in *Health and Disease: A Reader* (Open University Press, 2nd edn 1995; 3rd edn 2001).

until they become physically capable of fending for their own dependants. Thus, the differences in the sexes during adolescence may simultaneously enhance their own survival and that of their future offspring.

2.4.2 Menopause

Another specifically human characteristic is *menopause* in females. Starting at around age 45–50 years, female fertility gradually declines, menstruation becomes erratic and then ceases, secondary sexual characters such as breast-size may start to regress, and a variety of changes in **metabolism** occur (metabolism refers to all the biochemical reactions going on in the body), including the turnover of calcium in the skeleton. After menopause, women usually remain in good health and, in advanced industrial economies such as the UK, typically live for 30 years or more in the post-reproductive state. By contrast, female apes and monkeys continue to bear and rear young to the end of their lives, although the interval between births may increase a little with age; profound metabolic changes comparable to those that are observed in women do not occur in other primates.

The fertility of men (and male apes) declines with age no faster or more abruptly than the age-related decline in other physiological abilities, such as running speed or maximum grip strength. In Chapter 8, we return to the subject of the female menopause and ask what its evolutionary significance might be. We also consider its effect on women's health.[6]

2.4.3 Longevity

Seventy years seems to be an absolute maximum lifespan for most mammals other than humans, even for large species such as elephants, and few non-human primates live longer than 30–40 years, although it is very difficult to be certain about the maximum lifespan of any wild mammal.

● Can you explain why?

■ Elderly individuals are always a small proportion of natural populations, and their greater experience may enable them to avoid the attentions of intruding biologists more efficiently!

Despite this difficulty, it is clear that both the maximum and the average human lifespan are more than twice that of all modern apes. However, so far as can be determined, the average longevity of most female mammals is usually slightly greater than that of males, particularly in species such as baboons and polar bears where the adult males are much bigger than the females. On average, modern women in most societies live several years longer than men in similar conditions, a feature of the life history that we may have inherited almost unchanged from our primate ancestors.[7]

---

[6] The social and personal consequences of the menopause among women in the UK are discussed in *Birth to Old Age: Health in Transition* (Open University Press, 2nd edn 1995; colour-enhanced 2nd edn 2001), Chapter 9, which also speculates on whether there is a 'male menopause'.

[7] Countries where this female advantage is much smaller or absent are discussed in *World Health and Disease* (Open University Press, 2nd edn 1993; 3rd edn 2001), Chapters 3, 4 and 8.

Much effort has been directed to determining when, in hominid evolution, the peculiar features of human growth and longevity evolved. But since the analysis depends upon determining the age of hominid bones *independently* of their size and skeletal maturity, the subject is controversial, and there is little agreement beyond the conclusion that all the essential features of human growth and sexual maturation were in place by 1 million years ago. However, studies of tooth wear in skulls of Neanderthal people, an early subspecies (form) of *Homo sapiens* that lived in Europe between 130 000 and 40 000 years ago, suggests that few of them survived beyond the age of 40 years.

● What does this suggest about the experience of menopause in Neanderthal women?

■ Menopause must have been a relatively rare occurrence, until a few tens of thousands of years ago.

In most long-lived species (e.g. elephants), organs such as teeth, eyes, ears, etc. 'wear out' before the end of the maximum lifespan, and the failure of these structures often leads to starvation because individuals cannot chew the available food, or to increased vulnerability to predators through lack of awareness of danger, or failure to keep up with the running herd.

● Defects of teeth, vision and hearing are an almost inevitable consequence of old age in humans. How are the potential risks to life overcome in human societies?

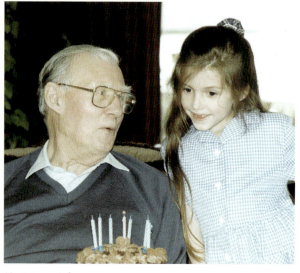

Human social organisation into extended family groups, usually spanning three or four generations, tends to protect its older members from threats to their health, e.g. from declining mobility and loneliness. (Photo: Mike Wibberley)

■ Technological advances in human evolution such as cooking, the cultivation of plants that yield soft foods, and the keeping of domestic animals for milk and eggs, reduce the rate of tooth wear and offset the impairment of function once the teeth are worn. Living in social groups in which children and elderly people are protected reduces the dangers that arise from defects of vision and hearing. In most present-day societies, manufactured tools such as spectacles, hearing aids and false teeth partially correct loss of function (as do walking sticks, wheelchairs, lifts, etc.).

All these aids and social habits greatly increase the life expectancy of older people; impairment of function generally has to be severe, even in 'archaic' tribal societies, before the risks of external causes of death (e.g. from starvation, predation and accidents) are substantially increased. Life expectancy for a few individuals in advanced industrial economies may also be increased by 'spare-part' surgery or cell therapy to replace diseased or damaged organs and joints, a subject to which we return in Chapter 9.

Increased longevity has its drawbacks, however. Many parasites and pathogens that affect humans are rare and infection depends upon a chance encounter. Obviously, a longer lifespan increases the chance of exposure to a greater variety of such organisms and increases the probability of repeated infection. The human immune system has to be efficient to cope with the wide range of parasites and pathogens that it may encounter in its long life. These topics, and how modern medicine has enhanced our ability to fight infection, are covered in Chapters 5 and 6 of this book.

2.5   The evolution of soft tissues

We turn now to consider the soft tissues of the body and how they appear to have evolved in hominids. This is a more difficult area for evolutionary biologists to research, because the brain and other organs disintegrate rapidly after death. So changes in soft tissues over thousands of years tend to be inferred from examination of skeletons and human artefacts, such as the remains of shelters, tools and clothing, or by comparing modern humans with modern apes.

2.5.1   Brain

The brain of the earliest hominids, as estimated from the volume of the brain case region of the skull, was about 0.4–0.5 litres, about the same size as that of modern apes such as gorillas (Figure 2.3, left), in a body that was a little smaller. For more than 2 million years, hominid brain size changed little, until about 2.2 million years ago when the two distinct lineages of hominids, *Homo* and *Australopithecus,* diverged. *Australopithecus* became taller and more massive than *Homo,* and evolved larger, stronger, more wear-resistant molar teeth (the grinding teeth at the sides of the jaw), but its brain volume changed very little from that of early hominids. By contrast, in *Homo erectus,* an extinct hominid that lived about 1.4–2.0 million years ago and is probably ancestral to modern humans, the teeth became smaller, the body lighter and more slender, and the brain larger than in early hominids (Figure 2.3, centre).

In *Homo,* the size of the brain relative to that of the body increased steadily for more than 1.5 million years, levelling off during the last few hundred thousand years at 1.0 to 1.6 litres (with an average of 1.36 litres in *Homo sapiens,* Figure 2.3, right) — more than double the brain volume of early hominids and modern apes. During the same period, molar tooth size decreased in *Homo.*

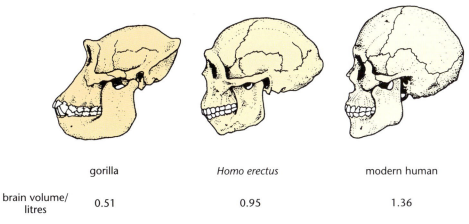

	gorilla	Homo erectus	modern human
brain volume/ litres	0.51	0.95	1.36

Figure 2.3   *Side views of three primate skulls. (Left) A modern gorilla, whose last common ancestor with humans lived more than 5 million years ago; the skull is similar to that of early hominids. (Centre)* Homo erectus. *(Right)* Homo sapiens, *modern human. Note that in* Homo sapiens, *the back of the skull enclosing the brain is taller and rounder than in* Homo erectus, *while the jaws are shorter and the face more flattened, with the eyebrow ridges greatly reduced. (Source: Open University S364 Course Team)*

Fossils of *Homo* and *Australopithecus* occur in the same sediments in eastern and southern Africa, indicating that, for at least a million years, the large-brained and smaller-brained hominids coexisted. About 1 million years ago, *Australopithecus* disappeared without descendants and *Homo*, the lineage that eventually evolved into modern people, began to spread to southern Europe and Asia as well as expanding its range in Africa.

●   What can you conclude from this information about the advantages of a larger brain?

■   The advantages did not emerge immediately. The large-brained hominids have only become dominant within the last 1 million years. Small-brained but muscular hominids with large, powerful teeth coexisted for a long time with the smaller, lighter species that had relatively large brains.

2.5.2 Hair and fat

One of the most obvious differences between humans and all other primates is the peculiar condition of the hair: it is sparse or absent over much of the body, but grows thick and long on the head and in a few other patches, notably around the genitals. Almost nothing is known about when this arrangement evolved, and there is much controversy about its function. One likely theory is that hair reduction is an adaptation to prolonged, strenuous exercise that enabled people to run far and fast on tropical plains without overheating. Consistent with this idea are the facts that human sweat glands are much more numerous than those of apes, and people — especially light-skinned people — sweat more than apes.

The onset of the Pleistocene glaciations (the Ice Age), about 100 000 years ago, and the colonisation of central and eastern Asia and of southern Europe meant that people began living in climates that were much cooler than those of Africa. There is no evidence that the body hair of such people became thicker or longer; instead, inhabitants of colder regions adopted the uniquely human habit of wearing the skins of other animals and, later, woven cloth.

Hair reduction reveals the skin and the tissues underlying it. Humans are almost unique among mammals in having pronounced, clearly visible sex differences in the distribution of fat (known to biologists as adipose tissue). These differences are minimal in children, develop rapidly at adolescence, are most pronounced in young adults and then regress in old age. The breasts of adolescent girls and non-lactating women (i.e. those not producing milk) consist mostly of fat; the arrangement of adipose tissue on the thighs and buttocks accentuates the sex differences in bones of the pelvis and thigh. The distribution, texture and colour of the hair and superficial fat indicate a person's social and sexual status (i.e. distinguishing children, adolescents, mature adults and elderly people), and also help in the recognition of individual people from a distance, which would have been very important for nomadic hunters. Such minor but conspicuous sex differences in hair and superficial fat may have evolved as result of *sexual selection* (this important evolutionary process is explained in Chapter 5).

2.6 Cultural evolution

Human **culture** can be defined as the habits, beliefs, values and knowledge transmitted between generations by observation and teaching, rather than by genetic inheritance. It incorporates the religious, artistic and technological practices and social expression of a group of people with a shared tradition. Almost all theories about cultural changes during human evolution are based on the study of manufactured artefacts such as graves, tools and cave paintings, which provide some indirect information about hunting methods, living conditions and religious beliefs. Very little data about cultural evolution can be obtained from the study of fossilised skeletons alone. It is impossible to pinpoint when cultural evolution began; deliberate human burials date from 100 000 years ago in Europe and Asia, and representational art and bone needles (suggesting manufacture of clothing) are known from about 40 000 years ago.

2.6.1 Tools

Manufactured tools are found only in association with remains of *Homo*, although earlier and contemporary hominids may have used sticks and unmodified stones as tools, as modern chimpanzees do. The first stone artefacts are dated at about 2 million years old, but manufacturing techniques and materials improved only slowly for the next 1.5 million years (see Figure 2.4). Nonetheless, such simple technology must have contributed greatly to hunting success, because the skeleton of *Homo* became less massive and the teeth smaller during this period, the opposite to expectations if teeth and brawn, rather than skilled manufacture and use of tools, determined hunting efficiency.

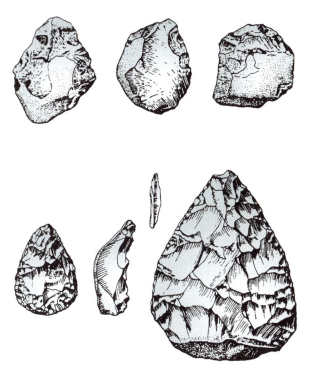

Figure 2.4 *Stone tools made by two different species of* Homo. *(Top row) Simple chopping tools found in South Africa that were made about 1.7 million years ago, probably by* Homo habilis, *the first hominid to make stone tools. (Lower row) More elaborate cutting and scraping tools made about 70 000 years ago by Neanderthal people, an early subspecies (form) of* Homo sapiens *living in western France. (Source: Open University S364 Course Team)*

●   Should we conclude from such finds that all tools were made only of stone?

■   No. People may have made tools and other artefacts (e.g. clothing) out of other materials such as wood, shell, bone and leather, but they have all broken or rotted away. Only those made from very durable materials such as stone and pottery have survived long enough for archaeologists to study them.

Beginning about 0.5 million years ago, technology started to improve rapidly. A greater variety of more finely made stone tools (axes, choppers, scrapers and arrow heads) appeared, together with barbed fish-hooks, spear-throwers and — only a few tens of thousand years later — bows and arrows, traps for catching fish and land animals, and tools for making tools. Some of these artefacts were composites of many different materials, including several kinds of wood and various grades of leather. In order to make such complex structures, people would have to plan ahead, assembling and preparing all the materials they would need to complete the article. It is possible that people obtained some of the rarer materials by trading with specialised suppliers, which gives us an important insight into the extent of cultural change taking place in this period.

It is important to emphasise that such elaborate artefacts are known only from the last 1–5 per cent of the time for which hominids have existed: they appeared *after* the brain reached its modern size and long after skeletal features such as erect posture, hands capable of fine manipulation, and reduced size of teeth were established.

2.6.2 Fire and cooking

The control of fire is a uniquely human achievement and is one of the major technological advances of the period in human cultural evolution termed the Palaeolithic (or Old Stone Age) by archaeologists. The Palaeolithic began about 2.6 million years ago in Africa before spreading to Asia and Europe. It is characterised by the development of stone tools and the complete absence of any form of agriculture.[8] Exactly when people acquired the ability to control fire is much disputed. Hearths have been found which are 0.5 million years old; human control of fires that started naturally (e.g. by lightning or volcanoes) may have begun as long ago as 1.5 million years, long before people learnt how to light fires for themselves. Almost all animals are instinctively afraid of heat and flame, so fires near shelters and camps deter large predators, such as wolves and lions, thereby reducing losses of both people and stored food.

The earliest use of fire was probably the deliberate burning of forests. This technique (which is still used) greatly increases the efficiency of hunting large animals by the creation and maintenance of open grassland, instead of scrub or forest in which prey are less plentiful and more difficult to see. Analysis of animal bones found near human settlements shows that hunting efficiency improved so much that, in many areas, some large mammals, including wild horses and mammoths, became extinct. Later people took to eating more small animals (e.g. birds, rabbits), fish

---

[8] Archaeological terms like the Palaeolithic and Neolithic (New Stone Age) refer to stages in human *cultural* development with particular characteristics, for example the manufacture of certain kinds of tools or pottery. These terms do not indicate exact dates in the past, because different social groups developed the cultural characteristics (e.g. of the Palaeolithic) at different times in different parts of the world.

and shellfish, and — increasingly — plants. The control of fire also assisted the permanent colonisation of colder climates, but its most far-reaching contribution to human culture was cooking.

● How does cooking modify plant foods?

■ Many plants, especially roots and seeds, that are tough, toxic or unpalatable when raw can be made appetising and digestible by cooking, e.g. chestnuts, acorns, cassava, potatoes, turnips, rice, wheat, maize, beans, cabbage and many more.

Cooking meat also makes it easier to eat, and destroys the infective stages of most potentially harmful parasites, such as tapeworms (segmented flatworms, e.g. *Taenia*) found in many large herbivores including cattle and pigs, and nematodes (unsegmented roundworms, e.g. *Trichinella spiralis*), which cause debilitating diseases such as trichinosis. At the end of this chapter, we will return to the origins of infectious diseases among humans.

However, cooking also degrades the nutritional quality of many foods. For example, early European explorers living off the land in the Arctic often suffered from scurvy, a disease caused by lack of vitamin C, characterised by anaemia, spongy gums and 'bleeds' under the skin.[9] Scurvy is almost unknown among the indigenous Inuit peoples (Europeans called them Eskimos), even though they never ate potatoes or citrus fruit, which contain vitamin C and therefore prevent scurvy, and indeed had no plant food at all except for a month or two in the summer. The reason is that vitamin C occurs in meat, but is easily destroyed by cooking, smoking or drying. The Inuit traditionally ate meat raw and so obtained sufficient vitamin C from it. However, they suffered from trichinosis, particularly if they ate polar bears or arctic foxes, in which the parasites are common. There are many other examples, some only recently revealed by modern chemical analysis, in which cooking improves or degrades the nutritional quality of foods. Clearly, the control of fire has far-reaching effects on both diet and health.

2.6.3 Clothing and shelters: evidence from fleas and lice!

Many early hominid remains are found in landscapes that include cliffs and caves, but it is far from certain that such shelter was any more essential to humans than it is to modern apes. Colonisation of cooler climates led to a profound change in human culture — the wearing of animal skins and, later, other forms of clothing, and the regular occupation of caves and (probably) other kinds of shelters. Leather and fur are rarely preserved, so there is little direct evidence about when or where human clothing first appeared, but the evolution of our ectoparasites tells us something about the change from naked nomads to fur-clad cave-dwellers.

Fleas are one such ectoparasite. They are wingless insects which, as adults, suck blood from mammals or, more rarely, birds, and attach themselves firmly to the host's fur (or feathers) by special hooks on the legs. Their flattened shape and remarkably tough outer covering enable them to scuttle quite fast through dense fur and to evade the most thorough grooming. The adults can live a long time between blood meals and can jump huge distances (relative to their minute size) from host to host. The eggs are laid in the host's 'nest', and the grub-like larvae

---

[9] The discovery by James Lind that citrus fruit could prevent scurvy is discussed in *World Health and Disease* (Open University Press, 2nd edn 1993; 3rd edn 2001), Chapter 11.

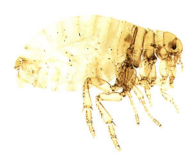

A human flea, Pulex irritans, *(4 mm long). Fleas parasitised humans when they migrated to colder climates and began wearing clothing and sleeping in semi-permanent shelters.*

feed for several weeks on detritus, dandruff and droppings deposited by the host. Nearly all mammals that breed or sleep in nests or dens are infested with fleas, often a unique species for each kind of mammal. However, nomadic mammals, including nearly all primates other than humans, do not have their own species of fleas, although adult fleas from other species may feed on them transiently. By contrast, humans are parasitised by a unique species of flea, *Pulex irritans*, that closely resembles the fleas that breed in the nests of badgers and foxes.

●   What can you deduce about human habits from these facts?

■   Humans have been occupying caves and other shelters regularly enough and for long enough for a species of flea that breeds only in association with humans to have evolved. The first human 'homes' may have been shared with, or formerly occupied by, ground-nesting mammals such as badgers and foxes. Early people were probably also more hairy or wore animal skins as clothes (or both).

Although their bite is little more than a nuisance, fleas, like other blood-sucking insects, can transmit disease-causing micro-organisms between species and from infected to uninfected members of the same species. Fleas that breed in the nests of other mammals, including those of rats, dogs and cats, often feed from each other's hosts, particularly when their normal host is absent. (You may have experienced bites from cat fleas.) Many of the great plagues of the Middle Ages were caused by bacteria transmitted to humans by rat fleas. Three (of more than 30) species of mouse, and later several species of rats, evolved their habit of living in and near human dwellings, where they raided people's food stores and accompanied them whenever they travelled with their baggage and provisions. The consequences of this association for human health have been profound, as past epidemics and modern outbreaks of plague exemplify.

Humans also harbour lice, another kind of blood-sucking insect that differs from fleas in many ways, among them the fact that the entire life cycle is completed in the host's fur. The human louse is similar to the species found on apes; we undoubtedly inherited the parasite from some distant common ancestor and have been troubled by their intensely irritating bites continually during the last 5 million years. The curvature of the louse's six legs closely follows that of its hosts' hair, enabling it to grip very tightly (and to resist combs and other forms of grooming). Each species is adapted to the shape of the hair of its own host. Humans have two kinds of lice; the head louse, *Pediculus humanus capitis*, which keeps strictly to the hair on the head, and the larger body louse, *Pediculus humanus humanus*, which seems happy to frequent, and lay its eggs upon, woven clothing and blankets as well as on body hair (e.g. pubic hair).

● What can you deduce from these facts about the evolution of human hair?

■ The texture of head hair has been different from that of body hair for a long time.

Lice are still common in many parts of the world, especially where people live in close contact with each other or share unwashed bedding or clothing. Modern head lice resist regular shampooing and are now common among children in Western countries, including the UK.

2.6.4 Agriculture and pastoralism

Agriculture (the growing of crops) and **pastoralism** (herding and controlled breeding of animals as a food source) began about 10 000 years ago and continues to the present day. Instead of foraging for wild food and materials (the method of subsistence in *hunter–gatherer* societies)[10], people began to grow crops and herd or confine animals from which they could obtain blood, milk, meat and non-edible products such as leather, fur, wool, horn, bone and (later) silk. Crops and livestock gradually became the main sources of nourishment, although many modern people still eat small quantities of wild food, e.g. wild mushrooms, truffles, berries, fish, shellfish and game.

Many scores of different plants, but fewer than 20 species of animals, have been *domesticated*, i.e. selectively bred in captivity for features and habits that suit human needs and desires. Agriculture and pastoralism have had profound effects on human diet, social organisation, health and the ecology of the organisms around human settlements; for example, many wild animals have been hunted to extinction, and natural habitats have been destroyed, to make space for agriculture and pastoralism. The process is by no means complete; as biological knowledge advances, more animals, plants and, increasingly, micro-organisms are being harnessed to human uses (for example by genetic and embryo manipulation, a topic we discuss in Chapter 9).

Grains (e.g. wheat, oats, barley, maize, rice), roots (e.g. taro, yams, manioc, potatoes) and pulses (e.g. peas, beans, lentils, soya) were among the first plants to be domesticated, and are still the most widely cultivated species. Such foods store very well, but must be cooked or otherwise processed before they can be eaten. They contain much more starch and starch-like nutrients, and much less protein than was normal in the diets of hunter–gatherers. Both wheat and maize lack certain nutrients that are present in pulses: long-established recipes and eating habits minimise the nutritional deficiencies of monotonous diets. Thus tortillas and beans, pea-soup and bread, and baked beans on toast are more satisfying and more nutritious eaten together than is either component separately. Comparisons of seeds and other plant remains found in and around ancient human settlements before and after the development of agriculture reveal a drastic reduction in the variety of food eaten, which was only reversed in Western countries during the twentieth century.

Animals and humans living in parts of the world where there are marked seasonal changes in climate face a severe problem; fresh food is abundant at some times of year but scarce at others. Some kinds of mammals (e.g. rodents such as squirrels,

[10] Hunter–gatherers and the consequences of the transition to agriculture and pastoralism are discussed in *World Health and Disease* (Open University Press, 2nd edn 1993; 3rd edn 2001), Chapters 5 and 11; the Reader article associated with Chapter 5 — 'Agriculture's two-edged sword' by Jared Diamond — is highly relevant to the discussion here (see *Health and Disease: A Reader*, Open University Press, 3rd edn 2001).

rats and mice) thrive on stored food such as seeds and dead leaves. Their bodies can synthesise many of the vitamins that would otherwise be obtained from a diet of fresh food.

● What basic habits of primates other than humans indicate that they could obtain plenty of fresh food at all times of year?

■ Nearly all primates, including all the apes, live in the tropics, where there is less seasonality of plant growth than at higher latitudes, and they are nomadic, moving between food sources, so they have continuous access to fresh plants and do not need the ability to survive on stored or dead plants.

Unlike other primates, humans have colonised virtually every land habitat. Especially in mountains and semi-desert areas, only a few plants can be cultivated efficiently and almost all crops are seasonal, so much of the harvest has to be stored, often for many months. Modern people are the only primates to store food in large quantities or for longer than a few days, and we cannot match the rodents' ability to compensate for absent or degraded vitamins and other essential nutrients in stored food.

The less nutritious diet probably contributed to the reduction in stature and robustness following the adoption of agriculture that has been observed among skeletons found in various parts of southern Europe and Israel. Farming men were, on average, 3 cm shorter, and women were 4 cm shorter, than their hunter–gatherer ancestors. Analysis of skeletons and tooth enamel in cemeteries shows that life expectancy after the age of 15 *declined* in many parts of the world after the adoption of farming.[11] Although it later improved gradually, average life expectancy did not reach pre-agricultural levels until the eighteenth century.

2.6.5 Effects of cooking and farming on health

Cooking and farming, particularly of cereals, also had other less direct, but equally profound, effects on people's well-being. The consequences of the new diet for dental health remain unsolved to the present day. Raw food, particularly leaves and nuts, are coarse and abrasive, and make the teeth wear rapidly, but the frequent abrasion prevents the accumulation on the teeth of the bacteria that cause dental caries (tooth decay). The teeth of ancient hunter–gatherers (and of some modern people who did not eat cereals, such as the Inuit) wore rapidly but rarely decayed. Grains such as wheat are among the stickiest of all foods, and, particularly when combined with sugar and fats, form a coating on the teeth that provides an ideal habitat for bacteria. Continual exposure to high concentrations of bacteria gradually corrodes the hard surface of the teeth. Dental caries are now so widespread in high-income countries that people regard them as inevitable, but they were very rare among pre-agricultural peoples and uncommon among the early farmers of ancient Egypt.

● How can we know so much about dental health in these ancient peoples?

■ Teeth are very durable and remain intact for thousands of years after burial. Surface scratches and cavities in teeth are easily identified in human remains, as is evidence of surgical extraction or natural loss of adult teeth. The practice of burying the dead in specially prepared tombs (first performed on a large scale by the ancient Egyptians about 5 000 years ago), further facilitates such studies.

[11] Some of the reasons are discussed in *World Health and Disease* (Open University Press, 2nd edn 1993; 3rd edn 2001), Chapter 11.

Cooking makes most foods easier to chew and more digestible and thus more suitable for infants and people who have lost most of their teeth. Babies in agricultural communities could be weaned onto cereal gruels and meat or vegetable soups at a much earlier age than was possible among hunter–gatherers, where the only soft food available was that pre-chewed by the mother. In humans, lactation partially (though not completely) inhibits conception, but once breast-feeding stops, a woman's fertility increases quickly.

● How would the development of cooking and cereal production have affected birth spacing and, in consequence, maternal health?

■ By facilitating early weaning, these practices promoted shorter average intervals between births, and hence increased the number of children born to each woman. But the physiological stress to the mother of each pregnancy and of caring for infants remained much the same, so the health burden of reproduction became greater for most women.

The development of dairy farming permitted even earlier weaning onto goats', ewes' or cows' milk, and further reduced the minimum time between births from about 4 years to less than 2 years. This reduction doubled the potential number of children a woman could rear in her lifetime (i.e. her **fecundity**), from 5 or 6 children in pre-agricultural societies to more than 10 in pastoral communities. Cereal gruels and animal milk are less easily digested by very young infants, and are often less nutritious than breast milk. The artificial diet is also much more easily contaminated with pathogens or pollutants, so infants weaned at a young age often suffer more ill-health and grow more slowly than breast-fed children. Consequently, infant mortality was probably higher among farmers than among hunter–gatherers, but the number of such deaths was more than offset by the greatly increased number of children produced. The total human population grew after the first Agricultural Revolution and numbers have never ceased rising.[12] This is a striking example of the power of cultural changes to impact on human health and disease.

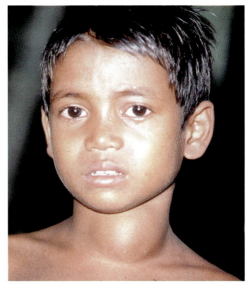

The reduced variety in the diet of settled communities compared with that of hunter–gatherers can give rise to nutrient imbalances and deficiencies, and to nutritional degradation from crop processing and storage. For example, iodine deficiency occurs in certain parts of the world where people live away from the sea (the main dietary source of iodine is fish and other seafood) and where iodine is lacking in drinking water from rivers, lakes and wells. In these regions, excessive growth of the thyroid gland can result (a condition known as goitre). The thyroid requires iodine to synthesise hormones involved in normal growth and development; in its absence the gland grows larger and attempts to increase its output. Goitre was common in Derbyshire before the early nineteenth century (where it was known as 'Derbyshire neck'), until the invention of the railways gave local people access to marine fish and whelks. Extreme iodine deficiency among children causes retarded growth and

The enlargement of the thyroid gland in this boy's neck is a response to the prolonged deficiency of iodine in his diet in inland Pakistan, away from iodine sources such as fish and other seafoods. (Photo: John Paul Kay, Peter Arnold Inc./Science Photo Library)

[12] The growth of the human population from the first Agricultural Revolution to the present, and projections of population size to the middle of the twenty-first century are discussed in *World Health and Disease* (Open University Press, 2nd edn 1993; 3rd edn 2001), Chapters 2 and 8.

irreversible brain damage leading to severe learning difficulties. The exploitation of the sea as a source of food became important several thousand years ago and led to settled communities close to natural harbours and fishing grounds.

2.6.6 Costs and benefits of working the land

Wherever hunter–gatherer and primitive agricultural lifestyles have been compared, the latter is much harder work, involving longer hours of strenuous physical activity, and more repetitive actions and unnatural postures (e.g. planting crops, grinding corn — using primitive stone tools), which involve physiological stress. For example, comparison of the incidence of arthritis in skeletons from pre-agricultural and post-agricultural deposits suggest that the disease is largely restricted to elderly people in hunter–gatherer societies, but becomes much more common in younger farming people.

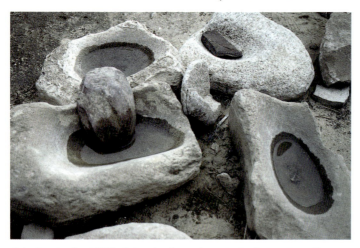

Grinding tools at Little Petra, Jordan, where agriculture was well established 8 000 years ago. Grain was ground, a handful at a time, in a hollowed-out bowl using hard stones such as the one in the left foreground, by the operator kneeling in front and pushing and pulling with both arms. Very similar apparatus was in use in remote areas until the middle of the twentieth century. (Photo: Caroline Pond)

To be able to reap where they have sown, farming people are much more sedentary than hunter–gatherers. Many forms of animal husbandry also require people to live in permanent settlements, although some pastoralists remain nomadic to the present day, moving between good grazing areas with their flocks and herds.

● How would sedentary habits affect the incidence of infectious diseases?

■ A settled community lives continuously near its own refuse and that of its livestock which, together with more disturbance of soil and water, promotes transmission of infectious diseases. A settled home also favours the breeding of ectoparasites such as fleas and lice, and stored food supports rats and mice, some of which may harbour infectious diseases.

On the other hand, agriculturalists came into contact with wild animals less frequently, so accidents and hunting injuries may have become rarer.

Therefore, compared with hunting, as we have said above, agriculture and pastoralism are much harder work and do not produce a healthier diet. Moreover, unforeseen and uncontrollable failures in supply are not so easily avoided, as the frequency of famines demonstrates. So why did people abandon hunting and gathering in favour of the new technology? The most plausible answer is that the practices enabled people to live at higher densities and, because one family could produce enough food for several others, more people were able to devote themselves full-time to activities unrelated to food acquisition, such as religion, arts, manufacturing, building, commerce and politics. Agriculture made possible the political infrastructure and labour needed to raise an army or undertake major projects such as building irrigation systems, ramparts, temples and pyramids.

Wherever they come into direct conflict, people living in such complex communities defeat hunter–gatherer groups who have no tradition of centralised political

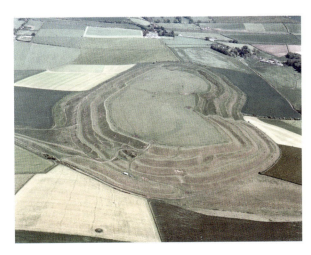

Maiden Castle near Dorchester in Dorset, England. This impressive structure, fortified with several rows of dykes and ditches, was built by people who became numerous and had established a highly organised society more than 2 000 years ago (long before the Romans invaded Britain). It may have been a religious centre or a military fort, or both, for the surrounding population, who kept sheep and other livestock, grew crops and made a rich variety of metal and wooden tools, pottery, clothes and ornaments. (Photo: London Aerial Photo Library)

leadership. For example, the main reason why the Inuit are confined to the Arctic tundra is that more numerous, better-armed and politically better-organised Amerindians could (and frequently did) defeat small bands of Inuit that entered the forested areas in search of wood. Except in Australia, all modern hunter–gatherers are confined to the Arctic, deserts, inaccessible rainforest and other areas which are useless for agriculture. In short, the cultural evolution of agriculture produced modern society and enabled the human population to increase very rapidly. It is estimated that there are now at least 1 500 times as many people as there were about 9 000 years ago, when agriculture and animal husbandry began.

Comparisons between the few remaining modern hunter–gatherer societies and agricultural societies suggest that, although the changes brought about by agriculture diversified and extended men's activities, on the whole they reduced the social status and opportunities of women. Ownership of agricultural land and other resources increased the importance of inheritance and hence of paternity, which restricted women's choice in marriage and promoted more severe penalties for infidelity and low fertility. More of their lives were spent pregnant or caring for small children, many of whom would die young; food production, preparation and storage became more onerous; women became more tied to the home and had less opportunity to collaborate with the men in artistic, commercial and political activities.

2.7   The origins of infectious diseases

As you will see later in this book (Chapter 5) many of the most dangerous and debilitating human diseases are caused by pathogens. They fall into two main groups: **endogenous human diseases** in which the pathogens are transmitted from person to person (e.g. dysentery, typhoid, cholera, syphilis) and **zoonoses** in which the pathogens either spend part of their life cycle in or on another species (the secondary host), or were originally diseases of other animals that incidentally or occasionally infected people. The prevalence of the endogenous human infectious diseases depends very much upon the habits of the people themselves, such as their mobility, hygiene and group size. The life cycles and abundance of zoonoses are largely independent of human population density, although our habits, particularly diet, may greatly influence their transmission from other species to humans.

While working as a vet at the London Zoo in the 1950s and 1960s, Richard Fiennes demonstrated **cross-infection** of parasites and infectious diseases between different species of animals and between animals and people, and developed the theory of the animal origins of many human infectious diseases. (The standard text is listed under Fiennes, 1978, in the Further sources list at the end of this book.) In the final part of this chapter, we will illustrate this theory in a brief review of some major infectious diseases, starting with those involving larger parasites, which are generally visible with the naked eye for at least part of their life cycle; most are mentioned again in Chapters 5 and 6.

2.7.1 Multicellular parasites

Most flatworms (which include tapeworms and flukes) and unsegmented roundworms (nematodes) cannot be transmitted from person to person, but require a secondary host to complete their life cycle. Most such life cycles are very complex and often variable. The following examples give you an idea of the number and variety of interactions between people and their biological environment.

Schistosomiasis (or bilharzia), a complex and debilitating disease, is caused by *Schistosoma*, a fluke for which the secondary host is a freshwater snail; river blindness and elephantiasis are caused by several species of nematode and are transmitted by various biting flies including blackflies (*Simulium* species) that breed in freshwater; the guinea worm, *Dracunculus medinensis*, is also a nematode that proliferates in a small freshwater shrimp-like animal. All these *macroparasites* (i.e. multicellular pathogens) also infect other mammals, including dogs, horses, cattle, apes and monkeys and have probably troubled hominids for millennia. But the parasites probably became more common when fish became an important food many thousands of years ago. People spent more time standing or swimming in freshwater (and defaecating in or near it) than would have been necessary when they hunted land mammals. More recently, artificial irrigation systems created additional habitats for the snails that serve as the secondary host for the *Schistosoma* fluke.

The adult stages of the tapeworm *Taenia* (and of the nematode *Trichinella*, mentioned earlier as a cause of trichinosis among Inuit peoples) occur only in mammals that eat the flesh of other mammals, so these parasites are very rare in non-human primates. They have probably been an occasional cause of illness ever since hominids became hunters, but *Taenia* infestation of humans did not become common until people began living in close association with domesticated pigs. The use of human and animal excreta as manure increases crop yields and reduces the need for chemical fertilisers, but it also facilitates the transmission of parasites. In fact, in rural China in the past, lavatories were sometimes built over pigsties, enabling the pigs to eat the freshly deposited human faeces. While these arrangements recycled the faecal nutrients as pig food and hence eventually as food for humans, they also maximised the transfer of tapeworm eggs from humans to pigs.

● How can the spread of the parasites from pigs to humans be limited?

■ Cooking the pork kills the infective stages of the tapeworm in the pigs' muscle, and thereby limits the spread of the parasite.

However, one meal of incompletely cooked meat is often enough to establish infection, so in practice a high proportion of people who eat pork from pigs reared in this way harbour tapeworms. People have probably been troubled by tapeworms for many thousands of years, but many parasites, some of which cause serious disease, have apparently spread into the human population quite recently, as a direct result of people's habits and their associations with domesticated animals.

For example, the *Toxocara* nematodes are normally parasites of dogs and cats. The larvae infest the lungs, liver, muscles and uterus (whence nearly all puppies and kittens acquire them from their mother before birth) and eventually migrate to the gut where they mature. The ripe eggs are eliminated with the faeces and may be eaten by a rat or mouse, in which they become larvae that burrow into the rodent tissues. Dogs and cats are normally re-infected by eating infested prey. Humans, particularly children, may acquire *Toxocara* eggs from contact with contaminated dog or cat faeces or from handling puppies and kittens. The resulting larvae wander through the human tissues, causing abdominal and muscular pains. More rarely, but more seriously, they infest the eye, and cause blindness. Clearly, the use of cats to kill the rodents that eat our stored food, and the keeping of cats and dogs as pets, greatly facilitate the transmission of *Toxocara*, increasing its abundance and turning what were formerly rare, isolated cases of cross-infection into a significant medical problem.

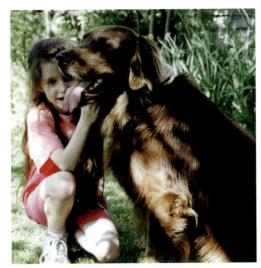

The intimacy of the relationships between people, especially children, and their domestic pets promotes the transmission of parasites. (Photo: Mike Wibberley)

Another example — psittacosis — is a disease derived from keeping birds as pets, or for racing, and is a kind of bird pneumonia that is common in pigeons (named after the Latin word for parrot, *psittacus*). It is important to emphasise that most pets and livestock pose little threat to the health of their owners, as long as basic rules of hygiene are followed, and the animals receive regular preventive treatment for worms, fleas and other parasites. The half a dozen cases of psittacosis each year may attract attention, but the rest of the millions of people who live for years in close contact with poultry, pigeons, budgerigars and parrots do not develop the disease (though such contact may contribute, along with smoking, to susceptibility to lung cancer).

2.7.2 Micro-organisms

Malaria and sleeping sickness are zoonoses endemic to Africa that we probably inherited from our primate ancestors. At least four different species of the single-celled organism, *Plasmodium*, cause malaria, and a virus causes yellow fever. These pathogens cannot pass directly from person to person but are transmitted by a *vector*, in both cases blood-sucking mosquitoes. Although the micro-organisms live for some time in the secondary host, their presence does no apparent harm to the mosquitoes, which continue to feed from any thin-skinned mammal they find, including humans. An opportunity for the pathogenic micro-organisms to invade another host is created each time an infected insect pierces a host's skin to take a blood meal. The malaria-carrying *Anopheles* mosquitoes breed in warm, stagnant water, so shallow pools and ditches created by artificial irrigation systems in the tropics provide ideal habitats for them. Malaria causes more than 1 million deaths per year in developing countries, mostly among children under the age of five.

Sleeping sickness is caused by several different kinds of another single-celled organism, *Trypanosoma*, which also parasitises many species of birds, reptiles, amphibians and mammals, including deer, horses, antelope, buffalo and cattle. *Trypanosoma* is transmitted by tsetse flies between people and between humans and other animals, many of which appear not to suffer any serious symptoms of disease. Because wild animals can harbour the pathogen for a long time without becoming ill, they act as a reservoir from which humans and their domesticated livestock can acquire the infection.

● Is it likely that sleeping sickness would have occurred among our hunter–gatherer ancestors?

■ Yes, probably. Hunters had frequent contact with the large mammals in which the pathogens occur, and people may have followed the herds, sleeping and eating near their grazing grounds, thereby exposing themselves to tsetse flies.

Diseases such as sleeping sickness and malaria are rare outside the tropics because their insect vectors cannot breed in cold climates. In contrast, rabies is a zoonosis that is transmitted by one mammal biting another and so is worldwide in distribution, even occurring among foxes and seals in the high Arctic. People can acquire the infection from many kinds of mammal, most often bats, foxes and dogs (but, curiously, not from other humans), and so this fatal disease almost certainly afflicted hunter–gatherers who shared the caves that these animals used as dens or roosts, and which they may also have killed for food.

Some bacteria and viral diseases that are now endemic to humans appear to have originally been zoonoses that underwent a physiological transformation, which enabled them to transfer directly from person to person. We will look at the evolutionary processes more closely in Chapter 5; here we focus on the interaction between human culture and the biological environment that increased the likelihood of transmission between people and other animals. Many of these infectious diseases originated in domestic animals and therefore must have spread to people only since the rise of animal husbandry.

For example, the microscopic structure of the measles virus closely resembles that of the canine distemper virus (which causes a 'flu-like disease in wolves and dogs), and the rinderpest virus, which causes debilitating disease in many kinds of hoofed mammals, including domestic cattle. Measles may have become a human disease after domestication of the dog about 12 000 years ago, or when people took up pastoralism about 8 000 years ago, but no serious epidemics of measles were recorded until the middle of the first millennium AD. It was a major cause of death among children in Europe and Asia until the middle of the twentieth century and remains a significant hazard among children in the low-income countries of the developing world, particularly in Sub-Saharan Africa.

Smallpox is probably a mutant form of cowpox, a relatively benign disease of cattle. The first recorded major smallpox epidemic occurred in the eastern Roman empire (Syria, Turkey, Cyprus) in the second century AD, and there were scores more outbreaks of the disease before its similarity to cowpox was exploited. Edward Jenner's experiments with vaccination using matter from cowpox pustules gave some protection in the eighteenth century against later infection with smallpox.[13]

Diphtheria is another major disease derived from cattle husbandry and milk drinking. It is caused by the toxins secreted by the bacterium *Corynebacterium diptheriae*, which proliferate on cow udders, producing ulcers but no serious disease in the cows. Diphtheria is a relatively new disease; it is mentioned in writings from the sixth century AD, but did not become widespread until the sixteenth century in

[13] The early history of vaccination (Jenner's term comes from the Latin *Vacca* for cow, the source of the cowpox vaccine) is described in *Caring for Health: History and Diversity* (Open University Press, 2nd edn 1993; 3rd edn 2001). The successful campaign to eradicate smallpox from the world in 1980 is discussed in an article by Strassburg, which appears in *Health and Disease: A Reader* (Open University Press, 2nd edn 1995; 3rd edn 2001), and is set reading for OU students during *World Health and Disease* (Open University Press, 2nd edn 1993; 3rd edn 2001), Chapter 3.

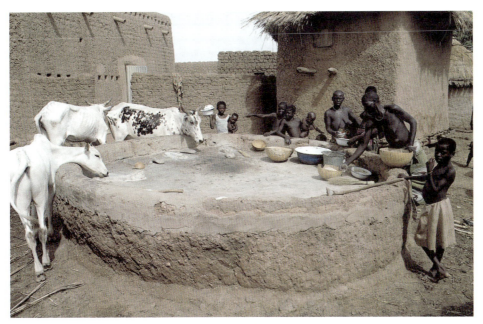

People and their domestic animals have lived in close proximity since animal husbandry started to replace hunting more than 8 000 years ago. Parasites and infectious diseases derived from, or shared with, livestock are very common in pastoral societies, like this one in the West African state of Burkina Faso, often affecting almost the entire population. (Photo: Jeremy Hartley/ Panos Pictures)

Spain, by which time it could be transmitted directly from person to person as well as from cattle to people. It remained common around the world until the antitoxin began to be used in treatment in Europe and the USA at the end of the nineteenth century. In Britain, diphtheria has declined to isolated cases since the mass immunisation of children began in the 1940s, but it remains a significant source of child deaths in the developing world.

Cattle (and many related hoofed animals) suffer from tuberculosis, caused by the bacterium *Mycobacterium tuberculosis bovis*. People who drink raw (i.e. unpasteurised or unboiled) milk risk infection with the bacterium, which enters the body via the bowel and thence travels to the spleen, kidneys, bones and joints, where it produces characteristic deformations. Such evidence for bovine tuberculosis is observed in a few Neolithic human skeletons from 7 000 years ago and in some Egyptian mummies. Much more recently, probably within the last 1 000 years, a new strain of bacteria called *Mycobacterium tuberculosis hominis* has appeared; it can live for short periods in air and so can be transmitted directly from person to person in their breath. This form of tuberculosis mainly affects the lungs (pulmonary TB) and has once again become a serious endemic disease in the twenty-first century.[14] We return to the physiological and evolutionary consequences of people drinking animal milk in Chapter 7.

Cattle have proved a source of a more recent infectious human pathogen. Several species of wild and domesticated animals carry unusual pathogens known as **prions**, which cause fatal neurodegenerative diseases (you will learn more about the nature of these agents in Chapter 5). In the case of cattle, a prion causes bovine spongiform

[14] Tuberculosis is the subject of a major case study in the first book in this series, *Medical Knowledge: Doubt and Certainty* (Open University Press, 2nd edn 1994; colour-enhanced 2nd edn 2001) , Chapter 4.

encephalopathy (BSE), and there is now substantial evidence that in the 1980s and 1990s it was passed to humans in several European countries, but predominantly in the UK. By the end of the year 2000, human prion infection in the UK had caused over 70 cases of neurodegeneration, termed variant Creutzfeldt–Jakob disease (vCJD). It is believed that the infective prion spread to UK dairy and beef herds through the use of contaminated feed, and then into the human food chain via beef and processed beef products. More than 175 000 cattle in the UK, primarily dairy cows, had died of BSE by the early 1990s, when the early slaughter programmes were introduced in an attempt to eradicate the disease. Although it is not yet known whether the number of cases of vCJD will increase in the coming years, the size of the cattle population affected by BSE suggests that the consequences for humans had not reached its peak by the turn of the new millennium.

Horses are the only animals other than humans to harbour the rhinoviruses ('nose' viruses) that cause the common colds. Rhinoviruses undergo frequent changes in microscopic structure and properties and numerous variant forms of the virus probably spread into the human population after horses were domesticated about 6 000 years ago. The large number of variants of rhinovirus means that people 'catch a cold' many times in their lives, as new variants are encountered.

Earlier, we mentioned plague and the association with rats living in human settlements, but we can take the story back even further in time. The plague bacterium (*Yersinia pestis*) originated among burrowing rodents and their fleas on the dry plains of central Asia. Gerbils were probably the original host, but the organism proliferates in dozens of related species, including ground squirrels, marmots, hamsters and rats. By 1940, it had been described in 34 different rodents and 35 species of fleas in the USA alone. Disturbance of the land by agriculture brought gerbils and their fleas into contact with the rats that lived in close association with people, eating their stored food. Where mammals mix, their fleas do as well, and thus plague became a disease of rats and then of people, probably during the first century AD. There were numerous outbreaks of plague, particularly in the densely populated agricultural areas of India, northern China, southern Russia, parts of Africa, and, from the fifth century AD onwards, in western Asia and Europe.

Typhus also originated from rodents, in this case mice. It is caused by a kind of very small bacterium called rickettsia. Mouse typhus is transmitted by lice and, although widespread, is not very dangerous to mice nor to people who, since ancient times, have sometimes contracted this form of the disease from mouse lice. Early in the fifteenth century, probably in Europe, a new form of the rickettsia arose that is much more lethal both to people and to the human lice that transmit it.

● What would be the consequences of the lice becoming ill?

■ They probably stop searching out new hosts and sucking their blood, thereby ceasing to be effective as vectors of the disease, and they may fail to breed.

Failure to feed and abnormal lethargy are probably the only ways that scientists know that the lice are adversely affected by infestation with the rickettsia. Lice infected with the typhus rickettsia never survive longer than a fortnight, and louse morbidity and mortality usually contribute more than human mortality to terminating epidemics of typhus that were (and in some areas still are) frequent and severe, especially in refugee and squatter camps, hostels, and among people displaced by warfare, famine or natural disasters. This example illustrates the *instability* of the balance between survival of the host species and survival of the

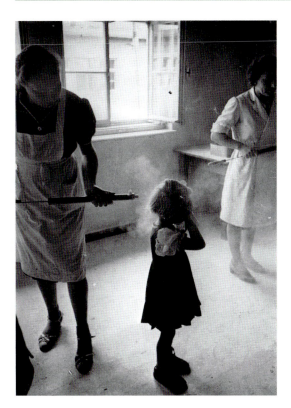

The human body louse flourishes where people are forced to live in overcrowded and insanitary conditions, e.g. in refugee and squatter camps, hostels for homeless people. Here a refugee child from Sudetenland is being deloused, 1948. As well as being an irritant, numerous lice can lead to epidemics of typhus fever, which took thousands of lives in refugee and army camps all over continental Europe at the end of World War II. (Photo: Hulton Getty Picture Collection)

pathogens that infest them. The constantly changing relationship between environmental conditions and the coevolution of pathogens and their hosts is discussed further in Chapter 5.

The hunter–gatherer way of life also brought with it risks from micro-organisms infecting their prey. Present-day tribal societies that live in partly settled communities remain at risk when they supplement their diets with 'bushmeat'. The most dramatic example of a human infectious disease originating in this way reached public attention in the 1980s, when AIDS (Acquired Immune Deficiency Syndrome) was first identified in the USA. The human immunodeficiency virus (HIV), which causes AIDS in humans, is believed to have originated in African monkeys, and may have been first transmitted to hunters via cuts and scratches from trapped or wounded animals. It is not known exactly when it first infected humans, but it is likely to have been several decades before it began to spread from person to person as a sexually transmitted disease, and later via infected blood, transmitted during medical procedures or between injecting drug-users. AIDS was responsible for the deaths of an estimated cumulative total of 16.3 million adults and children by the end of 1999, and a further 33.6 million were living with HIV infection or had developed AIDS worldwide (WHO/UNAIDS Report 1999).

2.8   Conclusions

Humans are primates and much of our anatomical structure and sensory abilities, our social habits and dietary needs, arise directly from that heritage. Some of the anatomical and physiological features that make humans unique among primates still have medical repercussions. The demands of giving birth to large-brained infants compete with those of bipedality and walking efficiency in shaping the pelvis. The hip and thigh of modern women are significantly less efficient for walking and running than those of hominids of 3 million years ago, and mechanical difficulties in giving birth are much more frequent and severe than in any other mammal for which there is adequate information.

It is important to realise that evolution cannot be arrested; human anatomy, physiology, reproductive habits and longevity will change in the future in ways shaped by agriculture, industrialisation, social organisation, modern medical practice and much more. The fossil record of humans and other species clearly shows that the rate of change of a structure usually accelerates when habits and habitat are changing rapidly. Human culture and technology are now changing faster than ever.

The course and incidence of infectious diseases are profoundly affected by our biological heritage and by interactions with other species, both ancient and recent. One striking feature of the biology of 'new' human infections is the variable, often very long, interval between their first appearance and becoming widespread or serious. Measles, tuberculosis, plague, and perhaps smallpox probably affected people occasionally for centuries, even millennia, before they became a cause of serious epidemics (and hence were mentioned in official records). The same may be true of AIDS.

The evolutionary processes described in this chapter (and expanded in Chapters 3 to 5) are still in operation and will continue in the future. Infectious diseases have been acquired from 'new' foods such as cows' milk, and from animals such as cattle, pigs, rats and domestic pets with which humans came into frequent contact only relatively recently in our history. Although most of these diseases are now controllable in countries with adequately resourced public-health systems, they are major causes of death in the developing world. New infections can, and probably will, emerge by similar mechanisms — as AIDS and vCJD testify. AIDs is just one of a long series of diseases that have arisen apparently *de novo*, and spread alarmingly rapidly through populations who are unused to dealing with them. We also add new components to our diet (e.g. novel foods, synthetic drugs and hormones) and acquire new stressful habits (e.g. driving fast cars in dense traffic).

However, there is no reason to conclude that humans are inherently more susceptible to disease than other animals. Human diseases have been far more intensively studied than those of any other species, so we know something about even very rare diseases that affect perhaps one person in a million. Among wild animals, only the commonest and most lethal diseases have been investigated scientifically; rare or chronic diseases go unnoticed among all the other causes of mortality such as starvation and predation. Other animals, particularly large, long-lived species, probably have similarly complex relationships with their biological environments, about which we know very little. Indeed, disturbance of such disease patterns may be behind the unexplained decline and extinction of some species.

Finally, we should avoid idealising primeval humans and should not underestimate the enormous benefits that agriculture, animal husbandry and other aspects of civilisation have brought to human health. You might consider whether you would swap a comfortable home for a damp, dark, smoky cave infested with lice, fleas and rabies-carrying bats and rats, in constant danger of injury from both large prey and other predators!

OBJECTIVES FOR CHAPTER 2

When you have studied this chapter, you should be able to:

2.1 Define and use, or recognise definitions and applications of, each of the terms printed in **bold** in the text.

2.2 Describe some anatomical and physiological similarities and differences between modern humans and other living kinds of primates, and comment on their possible consequences for human health and survival.

2.3 Outline the evolutionary origin and main implications for human health of: bipedality; enlarged brains; hair reduction; adolescent growth spurt; menopause.

2.4 Outline the main implications for human health of: the control of fire; living in caves and shelters; wearing clothes; cultivation of crops; animal husbandry.

2.5 Illustrate the interaction between human culture and the biological environment with examples of some zoonotic human diseases.

QUESTIONS FOR CHAPTER 2

1 (*Objective 2.2*)

Which features and habits of non-human primates are associated with the evolution of the following?

(a) large, forward pointing eyes, good colour vision and reduced sense of smell; (b) relatively small jaws and unspecialised teeth; (c) good balance, agile, flexible limbs and flat, blunt fingernails and toenails.

2 (*Objective 2.3*)

Describe in a few sentences the main changes to the pelvis and spinal column that have evolved in humans. How do these adaptations to locomotion affect the process of giving birth? How does the growth and mature shape of the female pelvis affect locomotion?

3 (*Objective 2.4*)

What adverse effects did (a) occupying caves and shelters, and (b) living permanently in one place, have on human health?

4 (*Objective 2.5*)

Describe in a few sentences the roles of: (a) insects, (b) freshwater animals, and (c) dogs, in the transmission of human infectious diseases.

CHAPTER 3

The story of life in a few pages

Study notes for OU students

This chapter is the longest and most complex in the book for those of you who have not studied biology before. It builds on the hierarchy of biological organisation, described in Chapter 9 of *Studying Health and Disease* (Open University Press, second edition 1994; colour-enhanced second edition 2001). There you also learnt about methods of viewing biological material through various kinds of microscope; these methods produced many of the photographs in the present chapter. The theory of evolution by natural selection and the biological meaning of 'adaptation' and 'fitness' were introduced in Chapter 5 of *World Health and Disease* (Open University Press, second edition 1993; third edition 2001), and are expanded here.

We introduce many new biological terms and concepts in this chapter, some of which (e.g. cell, protein, DNA) are in everyday use. We suggest that you read right through the *whole* chapter once (it will take 2–3 hours), and then return to re-read any sections that you feel uncertain about. In particular, you will need to study Sections 3.4 and 3.6 on DNA and protein synthesis carefully — later chapters frequently refer back to them. The TV programme 'Bloodlines: A family legacy', associated with this chapter, will help you to visualise DNA and understand its central role in evolution.

3.1   The time-scale of evolutionary biology

Biology is the study of living things. All living things — organisms — share two fundamental properties that distinguish them from inanimate objects. They have the capacity, first, for self-maintenance and, second, for reproduction. **Self-maintenance** refers to the fact that organisms grow, they have a limited capacity to repair or replace parts that wear out, and they can protect themselves to some extent against threats to their survival. **Reproduction** refers to the ability of organisms to leave progeny that are replicas of themselves. These properties are shared not only by all the organisms that coexist on Earth today, but also by every successful life-form that has ever existed. In this context, 'success' simply means that the organism survived long enough to reproduce.

This chapter introduces some basic biological concepts that provide a framework in which the **evolution** of large, complex animals such as ourselves can be examined. Evolution can be defined as:

> All the changes that have transformed life on Earth from its earliest beginnings to the diversity that characterises it today. (Campbell, 1993, Glossary, p. G–11)

In Chapter 2, we turned back the 'evolutionary clock' just a fraction, to the appearance of primates about 60 million years ago. But there is evidence to suggest that the Earth was formed very approximately 4 500 million years ago and that the most primitive life-forms evolved sometime within the next 1 000 million years. What happened in the unimaginably vast period between the first life-forms appearing and the evolution of modern humans, *Homo sapiens*? This time-scale may be easier to grasp if you think of the history of the Earth as being represented by a single year:

the Earth formed on the first of January and the earliest single-celled organisms appeared around the end of March, but it took until early November before simple, worm-like multicellular creatures evolved; reptiles appeared about the middle of December and humans at about teatime on New Year's Eve.

On this time-scale, we have some reasonably well-accepted theories (described in Chapter 2) about what went on in the last week of December, but little more than a number of interesting hypotheses about the nature or sequence of events for the first 95 per cent of the time for which life has existed on Earth. We begin this chapter by sketching in some of the ideas that are currently being discussed among evolutionary biologists, noting that it is highly unlikely that a definitive version will ever be agreed.

In describing the possible circumstances of the origins of life-forms, we inevitably have to use some new biological terms. Our intention in this chapter is first to 'tell the story' of the origins of life (in so far as we can guess at it) and then go back and unpack the important terms and concepts, piece by piece. The middle of the chapter describes a number of processes within living things that are so basic they occur in all organisms — from bacteria to people. Then we look at the kind of organisational features that accompany an increase in complexity, as multicellular (many-celled) organisms evolved from their single-celled ancestors. Finally, the chapter examines the meaning of such words as 'simple', 'complex', 'primitive' and 'advanced' in the context of evolution.

3.2   In the beginning?

As the crust of the newly formed Earth cooled, the surface seems to have been a slurry of muddy water which gradually formed into pools of liquid and expanses of soft clay. This has often been called the 'primeval soup'. The Earth's surface was subject to violent electrical storms, intense ultraviolet radiation, very high temperatures and volcanic eruptions on a massive scale. The surface layers contained a rich variety of molecules but — unlike the Earth today — neither the crust nor the atmosphere above it contained more than a trace of 'free' oxygen (oxygen that is not bound to other chemical substances).

As defined in Chapter 1, *molecules* are assemblies of *atoms*, which in turn are the basic units of matter from which each of the unique chemical *elements* (such as carbon, oxygen, hydrogen and nitrogen) are made. Some molecules are very simple and very small; for example, carbon monoxide (a constituent of volcanic vapours and of modern car exhausts) consists of just one atom of the element carbon (denoted by the letter C) and one of another element, oxygen (O), hence its chemical symbol, CO. Small molecules like this one may have been present in the interior of the newly formed planet and were thrown up by volcanic activity, or they may have arrived from outer space in meteors and the dust-tails of comets.[1]

We have limited knowledge of which molecules were actually dissolved in the pools and clays of the early Earth environment, or were part of its atmosphere. What biologists think may have been present has been deduced partly from observations of conditions on Earth today. For example, it is widely assumed that there must

[1] You do not need to know any more chemistry to follow the rest of this book; it is enough to know that each element has a unique symbol (such as C and O) and these can be used to write down a chemical formula for a molecule formed from those elements (as in CO, carbon monoxide or CO_2, carbon dioxide, where the subscript 2 denotes that there are two atoms of oxygen in the carbon dioxide molecule).

have been some simple compounds containing carbon and oxygen, such as carbon monoxide and carbon dioxide (CO_2), plus some nitrogen gas (two atoms of the element nitrogen joined together, N_2), lots of hydrogen gas (H_2) and some ammonia, sulphur dioxide and methane, because these gases are found in the emissions of present-day volcanoes. The other strand of reasoning has been to work backwards from the molecules found in present-day organisms and deduce how they might have been formed from simpler precursors, under the conditions believed to exist on the primitive Earth. From the 1950s to the present day, biologists have attempted to recreate the 'primeval soup' in laboratory apparatus; various mixtures of small molecules that were believed to be present in the earliest times have been subjected to heat, electrical activity and ultraviolet radiation to see if they would fuse to form larger molecules.

Under these conditions *organic molecules* can be induced to form; these are molecules containing mainly the elements carbon, hydrogen, oxygen and nitrogen, arranged in configurations that resemble the molecules of living organisms today. Organic molecules are the building blocks from which the cells, tissues and organs of all organisms are made, and they form the 'liquid' fraction inside and between cells, in which the chemical reactions necessary to sustain life take place.

Experimental manipulation of conditions in the test-tube have shown that these organic molecules can be induced to 'coalesce' into droplets (rather like tiny globules of liquid fat in water), creating a primitive structure that *may* have been the forerunner of the cell. Whether or not the laboratory experiments have actually recreated what went on 4 000 million years ago we shall never know, but the theoretical principle has been established: little molecules can be made to fuse into bigger ones which resemble the building blocks from which present-day organisms are made, and these in turn can form structures with a surface boundary that have a passing resemblance to cells. The 'giant leap' in the evolution of life on Earth was the formation of a cell with the ability to *replicate*, that is, produce more cells just like itself.

3.2.1   RNA: the first self-reproducing molecule?

Imagine that, by chance, small molecules assembled in the 'primeval soup' and combined to produce a large organic molecule with the potential to form part of a living structure. However, no progress towards the evolution of a cell could be made unless this large molecule had the capability to *reproduce itself*.

● Explain why this property was (literally) vital to the evolution of life on Earth.

■ In the chaotic world of random encounters between molecules, potentially useful assemblies would be demolished in the next electrical storm, *unless* some process developed that not only preserved the useful molecules but also made lots more. A useful molecule could only persist in an environment if it could reproduce itself, so even though some copies of the molecule would be destroyed, lots more could be made. They could thereafter contribute to the evolution of more complex structures such as living cells.

The prime candidate for such a key stabilising role in early evolution is a large organic molecule called **RNA (ribonucleic acid)**, which is a single strand of much smaller organic molecules called *nucleotides*, joined end-to-end like beads on a

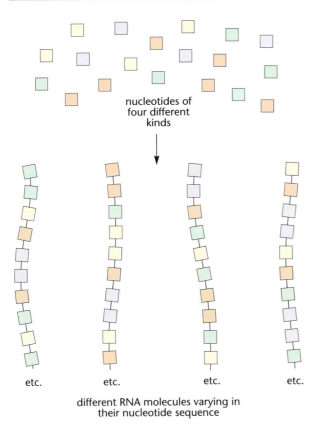

nucleotides of
four different
kinds

different RNA molecules varying in
their nucleotide sequence

Figure 3.1   *RNA consists of four different kinds of building blocks called nucleotides, which can join up in any sequence to form a huge number of unique variant RNA molecules.*

necklace.[2] RNA consists of only four different kinds of nucleotides, but they can join up in any order (see Figure 3.1), to form a strand of anywhere between a few hundred and a few thousand nucleotides long. The fact that nucleotides can be joined together in any order means that RNA molecules can be synthesised in a huge number of variants — each unique RNA molecule is made of the same four nucleotides, but they differ in their nucleotide number and sequence.

One of the most important points to remember about the very simple structure of RNA is that it lends itself to being *copied*. If whole molecules of RNA are placed into a test-tube with a mixture of separate nucleotides of all four types, then (under certain conditions) each of the original strands of RNA can act as a sort of 'template' or 'pattern' for the construction of new copies of itself, built from the nucleotides in the surrounding mixture. Thus a single strand of a particular RNA variant can rapidly 'reproduce' to give hundreds, even thousands, of identical copies of the parent strand. This process is known as **RNA replication**.

RNA is a vital component of all living cells today, because it contains within its structure the 'codes' that instruct cells how to make *proteins*.

[2] We describe the structure of nucleotides later in this chapter, when we discuss DNA, which is also made from nucleotides; for now, just think of them as the 'blocks' from which RNA is constructed.

3.2.2 Building on success: from RNA to protein to cell

All life-forms use **proteins** for a huge variety of tasks (we shall discuss some of them later). They are large organic molecules, made from smaller molecules called **amino acids**, which — like RNA — may have formed in early Earth environments. The ability to produce proteins with the help of RNA must have been an important stage in the evolution of an ordered living cell from a random molecular soup. Biologists don't know exactly how this happened, so what follows is simply the best guess around at the moment.

The four nucleotides from which RNA is constructed have a weak affinity for amino acids. In the present day, there are only 20 different kinds of amino acids in living things and (like the nucleotides in RNA) they can be joined together in long strings in any sequence. Since there are 20 different kinds, endless permutations are possible in a string of several hundred amino acids. Each unique sequence of joined-up amino acids constitutes a different *protein*, and each protein has a unique function. A tentative idea about how primitive proteins may have been formed with the help of RNA is summarised in Figure 3.2. The hypothesis runs thus:

- First came RNA in a huge number of variants, differing in the sequence of their nucleotides (part of a single RNA variant is shown in Figure 3.2).

- Each of these RNA variants attracted a particular, unique sequence of amino acids, which joined up with each other to give a unique protein (again, we have only shown part of one protein strand forming alongside the RNA molecule).

- Once the complete protein had formed (and it would be many hundreds or thousands of amino acids in length), it floated off into the 'soup', leaving the strand of RNA free to attract more of the *same* amino acids to join together in the *same* sequence, and hence make another copy of the *same* protein, and so on.

Some of the RNA variants would, in theory, be more 'successful' than others at attracting amino acids and, by the same token, some of the resulting proteins would be more useful than others in constructing primitive cells. Later in this chapter, we will look at the processes by which most biologists believe these more useful RNA variants might have been 'selected' and as a consequence made more and more copies of themselves, while other less useful variants died out. As you will see, this selection process is thought to operate not only at the level of molecules, but on whole organisms: you may have heard of it referred to as *natural selection* in the context of Charles Darwin's theory of evolution.

For the moment, we ask you to focus on the notion that a primitive molecule that has the ability to replicate itself and to 'instruct' the building of numerous different proteins is an essential component of the origins of life. Whether this primitive molecule was indeed RNA, we may never know. The next step in the story is even more clouded in speculation. Where did the other sorts of molecules found in life-forms, such as carbohydrates and fats, come from? They must also have been assembled from simpler molecules found in the 'soup'. Some of them may have required complex interactions with primitive proteins before this could take place.

Certain proteins in the modern cell have the property of aiding the fusion of small molecules into larger ones, or conversely breaking down larger molecules into smaller components. These proteins are called *enzymes* and we will give them more attention later, but you should get the general idea at this point that enzymes *might* have been produced in the primeval soup (along with other proteins), and these in turn *might* have helped to build carbohydrates, fats and all the other organic molecules needed to build a cell and perform all the functions of life.

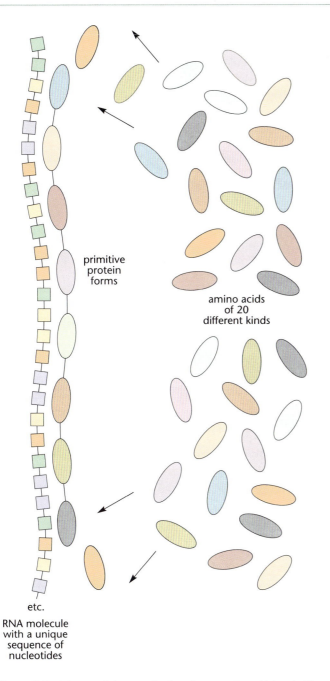

primitive
protein
forms

amino acids
of 20
different kinds

etc.

RNA molecule
with a unique
sequence of
nucleotides

Figure 3.2   *The possible organisational process by which primitive proteins were formed with the help of RNA. Amino acids exist in 20 different kinds; they are attracted to a particular RNA molecule and join together in a precise sequence, which is determined by the sequence of nucleotides in that variant of RNA. Thus, RNA carries in its structure the 'coded' instructions for making a particular protein.*

So, assuming that all the necessary building blocks of a primitive cell gradually appeared in the primeval soup and coalesced into droplets with a surface boundary, how did the first living cell arise? We have no answer to this except to say that the time-scale from 'soup' to cell may be 500–1 000 million years. In this vastness, primitive structures with some cell-like features may have evolved and died out many times, until by chance a variation on the theme arose which was stable enough to survive and, more importantly, *reproduce*.

The distinguishing features of living organisms are (as we said at the outset) self-maintenance and reproduction. The key to the reproduction of a whole cell is *DNA* (deoxyribonucleic acid), a molecule with certain similarities to RNA (and from which it may have evolved). Just as RNA contains the coded instructions for making certain proteins, so DNA contains the coded instructions for making whole new cells. You will find out later how it does this fabulous trick. Next, we look at the cell in some detail, since it is the building block from which all living organisms are made.

3.3   Cells

3.3.1   Variations on a common theme

Organisms are enormously diverse, but they also show uniformity; that is, they all share a number of features and fundamental properties that differentiate them from non-living things. As described above, all organisms are capable of self-maintenance and reproduction in appropriate environments. Another aspect of the uniformity of organisms is that they are all made up of similar basic units, called **cells**.

In this book, we are concerned primarily with human biology and evolution, including the interaction of humans with *pathogens* — other organisms that have the potential to cause us harm (we come back to them in Chapter 5). We can't get much further without stopping to look in more detail at the characteristics of the cells from which we are made, but note that the *basic* structure of all *animal* cells is very nearly the same, and they also have a great deal in common with (for example) the cells of all plants and fungi. In describing the basic features of a 'typical' cell, we have to introduce several new technical terms. This 'naming of parts' is one of the aspects of biology that many people find off-putting, but we have kept the terms to an essential minimum; they will come up again many times later in this book, so by the time you get to the last chapter you will be using them fluently!

Cells come in a huge variety of shapes and sizes (Figure 3.3), but a general rule is that the variations in structure reflect the specialised functions of that type of cell. However, the basic life processes carried out in every type of cell are remarkably similar. All cells are built on one of only two basic plans. The simpler of the two is found in all **bacteria** (Figure 3.3a), which are believed to have evolved before other cells. The more complex is found in all animal cells (Figure 3.3c) as well as all plants and fungi, and in single-celled organisms known collectively as **protoctists** (Figure 3.3b shows one of the best know types of protoctist, an amoeba). Protoctists are capable of independent life and, although most are harmless, they include several species that cause diseases in humans; for example some kinds of amoeba cause dysentery and other important protoctists cause malaria and sleeping sickness.

●   Compare the bacterial cell (Figure 3.3a) with the other cells in Figure 3.3. What are the most obvious differences?

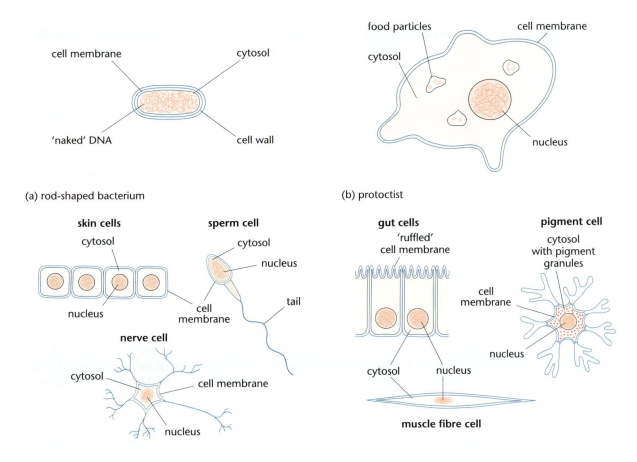

(a) rod-shaped bacterium

(b) protoctist

(c) animal cells

Figure 3.3 *Diversity in cell structure. (a) A bacterium (in this case a rod-shaped bacterium, but there are several other basic shapes). (b) A protoctist (in this case an amoeba), a single-celled organism capable of independent life. (c) Examples of animal cells illustrate the variety of shapes and structures evolved by cells with specialised functions.*

■ You probably noticed that the bacterium does not have a *nucleus* whereas all the other cells do, and that it is unique in having a protective *cell wall* outside the cell membrane.

You may have wondered why we left out **viruses**, but viruses are not true cells at all and are generally referred to as virus *particles*. They are minute 'boxes' containing little more than one or two strands of genetic material. They are not capable of independent life but survive by invading a true cell and taking control of the basic life processes going on in that cell, subverting them to produce new virus particles. (It is debatable therefore whether viruses can be described as 'living organisms'.)

Figure 3.4a shows the relative sizes of various types of true cells. Even if magnified 100 times, virus particles would be too small to see; look at the magnifications necessary to visualise the viruses in the photographs.

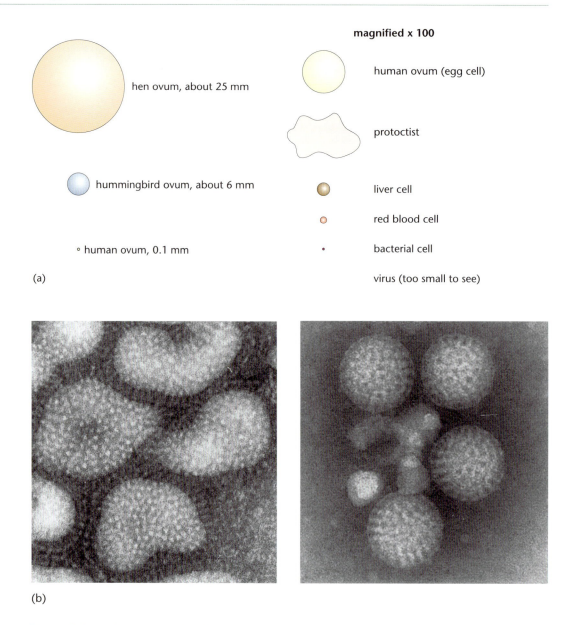

Figure 3.4 *(a) The relative sizes of various cell types; you may get some idea of the actual dimensions of these cells by considering that a fully grown human finger contains about one billion (one thousand million) cells. Even if magnified 100 times, virus particles would be too small to see. (b) Influenza virus particles (left) and rotavirus particles (right), photographed at a magnification of 350 000 with an electron microscope. The outer layer of virus particles generally displays a regular geometric pattern because it is formed from identical repeating structures, as shown in these examples. Rotaviruses are a common cause of diarrhoea in humans. (Photos: Heather Davies/The Open University)*

3.3.2 Inside the cell

A typical **animal cell** is shown in Figure 3.5; compare the drawing (a) with the photograph (b) and see if you can identify all the structures. All cells are bounded by an outer layer, the *cell membrane*. We will look at membranes in more detail shortly but, for the moment, it is enough to know that the cell membrane is a highly complex structure that allows the passage of certain substances *into* the cell and it also allows other substances pass *out* of it. The contents of the cell can be distinguished as the **cytosol**, a watery fluid rich in dissolved molecules, and a variety of solid structures called **organelles**, each bounded by a membrane very similar to the one around the outer margin of the cell. There are many different kinds of organelle; here we will do no more than point out some of the principal ones and give a 'thumbnail sketch' of their main functions (Box 3.1). You should be aware that this is a vastly simplified account: each of these organelles would have a whole chapter to itself in a textbook of cell biology.

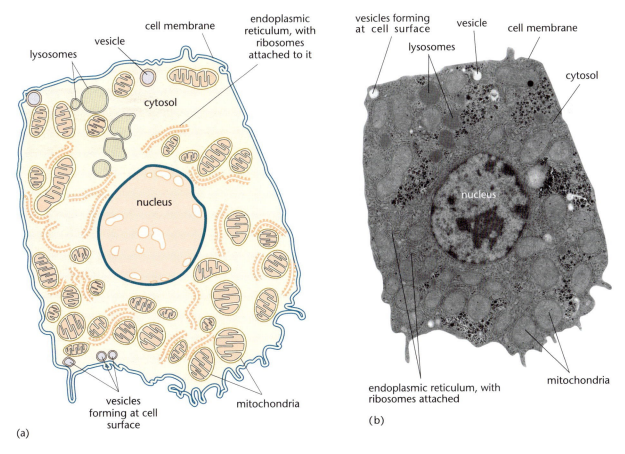

(a)

(b)

Figure 3.5   *(a) Schematic drawing of a typical animal cell, showing some of the common structural features. Compare this with (b) a photograph of a liver cell taken through an electron microscope and magnified 8 000 times. (Photo: Heather Davies/The Open University)*

Box 3.1 The principal organelles in animal cells (which are also found in the cells of plants, fungi and protoctists, but not in bacteria)[3]

The largest organelle in any cell is usually the *nucleus*, containing most of the DNA in the cell. Cells typically have one nucleus, though certain kinds of cell have more and others, e.g. the red blood cells of mammals, have none.

Ribosomes are where proteins are assembled from amino acids, with the help of RNA. They are often attached to the endoplasmic reticulum.

The *endoplasmic reticulum* is a vast canal system of membranes, on the surfaces of which an unimaginable number of chemical reactions takes place — some creating new molecules, others breaking down old ones.

Mitochondria are the sites where most of the energy is generated from chemical reactions to fuel all the processes going on inside the cell.

Lysosomes are fluid-filled 'bags' of membrane, containing organic chemicals that can break down complex molecules into their smaller constituents (e.g. they can release amino acids from proteins). Part of their function is to provide the cell with the simpler nutrients it requires, so they fulfil a similar role within the cell as the digestive system in our bodies; they also have a role in defence against infection, by breaking down invading organisms (Chapter 6).

Vesicles are also bags of membrane, containing substances being transported into or out of the cell. Lysosomes can fuse with these vesicles, emptying their chemicals into the 'bag' where they break down the contents.

If you look back at Figure 3.3, you might be surprised to learn that all the cells shown there have the structural features described above, because they *appear* to be so different. Certainly, they each have special characteristics that are reflections of the different lives they lead (or, put in a more biological manner, their structures reflect their functions), but these specialisations are superimposed on a common basic plan. What goes on at the chemical level inside these cells is also remarkably similar, as you will see shortly. First, we want to look more closely at an often neglected aspect of cell structure which is, in reality, crucially important.

3.3.3 Cell membranes: a dynamic interface

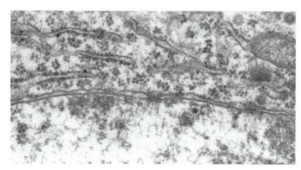

Figure 3.6 *Part of an animal cell, photographed at a magnification of 150 000 with an electron microscope, showing several internal membranes, which can clearly be seen to consist of a double layer. (Photo: Heather Davies/ The Open University)*

All the organelles mentioned above, as well as the cell itself, are bounded by **membranes**, which consist of a double layer of organic molecules (Figure 3.6). They give the cell its inner and outer organisation and act as the semi-solid 'platform' on which many of the chemical reactions inside the cell take place. In addition, as you will see from later parts of this book, membranes play a vital role in many life processes that affect the whole organism: for example, in the immune system which protects us against infection (Chapter 6) and in the digestive system which provides us with the nutrients required to sustain life (Chapter 7).

[3] If you are new to cell biology, you may like help in pronouncing the unfamiliar organelles in Box 3.1: ribosomes ('rye-boh-somes'); endoplasmic reticulum ('end-oh-plaz-mik ret-ik-you-lum'); mitochondria ('might-oh-kon-dree-a'); lysosomes ('lye-soh-somes'); vesicles ('vee-sickles').

Figure 3.7 shows a schematic diagram of the basic structure of the outer membrane of all types of animal cells (the membranes around the organelles within the cell are built on this same basic plan). Two parallel sheets of fatty molecules known as *phospholipids* form the regular framework of the membrane: you can see from the diagram that the 'heads' of these molecules are packed together to form the inner and outer layers of the membrane, with their 'tails' pointing towards each other like the jam in a sandwich. The two sheets are not fixed together, but can move laterally (from side to side), slipping across each other. This would be a highly unstable situation but for the presence of molecules of another fatty substance, *cholesterol*, which are dotted about between the phospholipids and stop the sheets from sliding too far.

Until now, you may only have thought of cholesterol as a harmful constituent of certain foods, which until quite recently was believed to be the main culprit in the causation of heart disease.[4] During the 1990s, this view was radically revised and it is accepted that for the great majority of people moderate amounts of cholesterol in the diet contribute to the construction of new membranes within and surrounding all cells. The high fat content of biological membranes also means that substances which can dissolve in fats can very easily pass into and out of cells; membranes also acts as reservoirs for fat-soluble substances, such as some vitamins.

Look at Figure 3.7 again. Bobbing about in the regular two-layer framework of phospholipids are lumps of *protein*, which can move laterally in all directions and can also 'bob up' so that sometimes they poke out of the membrane and at other times they 'bob down' below the surface. A vast number of small *carbohydrate* molecules also cover the outer surface of the membrane, standing up like trees in a forest; carbohydrates consist of strings of small sugar molecules (for example, glucose). On the inner surface, the cell membrane is in contact with contractile

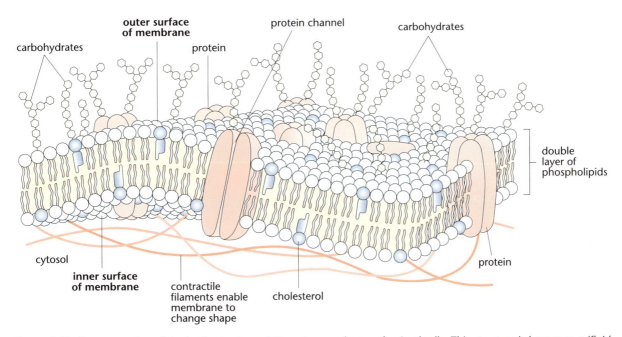

Figure 3.7   *Representation of the basic structure of the outer membrane of animal cells. This structure is known as a 'fluid mosaic'. Membranes surrounding the organelles within cells are also built on this basic plan.*

[4] The association of high blood levels of cholesterol and coronary heart disease is discussed in *Dilemmas in UK Health Care* (Open University Press, 3rd edn 2001), Chapter 10.

filaments — proteins that can contract and relax in a coordinated manner, changing the overall shape of the membrane. These filaments enable the cell to change shape, pulling it into folds or pushing it outwards, creating 'fingers' of membrane that reach out and can enclose material outside the cell. In some cells, this primitive musculature attached to the underside of the membrane can enable the cell to 'crawl' about over the surfaces of other cells. The highly mobile structure of biological membranes has been aptly named a **fluid mosaic**.

Biological membranes have three main functions, which can be thought of (metaphorically) in terms of a *barrier*, a *gate* and a *switchboard*. Membranes are barriers in that they prevent both the entry and the exit of certain substances, some of which are never allowed transit, but most are kept in or kept out only at certain times. When the 'internal world' of the cell begins to run short of a certain substance in order to maintain life processes, or when the concentration of waste rises too high, the barrier of the membrane turns into a highly selective 'gate' across which certain substances can enter or leave, while maintaining a barrier to others. It is also a 'switchboard' through which a great many chemical messages are transmitted to and from the cell.

3.3.4 Crossing a membrane

We will look first at the membrane as a barrier and as a gate. There are several different ways that substances can cross a biological membrane, but we will focus on three general methods, all of which will come up again later in the book. They are (a) *passive diffusion*, (b) *active transport* and (c) *endocytosis* and *exocytosis* (pronounced 'end-oh-sight-oh-sis' and 'ex-oh-sight-oh-sis'; *endo* signifies movement into the cell, and *exo* signifies movement outwards).

Passive diffusion

Passive diffusion refers to the free movement across biological membranes of molecules to which the membrane is *permeable* (that is, it cannot act as a barrier against them). These include very small molecules, such as water, oxygen, carbon dioxide and dissolved salts, and larger molecules that are soluble in fats (remember the membrane is formed from sheets of fats). Movement of these molecules into or out of the cell occurs by passive diffusion whenever the concentration of that molecule is greater on one side of the membrane than it is on the other (as in Figure 3.8). In this situation, a *concentration gradient* is said to exist; you could think of molecules 'rolling down' the gradient from the high side to the low side. Unless other forces oppose them, molecules will always 'spread out' or diffuse

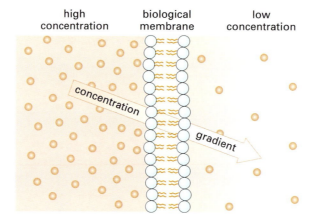

high concentration   biological membrane   low concentration

concentration gradient

Figure 3.8 *Schematic representation of a concentration gradient across a biological membrane.*

evenly through any available space (like a drop of ink in water) until any concentration gradient is abolished. This process is known as *passive* diffusion because it does not require the expenditure of energy.

● If there is a higher concentration of molecules of substance X on one side of a membrane than on the other (as in Figure 3.8), and the membrane cannot act as a barrier to those molecules, what will happen?

■ Molecules of substance X will move by passive diffusion across the membrane from the high concentration side to the low concentration side, until the concentrations are equal on both sides of the membrane. The molecules are then dispersed evenly through the available space.

Single-celled organisms, such as bacteria and protoctists, have a relatively large surface area of cell membrane in contact with the outside world, so they can get a lot of the water, oxygen and salts they need by passive diffusion of these substances into the cell from the external environment. As these vital molecules are used up by the cell, the concentration *inside* the cell falls lower than the concentration in the fluids *outside*; this creates a concentration gradient which 'sucks' more of these molecules across the membrane into the cell.

● What will happen to a waste product such as carbon dioxide, which builds up inside the cell as life processes go on?

■ When it reaches a higher concentration than the carbon dioxide in the outside world, it will leave the cell by passive diffusion across the cell membrane.

Multicellular animals have very few of their cells on the outer surface of the body, so they cannot rely solely on passive diffusion to supply the necessities of life, but it is still a vitally important method of exchanging molecules across membranes. For example, oxygen enters the bloodstream by passive diffusion across the membranes of blood vessels lying very close to the air-sacs (alveoli) in the lungs; as the oxygenated blood circulates around the body, oxygen leaves the bloodstream by passive diffusion out of the blood vessels into nearby cells. In Chapter 7 you will learn about digestion in the human gut and the absorption of small molecules, broken down from our food, which pass across the wall of the gut by passive diffusion into nearby blood vessels.

However, passive diffusion works only for very small molecules (like oxygen) to which biological membranes are completely permeable. What about the rest?

Active transport

One option for moving larger molcules is **active transport**, which relies on the proteins bobbing about in the membrane (look back at Figure 3.7). The function of many of these proteins is to transport across the membrane (in either direction) molecules which the membrane would otherwise exclude. This process requires the expenditure of energy, hence it is called *active* transport.

Transport proteins either form 'channels' through which the transported molecule can pass, or they act as 'carriers' by binding temporarily to the molecule and moving it physically through the membrane. These transport proteins are highly selective: each one will only transport a certain kind of molecule. For example, in mammals excess glucose molecules are 'mopped up' from the bloodstream for storage in the liver with the help of transport proteins in the outer membranes of liver cells; these proteins are so selective that they cannot transport other sugars into the liver cell, even those that are structurally very similar to glucose. (You will learn more about the regulation of blood glucose levels in Chapter 7.)

Before moving on, you should note that although we have discussed passive diffusion and active transport mainly in terms of the *outer* cell membrane, these processes are also going on across all the membranes *inside* the cell. Every organelle, including the nucleus, is bounded by a very similar membrane and molecules cross these membranes just as described above.

Endocytosis and exocytosis

The third method of getting molecules across biological membranes also illustrates the extreme fluidity of membrane structure. In **endocytosis**, the outer membrane of the cell is thrown into a cup-shaped depression, which gradually closes over and seals within itself a portion of the 'outside world' (see Figure 3.9a and photographs 1–4). This bag of membrane is called a *vesicle*. It separates from the cell surface and drifts into the interior of the cell. It may simply contain water and dissolved nutrients, or it may contain very large molecules such as certain proteins which are too big to get in by active transport. It may even contain whole cells: certain kinds of cell in the immune system can engulf bacteria and protoctists by endocytosis, drawing them into the cell for destruction (a subject we return to in Chapter 6).

In the opposite process — **exocytosis** — substances are transported *out* of the cell by first packaging them in a vesicle (bag of membrane), which travels to the cell surface and fuses with the outer membrane of the cell. The contents of the vesicle are then ejected outside (Figure 3.9b). The contents might be waste products, but this is also the method used by cells to *secrete* many essential molecules into the environment outside the cell. Examples of major groups of molecules which are secreted from cells by exocytosis include:

hormones, signalling molecules transported in the bloodstream in many animal species;

neurotransmitters, signalling molecules that pass between active nerve cells and between nerves and muscles (both of which are mentioned again later in this chapter);

enzymes, proteins that speed up the construction and breaking down of other molecules in all the chemical reactions taking place in living organisms (to which we return shortly);

antibodies, proteins produced by cells in the immune system as part of our defence against infection (discussed further in Chapter 6).

Note that all enzymes and antibodies are proteins, and so are some hormones and neurotransmitters.

Figure 3.9   *(a) The basic sequence of events in endocytosis, by which material is taken into a cell enclosed within a vesicle of membrane. The electron microscope photographs 1–4 relate to the stages in endocytosis numbered on the diagram. (Photos from: Perry, M. M. and Gilbert, A. B., 1979, Yolk transport in the ovarian follicle of the hen, Journal of Cell Science, **39**, p. 266) (b) The events in exocytosis, which culminate in material being ejected or secreted from the cell. The electron microscope photograph is of a secretory vesicle emptying its contents outside the cell (stage iii in the diagram). (Photo from: Herzog, V., Sies, H. and Miller, F., 1976, Exocytosis in secretory cells of rat lacrimal gland, Journal of Cell Biology, **70**, p. 698; reproduced by copyright permission of the Rockefeller University Press)*

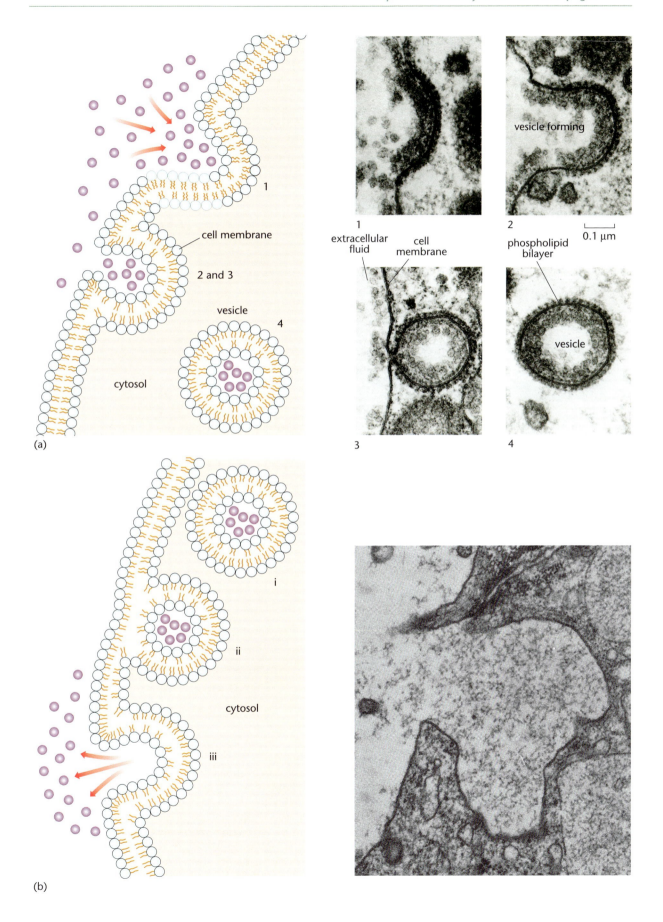

(a)

1

cell membrane

2 and 3

vesicle   4

cytosol

extracellular fluid   cell membrane

vesicle forming

phospholipid bilayer

0.1 µm

vesicle

1

2

3

4

(b)

i

ii

cytosol

iii

3.3.5 Lock-and-key interactions in membranes

Thus far, we have discussed the function of biological membranes in terms of barriers and gates, which leaves the other main function: the switchboard. Membranes act as switchboards in a communication network of daunting complexity. Cells are constantly sending and receiving signals across the outer cell membrane, which either modify the activity inside the cell or change the conditions outside; membranes around organelles inside the cell act similarly. You will meet examples of highly specific communication pathways later in this book, so here we will simply sketch in the basic principles.

As described above, cells can secrete a variety of different **signalling molecules**, such as hormones and neurotransmitters, into the fluid outside the cell. Each of these molecules has a highly specific three-dimensional shape, part of which is known as the *active site* (Figure 3.10a). It exactly fits a 'mirror image' of itself known as the *binding site* on the surface of a **receptor molecule** (often shortened simply to 'receptor', Figure 3.10b). The two surfaces fit together so precisely that — like a key in a lock — no other combination will result in the transmission of the correct signal. These events are commonly known as **lock-and-key interactions**.

Many of the proteins that bob about in the outer membrane of every cell, and most of the carbohydrates that stick out into 'space', are actually receptor molecules. When a receptor encounters a signalling molecule to which it can *bind* (that is, form a very close, though transient contact), the binding event sets off a chain reaction which leads ultimately to a change in the activity of the cell displaying that receptor (Figure 3.10b). In this example, only the receptor molecule is part of the structure of a membrane and the signalling molecule is 'free-floating'. However, *both* receptor and signalling molecule can be embedded in a membrane and this provides a mechanism to transmit messages back and forth between adjacent cells — a process called *cell-to-cell communication* (Figure 3.10c).

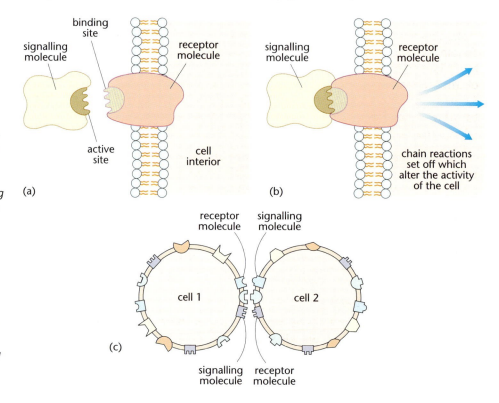

Figure 3.10 *(a) and (b) Stages in a lock-and-key interaction between the active site of a 'free-floating' signalling molecule and the binding site of a receptor protein embedded in a cell membrane. (c) Cells in close contact can send and receive signals simultaneously when signalling molecules in the membrane of each cell bind to receptors on the other cell. There are many different signalling molecules and receptors on the same cell.*

● Can you recall an example of a lock-and-key interaction mentioned a little earlier in this chapter?

■ The transport protein that picks up excess glucose from the bloodstream and carries it across the outer membrane of liver cells will transport only glucose; it cannot transport any other sugars. The transport protein appears to 'select' glucose from among a host of other molecules, but in reality its selectivity relies on an accurate lock-and-key fit between part of the transport molecule and part of the glucose molecule.

This glimpse into the 'working life' of a biological membrane should have convinced you that membranes are essential to maintain not only the structure but also the correct functioning of every living cell, from the simplest bacterium to the most complex animal cell, and hence are vital to the life of the whole organism. Several fast-acting poisons, such as the toxin produced by cholera bacteria, work simply by disrupting the 'traffic' across cell membranes, and medical science exploits the highly selective transport mechanisms across membranes in the delivery of certain drugs.

3.3.6 Cell metabolism

The unimaginably vast number of *molecular interactions* occurring on (and through) cell membranes and 'free' in the fluid-filled interior of the cell (the cytosol), are known collectively as **cell metabolism**. The term covers all the chemical reactions that go on from moment to moment, either building up molecules or breaking them down. In an organism made up of many cells (such as a human) it is conventional in biology and in medicine to speak of 'the metabolism' or 'metabolic activity', meaning the sum total of all the chemical reactions going on in all the cells of the body.

The metabolic activity of a cell has varying time-scales. Interactions between very small molecules, such as the fusion of water (H_2O) and carbon dioxide (CO_2) to make simple sugar molecules such as glucose, take place in fractions of a second. To join together these simple molecules into a long chain (called a *polymer*) takes much longer; for example, it can take many minutes to string together the hundreds of small sugar molecules required to make a long-chain carbohydrate such as starch. Similarly, individual amino acids can be made in seconds, but joining them together to make a coherent protein can take hours. You may get an insight into why it takes a relatively long time to make a protein if we give a specific example.

Haemoglobin, the substance that makes our blood red and carries oxygen around the body, is a protein molecule which (in the commonest form found in adults) is made from 574 amino acids linked together in a precise sequence. One critical amino acid out of place and it ceases to function properly as haemoglobin (as you will learn in Chapter 4). The scale of the 'manufacturing output' of just this one type of protein gives some idea of the total metabolic activity going on in the human body: your body contains about six thousand million million million (6×10^{21}) molecules of haemoglobin, which are constantly being used up and replenished.

Fuelling metabolic activity

All cells require *energy* to fuel the huge number of chemical reactions necessary to maintain life. In Chapter 7, we will spend some time looking at the breakdown of food molecules (particularly carbohydrates and fats) that yield energy, but at this point we simply want to emphasise the fact that all cells that live in an oxygen-rich environment get their energy in much the same way. Carbohydrates and fats, which are large and complex chains of smaller molecules, are broken down step by step in a complex sequence of hundreds of individual chemical reactions, yielding carbon dioxide, water and energy. The energy is 'trapped' in the structure of a molecule called **ATP** (adenosine triphosphate, a name you need not remember). ATP can be transported anywhere in the cell and energy can be released from it in controlled amounts wherever energy is required to drive a chemical reaction.

Enzymes

Millions of different interlinked reactions are taking place in every cell all the time. If you tried to draw a map of all these chemical reactions (biochemists have done this) it looks a bit like the bus, rail, road and underground networks of the London transport system superimposed on top of one another. You may be wondering what *regulates* these complex chemical reactions. The short answer is **enzymes**. These are proteins that catalyse (speed up) biochemical reactions in living organisms. As a general rule, each enzyme can only catalyse a specific reaction (as in Figure 3.11) and the presence or absence of the enzyme acts as a regulator on the extent to which that reaction occurs.

In Chapter 7, you will meet a real-life example in the enzyme *lactase,* which regulates the breakdown of *lactose,* the principal sugar found in milk. Each enzyme is restricted to act on a given biochemical reaction because an essential step in the catalytic process involves a lock-and-key fit between the enzyme and the other molecular participants in the reaction. We are used to thinking of enzymes digesting food in the cavity of the gut (this also described in Chapter 7), but the fluid interior of all cells (the cytosol) is rich in enzymes and some of the proteins embedded in the cell membrane and in the membranes surrounding organelles are also enzymes, each one regulating a highly specific biochemical reaction inside the cell.

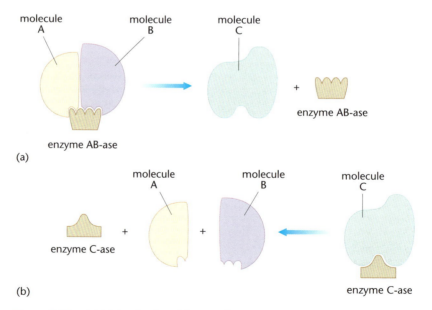

Figure 3.11 *(a) Molecules A and B can only combine to form molecule C at a biologically useful rate with the help of a highly specific enzyme, which we have called AB-ase (enzymes are named after the constituents of the reaction they speed up and all names end in the syllable 'ase'). (b) The reverse reaction, in which molecule C is broken down into A and B again, requires a different enzyme, this time called C-ase. Note that in both these reactions the enzyme is not used up and is released unchanged to participate in another identical reaction.*

Other proteins

Enzymes are just one category of proteins found in the structures of cells, or in the fluids between them in multicellular animals. In passing, we have mentioned several other categories of protein molecules earlier in this chapter.

● Can you recall any examples?

■ Transport proteins, some hormones and neurotransmitters, antibodies, haemoglobin and certain receptor molecules in cell membranes have all been mentioned.

There are a great many other types of protein, which we shall not attempt to catalogue, but you should keep in mind that much of the variation between cells of different types stems from *differences in the nature of the proteins they contain*. Although many of the metabolic processes are very similar in all cells, the end-products may have characteristic differences. So, for example, a 'cell-specific' protein with a familiar name is the hormone *insulin*, which is made only by certain cells in the pancreas (more on this follows in Chapter 7).

So, in one sense, proteins hold the key to the unique character of each living cell, both in terms of the cell's structure and functions, and (crucially) in the nature of its enzymes and hence the whole of its metabolism. Yet if you think back to our speculative account of how life may have begun on Earth, you will recall that proteins are assembled according to a 'template' carried in the structure of *RNA*. Amino acids do not join together in the absence of RNA, much less join up in the precise sequences that give each protein its characteristic form and function. So should we rewrite the first sentence of this paragraph to read 'RNA holds the key to the unique character of each living cell'? In fact we have to step back one stage further and look at the molecule that directs the production of RNA, its larger and more complex molecular 'cousin', DNA.

3.4   DNA: the double helix

Perhaps the most important aspect of the uniformity of all true cells is that they all possess the same genetic material, **DNA** (deoxyribonucleic acid). This very large organic molecule holds the key not only to RNA production (and hence to the assembly of proteins), but also the key to *inheritance*: the passing on of meaningful instructions about making RNA (and hence proteins) from one cell to another, and from one generation of organisms to the next. DNA plays a fundamental role in life on Earth, providing the 'instructions' by which all organisms develop, grow, survive and reproduce; hence, it is often referred to as the 'genetic code', or the 'blueprint' of an organism.

You may already have noticed that biologists with an interest in the early evolution of life on Earth are faced with a 'chicken-and-egg' conundrum about the relationship between DNA and RNA. Most believe that RNA evolved *first* (as we suggested at the start of this chapter), but in modern cells RNA is made *under the direction* of DNA. The solution to this puzzle may lie in the discovery that some variants of RNA can act like enzymes, speeding up the construction of much bigger molecules which resemble DNA. Maybe these early RNA 'catalysts' were involved in assembling primitive molecules of DNA, which in turn directed the assembly of more variants of RNA? These RNA molecules might, in their turn, have helped to make more DNA, and so on, until the DNA structure we recognise today was produced. This circular argument may reflect a circular process taking place over thousands of millions of years. Although biologists can only make plausible guesses about the sequence of events, the end-product, DNA, has been more extensively researched than any other organic molecule.

3.4.1 The structure of DNA

No twenty-first century adult should consider themselves literate without some knowledge of how DNA works; fortunately, the essential aspects of the 'story' are fascinating and relatively straightforward. DNA is a remarkable molecule, breathtakingly simple in its structure and yet capable of directing all the living processes of a cell, including the reproduction of new cells and new generations of organisms, for all the millions of species of animals, plants, fungi, protoctists and bacteria on Earth. Some viruses also have their few genes encoded in DNA (the rest use RNA). You will see as we progress through the story of DNA why it lends itself to being an ideal genetic material.

In all cell types, most of the DNA is in the nucleus, coiled around cores of protein in structures called **chromosomes** (you might like to glance ahead to Figure 3.20b to see what they look like; they are described in a little more detail later in this chapter and are a major topic in Chapter 4). Each species has a characteristic number of chromosomes in its cells; there are 46 of them in most human cells and 48 in the cells of chimpanzees, whereas rice has 12, corn 10 and the fruit-fly 4. The DNA of most bacteria is stored as a single chromosome. If all the DNA in the nucleus of a single human cell were uncoiled and stretched out straight, it would measure about two metres (see Figure 3.12, which is actually the DNA of a bacterium). If all the DNA in all of the cells in your body were stretched out end-to-end, it would reach to the Moon and back about 10 000 times!

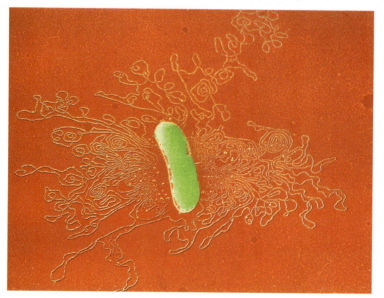

Figure 3.12   *A single strand of DNA released from a bacterium,* E. coli, *photographed at a magnification of 12 500; the colour has been added artificially. (Photo: Dr Gopal Murti/Science Photo Library)*

Since the helical structure of DNA was worked out by James Watson and Francis Crick in 1953, the study of all branches of biology and the scientific understand-ing of the nature of living processes have been revolutionised. The speed at which research on DNA has progressed is due to innovations in laboratory techniques for analysing and manipulating DNA, an achievement which is highlighted by the success of the **Human Genome Project** (HGP) less than 30 years after Watson and Crick built the first model of the double helix from test-tube clamps and bits of laboratory hardware. (You will learn much more about the HGP later in this book.) In order to understand how this revolution has come about, we must briefly describe the structure of DNA and its most important properties.

The basic structure of DNA is provided by two helical strands (like two interwoven spiral staircases), each coiled around one another — hence its name 'the double helix' (Figure 3.13a). The two strands are linked by cross-pieces like the rungs of a ladder; Figure 3.13b shows a tiny fragment of the double helix straightened out and 'laid flat' so we can more easily describe its chemical composition. Like RNA, each molecule of DNA is constructed from building blocks called nucleotides; now is the time to describe them in more detail.

There are just four kinds of nucleotide in DNA. They differ from those in RNA in ways that need not concern us here, but which makes them more stable. A single DNA **nucleotide** (Figure 3.13c) consists of three linked components; a phosphate, a sugar and a base. Together, the sugar and the phosphate form part of the 'backbone' of a DNA strand (like the handrail of a spiral staircase), whereas the base points into the space in the centre of the helix (Figure 3.13b). Each of the two strands of DNA in the double helix is a relatively stable polymer (i.e. a long chain of smaller molecules, in this case nucleotides) and the two can be 'peeled apart'. What holds the double helix together is an attractive force between the bases, rather like the poles of a magnet which can attract each other but which can be easily separated. Thus the double helix is rather like a zip fastener, which can be opened and closed — an important property as you will see shortly.

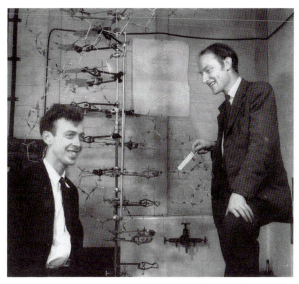

The American James Watson (left) and the Englishman Francis Crick in 1953 with the 'double-helix' model of DNA which they built to help them determine its three-dimensional structure; the model was assembled from metal clamps used to hold test-tubes and other bits of laboratory apparatus. (Photo: A. Barrington-Brown)

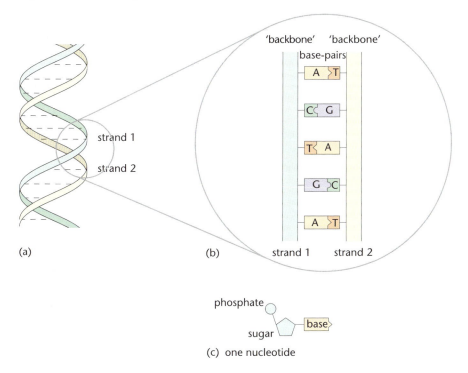

Figure 3.13 *The structure of DNA. (a) The DNA molecule consists of two helical strands coiled around one another; (b) A section of the double helix has been 'uncoiled' to show the two strands linked together by pairs of molecules called bases, of which there are four types, denoted by the letters A, T, C and G. (c) A single nucleotide, the 'building block' from which DNA is constructed; the 'backbone' of each strand consists of alternating sugar and phosphate molecules.*

The important feature of the DNA double helix from our viewpoint is that each 'rung' of the ladder holding the two strands together consists of a *pair* of different bases. The bases are what distinguish the four kinds of nucleotides: they are known by the initial letters of their chemical names: A (adenine), C (cytosine), G (guanine) and T (thymine). There is no need to remember these names; all you need to know is that the pairs of bases are not arranged randomly. The rungs across the DNA ladder are formed from *unvarying pairs* of bases: A can only bind to T, and C can only bind to G. This specificity is determined by the shape of the molecule, thus A and T have complementary shapes and attract each other, as do G and C. This property is known as the **base-pairing rule** and, as you will see, it gives the DNA molecule its unique ability to replicate exact copies of itself.

3.4.2 DNA replication

Watson and Crick ended the research paper in which they published the long-sought after structure of DNA with a classic understatement:

> It has not escaped our notice that the specific pairing we have postulated immediately suggests a possible copying mechanism for the genetic material. (Watson and Crick, 1953, p. 738)

To understand this statement fully, let us briefly reflect on how multicellular organisms such as humans grow from a single fertilised egg cell to an adult consisting of many billions of cells. In order to grow, an organism's cells must increase in number. Cells reproduce by dividing into two (you don't need to know the details of this now and we come back to it later), and each of the new cells must receive a full set of its genetic instructions. So before it divides, a 'parent' cell must copy its entire store of DNA and for a brief time it has *twice* the normal amount — two complete sets of genetic instructions on how to be a functioning cell. Then, as the 'parent' cell divides and becomes two cells, the two sets of DNA are shared out between them, so each receives a complete set of genetic instructions for sustaining life. This copying process is known as **DNA replication** and, as Watson and Crick pointed out, the structure of the double helix provides an elegant way for this copying to occur.

When a molecule of DNA makes copies of itself (replicates), the two strands of the helix separate (Figure 3.14), by pulling apart the bases which form the rungs of the ladder (like opening a zip fastener). This leaves *exposed* bases on each of the separated DNA strands, which then pair with 'free' nucleotides present abundantly in the fluids inside the cell nucleus. Each of these nucleotides has one of the four bases (A, T, C or G) as part of its structure; an exposed base on the original DNA strand can only attract and bind to a free nucleotide with the 'correct' partner base in its structure, in accordance with the base-pairing rule.

●   Suppose that, at a particular point on the separated DNA strand there is an unattached base of type C. What kind of nucleotide is attracted to it?

■   One containing the base G (remember the base-pairing rule is that C can only bind to G, and vice versa).

As the bases on the original DNA strand bind to the 'free' nucleotides they have attracted, a second new DNA strand begins to form alongside the original one, using it as a 'template'. When the new strand is complete and the two strands coil around one another, the result is a double helix, a complete DNA molecule in

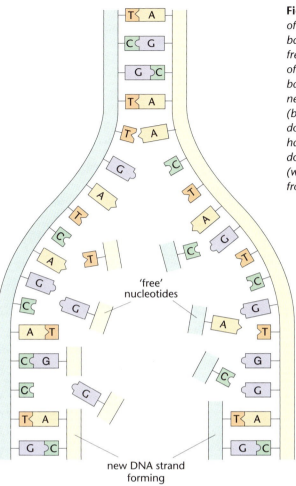

Figure 3.14   *Diagram of DNA replication. A molecule of DNA separates into two strands, exposing unpaired bases (top of diagram). Each exposed base attracts a free nucleotide containing the 'opposite' base (centre of diagram), to which it binds in accordance with the base-pairing rule (A pairs with T; C pairs with G). Two new DNA strands form alongside the original strands (bottom), leading to the formation of two identical double-helix molecules of DNA. Notice that when DNA has completed replication, each of the two resulting double-helix molecules is formed from one 'old' strand (which formed the template) and one 'new' strand, built from free nucleotides.*

'free' nucleotides

new DNA strand forming

which one strand is 'original' and the other is 'new'. Exactly the same process occurs alongside the *other* original DNA strand, so that ultimately there are two DNA double helices where formerly there was only one.

● How does the sequence of bases in these two DNA molecules compare with that in the original one?

■ They are each identical to it, because of the base-pairing rule that restricts the assembly of the new DNA strands; the order along one strand exactly defines the order on the other; the new strand is a kind of 'inverse image' of the original strand (look at Figure 3.13b again if you are unsure).

The DNA replication process occurs very rapidly within cells because it is assisted by enzymes. As these enzymes link nucleotides together they generate *polymers* of DNA nucleotides (and are therefore called DNA polymer-*ases*) at staggeringly fast rates, joining thousands of nucleotides per second! You will see later how DNA replication is regulated to coincide with cell division. This regulation ensures that at the appropriate time, DNA polymerases and other enzymes and free nucleotides are present for DNA replication to occur.

● Why is the ability of DNA replication always to generate two identical copies from one original double helix vitally important for the survival of the organism, and ultimately of the species of which it is a member?

■ DNA contains the genetic code that directs all the cell's metabolic processes; by maintaining the integrity of the genetic information when DNA replicates, the code can be transmitted accurately to new cells as the organism grows. And when DNA replicates in eggs or sperm cells, the preservation of the code ensures its accurate transmission to the next generation.

The integrity of DNA replication ensures that changes are not normally introduced into the DNA sequence, but as you will see later, occasionally copying errors do occur — errors which play a central role in evolution. The accumulation of DNA errors in replication is also an important factor in the development of cancers, the incidence of which increases with age, and DNA errors may also play a role in the ageing process itself — both subjects we return to in Chapter 8.

3.4.3 Infinite variation in DNA sequences

The *sequence* of nucleotides from which each molecule of DNA is constructed is infinitely variable, which enables it to act as a form of coded message. We have already said that DNA is constructed from four types of nucleotide, each characterised by the nature of its *base*. Analysis of the *linear* sequence in which the nucleotides occur in a single DNA strand reveals that they can be arranged in any order. The linear sequence can be written down as a series of letters corresponding to the four bases, 'read' from one end of the strand to the other. For example, an extremely small sequence of only 18 nucleotides might 'read'

AAGATGCCGAGTTAAGAT

but it could equally well exist in any other sequence you care to think of.

● How many different permutations of four nucleotides in a series of 18 'items' do you think there are?

■ If you have a powerful enough calculator you may have worked out that the answer is 68 719 476 736 (or 4 to the power of 18), not far short of seventy billion (thousand million) possible different permutations of four nucleotides in a sequence of DNA that is only 18 nucleotides long.

The nucleus of most of your cells contains 46 molecules of DNA (one in each chromosome), which together contain about 6.5 *billion* nucleotides (6.5 thousand million), each base paired with its opposite number. It is impossible to imagine the possible different permutations of 6.5 billion nucleotides, arranged in linear sequences in your chromosomes. This immense capacity for variation gives DNA one of its crucial properties; it can exist in an infinite number of different forms, each one specified by the linear sequence in which the four bases appear along each strand. The variation in DNA sequences that can exist give this unique molecule the flexibility to contain the coded instructions for all of the metabolic processes and cellular interactions that go on inside organisms, and create the variation we see between species and individuals.

3.4.4 A universal genetic code

Before we proceed further with the story of how genetic information is expressed within a cell, we will take a short detour to look at the universality of DNA. This unique molecule acts as the genetic information for virtually all organisms on Earth, from the smallest bacterium to the largest Canadian redwood tree (there are a few viruses which only have RNA). The fact that DNA is a universal genetic code suggests that, as life developed from the primeval soup, DNA became the prime method of storing genetic information.

Although the chemical composition and structure of DNA appear to be universal, the *amounts* of DNA in different organisms is very variable. Since DNA carries the codes from which to build cells, you might have predicted that a large complex organism would have more DNA in one of its cells than occurs in a single-celled organism, and generally speaking this is true; human cells have considerably more DNA than bacterial or yeast cells. But Table 3.1 shows that the amounts of DNA present in a single cell from a variety of organisms varies by over a thousand fold. These amounts constitute what geneticists call an organism's **genome**. The term refers to the total amount of DNA (i.e. the number of nucleotides) that between them carry the codes for all of the organisms' unique set of genes.

You may already have spotted that earlier we said that the 46 DNA molecules in a human cell contain *6.5 billion* nucleotides, but Table 3.1 shows the human genome as being *3.25 billion* nucleotides — exactly half the number. The reason for this discrepancy is that you (like all animals) have *two* copies of every gene: one inherited from each of your parents. So your *genome* — your unique set of genes — contains half as many nucleotides as your DNA.

Table 3.1 Amount of DNA in the genome of various organisms.

Organism	Amount of DNA (millions of nucleotides) in its genome	Organism	Amount of DNA (millions of nucleotides) in its genome
E. coli bacteria	4	chicken	2 400
baker's yeast	13	mouse	2 700
cress	70	human	3 250
flatworm	80	corn	7 800
fruit-fly	140	tobacco	9 600

Obtaining the precise order or sequence of the four nucleotides in the DNA of a variety of organisms, (biologists call this 'DNA sequencing'), has been a major goal of molecular research for several decades and during the late 1990s it became a reality. The precise methods used to work out a genome sequence are beyond the scope of this book, but it takes a lot of time, effort, patience and money! In 1995, the first genome of a free-living organism, that of the bacterium *Haemophilus influenzae*, consisting of just 2 million nucleotides, was published; it had taken a team of scientists just over a year to complete. Since then, the techniques used to decipher DNA sequences have improved rapidly and scientists have now decoded the complete genome DNA sequences of several of the organisms listed in Table 3.1, including baker's yeast, a flatworm, fruit-fly and cress. Over 600 genomes had been 'sequenced' by the end of 2000, including a working draft of the *human* genome. In spring 2001 this working draft was finally completed.

You will see in Chapters 5 and 6 how knowledge of the complete genome sequences of human pathogens (organisms that infect or parasitise humans) is having a major impact on the development of therapeutic treatments. In Chapters 4 and 9 we explore how knowledge of the human genome sequence can help identify individuals with DNA changes that predispose to, or cause, human diseases — an advance in scientific understanding that has far-reaching consequences for human societies as well as for personal choices.

3.4.5 Genes, mutations and variation

Within the millions of nucleotides in the DNA of cells from species throughout the world, there are 'meaningful' sequences which biologists call **genes**. A gene can be defined in two ways: either *chemically*, as a sequence of nucleotides which contains the coded instructions for making a specific *protein*; or it can be defined in *evolutionary* terms as a 'unit of inheritance', coded information about making a protein that can be passed on to future generations of cells or organisms. When biologists talk about a gene 'coding for' a certain protein, they are using a shorthand way of saying 'the sequence of nucleotides which contains the information to make' a certain protein.

The number of genes buried within the genomes of organisms is also variable. For example, the bacterium *E. coli* has 4 000 genes, baker's yeast has 6 000, the fruit-fly has 13 500 and the human genome is estimated to contain about 38 000 genes. However, the *proportion* of the total available DNA that carries these genes is rather small; in humans, only 5 per cent of the 3.25 billion nucleotides in the human genome contributes to our genes. The rest of the DNA is believed to contribute to maintaining the structure and integrity of the genes and the chromosomes, rather like an office filing cabinet which holds the important files (or genes).

Later in the chapter we will look at how a sequence of DNA nucleotides which *does* form a gene can be 'translated' into a sequence of amino acids to give rise to a specific protein; you already have most of the story, so just a few additional details are required to complete it. In Chapter 4, we reveal how genes are passed on from parent to offspring, and how the proteins 'encoded' by those genes affect the way that the offspring turns out. First we turn to how variants or *mutations* actually arise in DNA and how this leads to changes in the proteins coded for by the mutated genes.

Let us return to the primeval soup and the speculative story of how life might have evolved on Earth. Imagine that a primitive cell has formed, which contains molecules of some ancestral form of DNA, busily replicating more copies of itself (as in Figure 3.14). The environmental factors that probably helped DNA to form in the first place, like radiation, high temperature or lightning, are also likely to produce *random changes* in the sequence of its nucleotides, that is to produce **mutations**. We can have some confidence in this hypothesis because ultraviolet light, X-rays and other forms of radiation are among the factors known to produce mutations in DNA today; they are *mutagens*.[5] If you have ever had an X-ray, you are probably aware that considerable precautions are taken to protect your reproductive organs, and those of the radiographer, from the mutagenic effects of X-rays. This is primarily to prevent mutations occurring in the DNA of your sperm or egg cells, which might be passed on to future generations.

[5] Chemical mutagens, radiation and the thinning of the ozone layer are discussed further in Chapter 10 of this book.

There is currently much concern about the mutagenic effects of increased levels of ultraviolet light resulting from the thinning of the ozone layer, which is predicted to cause an increase in skin cancers. Far more extreme conditions existed when ancestral DNA molecules first appeared on Earth, so we can predict that random changes to the structure of primitive DNA molecules could have happened very frequently.

Mutations can be of four general kinds:

1   A section of DNA double helix might mutate by acquiring an additional pair of nucleotides, inserted into the original sequence. For example, a section of DNA with the following base-pairs (across the 'rungs' of the ladder):

A ... T

G ... C

T ... A

might acquire an additional pair of nucleotides to become

A ... T

G ... C

C ... G

T ... A

It is still DNA, but it is a *different version* of DNA, which nonetheless retains the essential property of exact self-replication. When the mutant version of DNA replicates, it will copy the additional pair of bases along with the rest. Mutation is a source of new *heritable* variants of DNA (there are other sources of variation, which are discussed in Chapter 4), and heritability is essential to evolutionary change, as you will see shortly.

2   The reverse process might equally well occur; a section of DNA might *lose* a pair of nucleotides. In fact, mutation might result in more than one pair of nucleotides being lost or gained.

3   One nucleotide might be replaced by another. For example, a base of type G might change to a T on one strand during replication. This would lead to an A being introduced on the other strand.

4   Alternatively, a section of DNA might be chopped out of the sequence and stuck back in elsewhere, that is, some nucleotides might be *relocated* in the DNA molecule.

Each time a mutation takes place, a different version of DNA is created. The variants might have slightly different properties from each other. Suppose that a new DNA variant, created by mutation, has the property of being able to replicate faster than the original version of DNA. For any DNA molecule to be able to replicate, it needs raw materials in the form of nucleotides. That version of DNA which could assemble the necessary nucleotides fastest and thus replicate fastest would, over time, produce more copies of itself, and they will survive to replicate faster in their turn than the slower-replicating versions. In other words, if there was *competition* among DNA variants for the resources that they required in order to replicate themselves, then a consequence of this competition is that certain versions would become more numerous than others. This, in essence, is what *natural selection* is all about. Mutation and natural selection are essential driving forces behind the evolution of all the diverse life-forms we see on Earth today.

3.5   Natural selection and DNA

Most people think they know what **natural selection** is about and will express it using such phrases as 'the survival of the fittest' or 'nature red in tooth and claw'. In fact, such phrases are misleading in many ways. The theory of natural selection, as set out by Charles Darwin, is a series of logical statements that explain how, over the course of a number of generations, the form of a given species can change.[6] The species might be a mouse or it might be a mango, or even a particular type of molecule. As our story of life is still focused on molecules, we set the theory out as it would apply to ancestral molecules of DNA, but the same arguments hold true for any organism.

There are four propositions in the theory of natural selection:

1   Reproduction generates more individuals than are able to survive until they themselves reproduce, because there are insufficient resources for all individuals to survive and reproduce.

2   There is a 'struggle for existence', because of the disparity between the number of individuals generated by reproduction and the number that can survive.

3   Individuals are not identical; they show variation one from another, arising at least partly from mutations in their DNA. Those variants with advantageous features have a greater chance of survival in the struggle for existence and thus have a greater chance of reproducing. There is thus *selection* of those molecules (or mice or even mangoes) that have greater *fitness* than others. **Fitness** is used here with a precise biological meaning: within a population of individuals, the one that produces the largest number of offspring who, survive to reproduce in their turn, is said to have the highest fitness. However, you should note that it is a *relative* term — the fittest organism is the best adapted to survive *under the conditions that prevail at that time*; if the conditions change, it may no longer be the fittest.

4   Since the fittest varieties of molecules, mice or mangoes, tend to produce offspring that are similar to themselves (that is, the advantageous variations are *inherited* by their offspring), these better-adapted varieties become more abundant in subsequent generations. As a result, over many generations, the characteristics that gave them an advantage spread throughout the population. Conversely, less-well adapted varieties are at a disadvantage in the competition for resources, and so will produce fewer offspring with that inherited 'defect', who in turn are also disadvantaged by it; in time and over many generations, the maladaptive characteristic will disappear from the population.

The conditions under which natural selection occurs — reproduction, variation, competition for resources and inheritance — existed in the environment in which life-forms first evolved on Earth. DNA molecules reproduce by replication, they vary because the order of base-pairs can change, they compete because they need smaller molecules in order to make copies of themselves, and they show inheritance because they can replicate themselves exactly. Thus, the natural selection of increasingly useful variants of DNA could take place and, with them, increasingly complex forms of life on Earth evolved.

---

[6] The theory of natural selection and the biological meaning of 'adaptation' and 'fitness' were introduced in Chapter 5 of *World Health and Disease* (Open University Press, 2nd edn 1993; 3rd edn 2001).

As we said earlier, ancestral DNA molecules would have been exposed to an environment which was highly likely to cause mutations (changes in the sequence of nucleotides) and hence increase the number of different variant forms of DNA. While some mutations would inevitably produce more successful (fitter) forms of DNA, others would have been deleterious, and thus would have produced forms of DNA that were less successful. This variation is the 'raw material' on which evolution by natural selection acts. As Steve Jones, a leading British geneticist, says:

> If everything was perfect, we'd still be living in the primeval ooze, because you know without mutation ... most of which is inevitably damaging, we couldn't evolve. (Quoted from an audiotape recorded for a previous edition of this book)

● Explain this statement, based on your understanding of natural selection.

■ It involves competition between variants (whether they be different molecules of DNA, or mice, or mangoes), created by mutation, which results in only the best adapted to survival under the prevailing conditions being able to reproduce and thus expand their numbers in the next generation.

We have one more stop to make on this tour round the structure and functions of DNA, to fill in a blank we left earlier in the chapter. How does the cell make all the various proteins it either needs for its own maintenance and reproduction, or pumps out into the surrounding fluid to fulfil other functions at a distance in the organism's body? You already know a great deal about the three molecules involved: DNA, RNA and amino acids, so it should not take much more effort to piece them together.

3.6   Protein synthesis and the genetic code

First a reminder of the story so far: there are 20 common amino acids which, when linked together in specific combinations and sequences, form specific proteins. The instructions about which of the 20 possible amino acids contribute to a given protein, and in what sequence they are joined together, are contained in a coded form in the structure of DNA. We mentioned earlier that the human genome contains about 3.25 billion nucleotides, and that only about 5 per cent of these sequences contain instructions about how to make a protein. Those sequences that can be 'translated' into functioning proteins are termed *genes*, and all the genes that an organism contains in its DNA are collectively referred to as the **genotype** of the organism.

3.6.1 Same genes: different cells

Nearly all the cells in an organism's body contain *exactly the same genes*; the principal exceptions are sperm and egg cells, and certain cells involved in the immune system of complex animals such as ourselves.[7] This raises an interesting question: if nearly all our cells contain the same genes, how is it that we have such a huge variety of different kinds of cells?

In an earlier part of this chapter, we stated that variation between cells of different types stems from differences in the *nature of the proteins* they contain. Genes contain the coded instructions for making proteins and each unique gene carries the

---

[7] The production of sperm and egg cells and the reasons why their DNA differs from that in all other cells in the body are discussed in Chapter 4 of this book. The cells of the immune system are described in Chapter 6.

specification for a unique protein. To use the shorthand of genetics, human DNA contains a 'gene for haemoglobin' and a 'gene for insulin', and so forth — about 38 000 different genes in all, each one unique. But they are not all active all of the time: there are mechanisms for switching genes on and off. A switched-on gene is actively engaged in the production of whatever protein it 'codes for', and synthesis of that protein ceases when the gene is switched off. The protein is often described by biologists as the **gene product**, that is, the *product* of the active gene.

● Can you suggest how the same set of genes can determine the variety of structures and functions of all the different cell types found in a human body?

■ The kinds of protein that a cell contains can be altered by switching on certain genes and keeping others switched off; for example, the gene containing the code for insulin is switched on in the hormone-producing cells in the pancreas, but switched off in all other cell types.

So, most cells in an individual carry the same set of genes, but not all of the genes are active all of the time. Differences in the structure and functions of cells of different types result from differences in which genes are switched on (actively engaged in producing certain proteins) and which genes are switched off.

3.6.2 From active gene to functioning protein

We will follow through the events that occur when a gene becomes active and its protein product is synthesised; the process from start to finish is known as **protein synthesis**. The following account of how the DNA code in a particular gene is 'translated' into a specific protein is greatly simplified, but you need only remember the general idea.

DNA is a huge molecule, containing about 38 000 different genes in humans, which remains in the nucleus throughout the cell's life; the amino acids from which all the proteins are constructed are found *outside* the nucleus, in the cytosol of the cell. How is the coded instruction from just one gene to be carried from the DNA out to the cytosol where the protein can be made? The answer is that *RNA* carries the message from nucleus to cytosol. In order to generate specialised cells, different subsets of genes must be expressed in different cells.

From DNA to RNA: transcription

You saw earlier how the 'unzipping' of the DNA helix before a cell divides leads to DNA replication. Once the cell has divided, each of the 'daughter' cells needs to grow, a process that requires the synthesis of particular proteins, which have their DNA codes stored in particular genes. Rather as we described for DNA replication, the process is initiated by the unwinding of the DNA helix, but instead of occurring along the whole length of the DNA molecule, it just 'unzips' at the gene required (see Figure 3.15; in fact, the gene 'unzips' in several places at once, but we have simplified the story here).

As the DNA within a gene 'unzips', the bases that contain the coded instructions for the particular protein are exposed. The sequence of nucleotides in the 'unzipped' section of DNA is now used as a template against which a new strand of RNA is built (using the kinds of nucleotides unique to RNA). Similar sorts of base-pairing rules apply when the exposed DNA bases attract RNA nucleotides, as those described earlier when DNA replicates. As a consequence of these DNA–RNA base-pairing rules, the new molecule of RNA reproduces in its structure the coded instructions that existed in the original section of DNA (the gene); the code has simply been 'transcribed' into a slightly different RNA nucleotide 'language'. Appropriately enough, this type of RNA is called *messenger RNA* (or mRNA for short).

An important feature to note in this process — which is called **DNA–RNA transcription** — is that the cell can make as many RNA copies as it requires from the single original DNA template. For example, a cell producing insulin will make many mRNA copies of the insulin gene. The details of the mRNA code need not concern us here; it is enough to note that it carries the DNA 'message' out of the nucleus to the organelles where proteins can be assembled. (These organelles are called *ribosomes,* and you can just about see some if you look back at Figure 3.5b.)

From DNA code to protein product

We should now spend a moment looking at the relationship between the original code in the DNA and the structure of the resultant protein, ignoring the intervening messenger RNA for simplicity. Rather like Morse code, where a series of dots and dashes each represent letters, the order of the bases carries within it the code for protein synthesis. The DNA, therefore, represents an encrypted message, which is transcribed into messenger RNA and then translated into a meaningful message in the cell. So what is the code made from? Imagine that a sequence of DNA bases in a tiny part of a gene has been exposed on one of the two 'unzipped' DNA strands (as in Figure 3.15). The letters that represent the bases in that section of DNA could be written down, reading along the strand from left to right:

ATGAAGCCGAGTTAAGAT

In the cell, the 'message' is actually formed from a series of three-letter 'words', again read from left to right; in this example they would be:

ATG–AAG–CCG–AGT–TAA–GAT

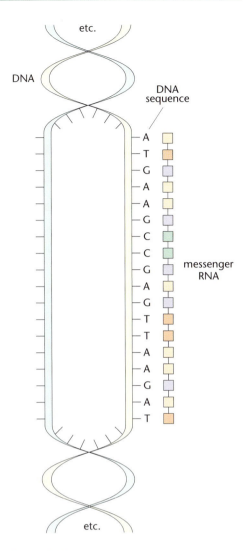

Figure 3.15 *A simplified version of the first stage in protein synthesis. The DNA sequence corresponding to a gene 'unzips' and becomes the template against which a new strand of messenger RNA is built. (In reality, a single gene would contain thousands of nucleotides, not the few shown here.)*

Biologists call these groups of three DNA bases **codons** (you will occasionally see them called *triplets* alternatively) and they sometimes refer to the genetic code as being 'written in codons'. Each unique codon can be thought of as a command-word, which tells messenger RNA to 'get a certain kind of amino acid'. For example, the DNA codon formed from adjacent nucleotides with the bases ATG (the first three bases in the sequence above, and in Figure 3.15) is an instruction to get an amino acid called *methionine*, whereas the next three bases along, AAG, is an instruction to get a different amino acid, *lysine*. (Don't try to memorise any triplets or their corresponding amino acids — the general idea is all that is required.) There are 20 types of amino acids, so there have to be at least 20 different DNA codons to code for them.

● How many different possible combinations of three nucleotides are there in DNA, assuming that each nucleotide can occur once, twice or three times in a codon? (Remember there are 4 nucleotides, A, C, G and T).

■ There are 64 combinations. The first base of the codon can be any one of the four bases A, C, G or T; this is true of the second base (giving 16 combinations) and the third (giving 64 combinations).

Only 20 unique codons are required (one for each amino acid), so there are plenty to spare; (in fact these spare codons act as additional codes for specific amino acids; for example, CAG and CAA both code for the amino acid *glutamine*).

Finally, think of the sequence of codons in the gene as instructions to join particular amino acids together in a particular order as specified in the gene. Thus, the first two amino acids to be joined together in the hypothetical protein we have been 'building' in this discussion would be methionine and lysine.

DNA makes RNA makes protein

Figure 3.16 summarises the process we have been building up, step by step. Because DNA cannot leave the nucleus, the first step towards producing a protein is to 'transcribe' into the structure of mRNA a complete set of instructions on how to make a particular protein. Hundreds of mRNA copies of the gene can be produced, and they pass out of the nucleus and attach to the ribosomes — the site where proteins are assembled. Amino acids are brought to the ribosomes alongside the mRNA and joined together in the appropriate order matching the order specified in the original DNA molecule.

As the protein is formed, amino acid by amino acid, the growing polymer forms into a specific shape, which is determined by the order of amino acids. Hence the DNA code also determines the shape of the final protein molecule. When the protein is complete, it is released from the ribosome and the mRNA is freed to act as a template on which to make another protein molecule with exactly the same structure.

This whole process of events is often abbreviated to 'DNA makes RNA makes protein' and it more or less brings us back to where we started in this chapter. Take a look back at Figure 3.2 and you will see that we have gradually built up a more detailed picture of the way in which proteins are made in cells. Remember that the ability to synthesise thousands of different proteins is the key to the variety and complexity of modern cells and hence the variety and complexity of present-day organisms.

Mutant genes make mutant proteins

You saw earlier (Section 3.4.4) how changes or mutations in DNA can occur. These changes inevitably lead to alterations in the instructions to make the encoded protein because the message in the codons has been altered. For example, if we return to the example of a DNA sequence given above, and mutate the *fifth* base in this stretch of DNA, changing it from an A to a T, thus:

ATG–AAG–CCG–AGT–TAA–GAT

would become:

ATG–ATG–CCG–AGT–TAA–GAT

● What effect would this have upon the structure of the protein manufactured according to the mutated instructions? (Look back at the earlier example.)

■ The mutation has altered the second codon from AAG (the code for lysine) to ATG (the code for methionine). The mRNA will now direct the incorporation of a methionine in place of the original lysine.

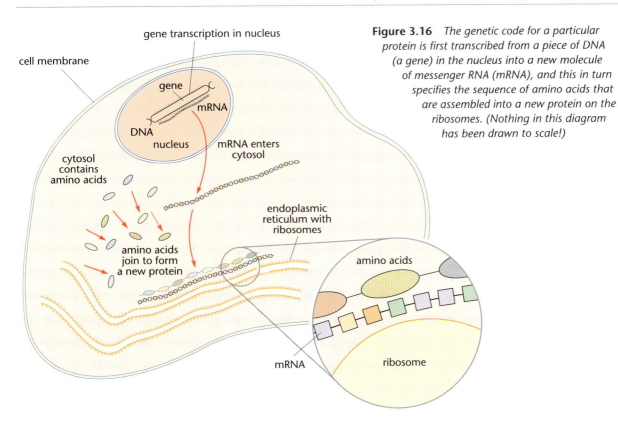

Figure 3.16 *The genetic code for a particular protein is first transcribed from a piece of DNA (a gene) in the nucleus into a new molecule of messenger RNA (mRNA), and this in turn specifies the sequence of amino acids that are assembled into a new protein on the ribosomes. (Nothing in this diagram has been drawn to scale!)*

Such small changes in DNA, which lead to alterations in the structure of proteins, could affect the functions of the cell or even the whole organism (as you will see later when we consider DNA mutations in human disease). But remember the quote from Steve Jones — without mutations we would still be back in the primeval soup. Some of the mutant proteins will be *better adapted* to perform their function in the cell, and as a result the organism in which the mutation occurred will have increased fitness and a better chance of surviving to reproduce and pass on its mutant gene.

3.6.3 Conservation of DNA throughout evolution

● Over millions of years of DNA mutation and evolutionary change, would you expect humans to have any DNA sequences in common with other organisms?

■ We have many DNA similarities within genes with our closest evolutionary 'relatives' such as chimpanzees (you may have heard that we have over 98 per cent of our genes in common with them), but in fact we share a great deal more of our genes with other organisms than anyone had originally thought.

● Can you think why this might be the case?

■ Many of the cellular processes which are performed by proteins are very similar in many organisms, for example, the transport proteins in cell membranes, hormones and other signalling molecules are all common to many animals.

The structure of a protein will have an optimal 'shape' or *conformation* in order to perform a particular function (think back to the lock-and-key interactions discussed earlier). Remember that the shape of a protein is determined by the order of the amino acids, which are themselves determined by the order of codons in the DNA. Thus the genes encoding the *same* protein in organisms from different species (e.g. mice and mangoes) will have very similar nucleotide sequences. For example, when proteins are constructed along mRNA templates on ribosomes, the process by which it is done in a bacterium, yeast, plant or in humans is very similar because every organism has to perform this task in each cell continually. In fact, throughout evolution this process has not changed a great deal and you might expect the genes that code for components of the ribosomes to be very similar, which indeed they *are* across many species.

As the nucleotide sequences in the genomes of more and more organisms have been worked out, it is clear that the same gene from many organisms can look very similar. In fact, over 40 per cent of the genes in the flatworm are recognisable in humans. Comparing the DNA sequence for the same gene between different species gives some idea of how closely or distantly related they are in evolution.

3.7   A brief reflection on immortality

It is worth pausing for a moment to reflect on the fact that an understanding of how DNA works can affect our perception of life. You have just read a quite detailed account of protein synthesis, though you should be aware that it is a greatly simplified one. Why is DNA so important, and why has the discovery of its structure and properties had such a profound effect on the study of biology?

It must be obvious that understanding the substance that controls the way that our cells, and hence our bodies, are built and function is pretty important in itself, but we can go further than that. At some stage in the evolution of early life-forms, DNA acquired the property of making proteins, which in their turn protected the DNA to some extent as it became 'packaged' ever more securely within cells. This enhanced its chance of survival. The evolutionary biologist Richard Dawkins, in his book *The Selfish Gene*, calls organisms 'survival machines'. Organisms are mechanisms, he argues, built by DNA to promote its own survival and reproduction; organisms are DNA's way of making more DNA. In terms of the old chicken and egg problem, a chicken is an egg's way of making more eggs. Such a view of living things places DNA at the very centre of our understanding of evolution.

It may come as a surprise to learn that a very small fraction of your DNA is *potentially* immortal and could continue to contribute to human evolution until humans become extinct, whereas the bulk of your DNA will die with you. The DNA with a chance of immortality is referred to by biologists as **germline DNA** and is contained in the *germline cells*; these are the **gametes** (sperm or egg cells) and the cells in the testes or ovaries which give rise to sperm or eggs. Some of your germline DNA will be passed on to the next generation in a sperm or egg if you have a child, and your offspring's gametes will contain some of *your* germline DNA, which could be passed on to your grandchildren, and so on from one generation to the next. By the same token, you inherited your germline DNA from your parents, and they got it from *their* parents, and so on back in time.

All the other cells in your body are collectively called **somatic cells** (from the Greek word 'soma' meaning 'the body') to distinguish them from the gametes and gamete-producing cells; the DNA in these somatic cells is called **somatic DNA** and it is not passed on to your descendants. Later in this chapter, we will describe how somatic cells divide to make more somatic cells for growth and repair of the body. In Chapter 4, we describe the rather different process by which germline cells divide to make sperm and egg cells.

3.8 Self-maintenance and reproduction

We can now return to the speculative story of the evolution of life on Earth and identify some of the features of present-day organisms that must have evolved early in the history of living things. As the newly formed Earth cooled and the crust solidified, varieties of DNA may have evolved within self-made 'jackets' of protein and, somewhere about 4 000–3 500 million years ago, the first truly independent, replicating, single-celled organisms appeared. Biologists generally believe that these early organisms were something like the bacterial cells we see today.

3.8.1 Cell movement

Some time later, single-celled organisms with a nucleus evolved, perhaps resembling the *protoctists* that generations of schoolchildren dredge out of stagnant pools and examine under simple microscopes. A feature of many protoctists is that they possess diverse means of moving about in their environment. An amoeba moves by altering the shape of its body using contractile filaments as described earlier in the section on membranes, but many other protoctists have various appendages which they can wave or vibrate and so push themselves along (Figures 3.17a and b).

● Why do you think the capacity for independent movement might have been an important stage in the evolution of life on Earth?

■ It meant that organisms could maintain themselves to some extent in *optimal* conditions. If the surrounding environment is hostile, they might be able to move to somewhere more hospitable.

Another important development in a hostile world is the ability to keep the conditions *within* the cell more conducive to life than the environment *outside* it. For single-celled organisms, the key to this vital property is the cell membrane, their interface with the outside world.

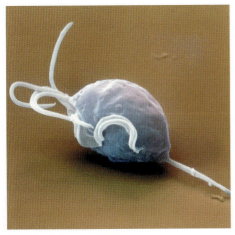
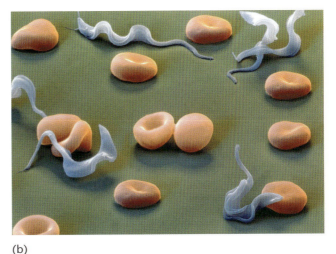

(a)   (b)

Figure 3.17   *Movement in protoctists (the colours have been added artificially). (a)* Trichomonas vaginalis, *a sexually transmitted protoctist, which causes irritation in the reproductive tract, moves by lashing four whip-like filaments called flagella. (Photographed at a magnification of 4 500.) (b)* Trypanosoma brucei, *an African trypanosome, moves in human blood by 'thrashing' a long filament extending the length of the organism and projecting from one end; several trypanosomes are shown among red blood cells. (Photographed at a magnification of 2 000.)* Trypanosoma *are transmitted by tsetse flies and belong to several different species which cause sleeping sickness in humans and severe diseases of domestic cattle. (Photos: Eye of Science/Science Photo Library)*

3.8.2 Homeostasis: regulating the internal environment

As you already know (Section 3.3.3), the cell membrane is a complex structure which has the capacity to control what passes into and out of the cell. As a result, the cell can, to a large extent, regulate its internal state. It can maintain such parameters as the concentration of essential nutrients and waste products in its cytosol, and achieve this with a degree of independence from the concentration of those substances *outside* the cell. This phenomenon of self-regulation is called **homeostasis** ('home-ee-oh-stay-sis'). Homeostasis literally means 'standing still' and is defined as the maintenance of a stable state close to the optimum conditions for maintaining life.

The principal process by which homeostasis is maintained is called **negative feedback**.[8] Figure 3.18 illustrates in general terms how it works. An organism that can maintain homeostasis must be able to make a comparison between the *actual* state of its 'internal world' and the desired *optimum* state, and then take action to reverse any drift away from that optimum. In order to achieve this, the organism has to have *sensors* that monitor the current state of the system and compare this with what the optimum state should be. Any difference between the two (the 'error') is then reduced; action is taken by *response mechanisms* that reverse the drift away from the optimum state. This process is called *negative* feedback because the action taken reverses any change that has occurred in the system; that is, the error is negated.

A good analogy is the thermostat in a central heating system, which uses a negative feedback circuit to keep the temperature in the house close to the optimum set by the inhabitants. When the temperature falls below the desired level (the set point), the thermostat (sensor) switches on the heater (response mechanism); conversely, when the temperature rises too high, the thermostat switches the heater off. Look closely at the bottom of Figure 3.18 and notice that the arrows leaving the 'response mechanisms' box *cross over* each other. This is an essential feature of any negative feedback circuit diagram.

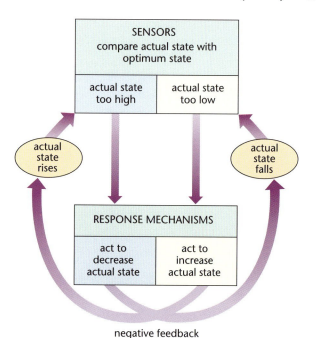

Figure 3.18 *Schematic diagram illustrating the basic principles of homeostasis, with particular emphasis on regulation via negative feedback.*

[8] Negative and positive feedback loops also exist in human social organisation, where a particular behaviour can either accelerate and magnify (positive feedback) or throw into reverse (negative feedback) the changes following a particular event. An example was discussed in terms of the Bangladesh famine of 1974 in *World Health and Disease* (Open University Press, 2nd edn 1993; 3rd edn 2001), Chapter 7.

- Use the analogy of the central heating system to explain the function of this 'cross-over' in the circuit, starting from the moment when the temperature in the house falls below the set point.

■ The thermostat senses that the temperature is below the set point and switches the heating on; the house warms up, but the rising temperature will *overshoot* the set point because the thermostat can only detect 'too much' or 'too little' heat. The arrows cross over each other in the circuit diagram to show that the overshoot will trigger action to *reverse* it, in this example, by switching off the central heating. The temperature drifts downwards, overshoots the set point, and the sequence starts all over again.

Homeostasis is an essential process in self-maintenance, one of the two fundamental properties of living things that we identified in the first paragraph of this chapter. Even in a hostile external world, cells may be able to survive because they can keep their internal world stable. We will return to the subject of homeostasis a little later, when we focus on the maintenance of a stable internal state within large multicellular organisms such as ourselves.

3.8.3 The cell cycle and cell division: mitosis

Another mechanism of self-maintenance, which *also* enables single-celled organisms and bacteria to reproduce, is the ability to split one cell into two, in other words, to make new cells.[9] New *somatic* (body) cells are formed by a process celled the **cell cycle**. In essence, a cell enlarges and makes copies of everything it contains; it then divides to give two 'daughter' cells, each of which receives a complete set of all the molecules and organelles that the 'parent' cell contained (Figure 3.19). The new cells rest for a time before the cycle starts again.

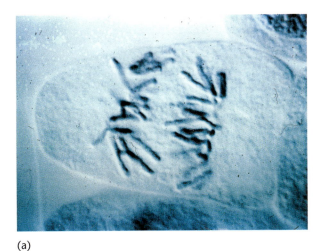
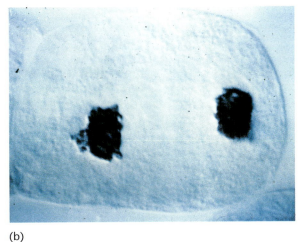

(a)　　　　　　　　　　　　　　　　　　　　　(b)

Figure 3.19 *Photographs of plant cells in late stages of cell division (the process is the same in animal cells but is particularly easy to see in plants). (a) The cell contains two sets of chromosomes (the dark shapes), each set carrying a copy of the DNA which the cell contained before it began to divide. (b) Two new nuclei have formed and a new cell membrane will soon develop between them, dividing the original cell into two. (Photo: S101 course material/The Open University)*

[9] Note that some protoctists and bacteria can also reproduce by combining genetic material from different individuals, in a form of sexual reproduction.

An essential part of cell replication is the assembly of identical copies of the DNA molecules in the cell so that they can be shared out between the daughter cells. This sharing out of two sets of identical DNA is called **mitosis** (pronounced 'my-toe-sis'). The complete cell cycle is a continual process but is usually represented as a series of phases as shown in Figure 3.20.

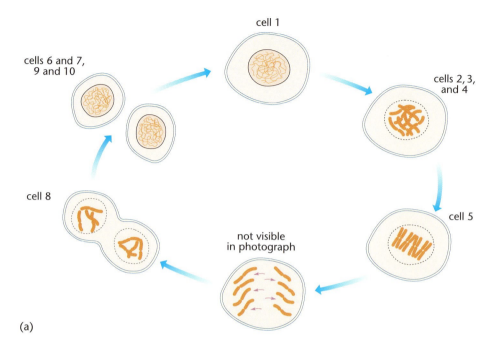

(a)

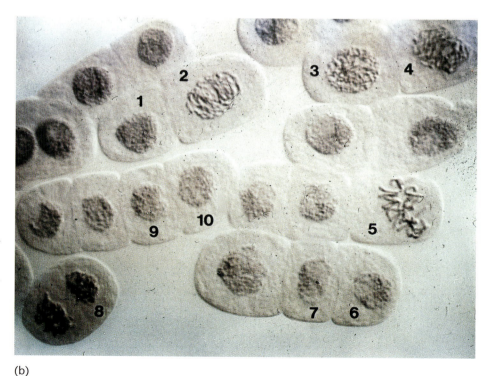

(b)

Figure 3.20 *The essential features of the cell cycle, illustrated (a) in diagrammatic form, numbered to identify corresponding cells in (b) a photograph of plant cells at various stages in the cell cycle. The phases are described in the text. (Photo: S101 course material/The Open University)*

In the first phase of cell division, the DNA in the 'parent' cell *replicates*, that is, each original molecule of DNA acts as a template against which a new molecule of DNA is constructed (cell 1). These DNA molecules gradually compress (like a spring collapsing) and begin to be visible as a tangle of *chromosomes* when viewed through a microscope (cells 2, 3 and 4); this is the start of mitosis. The cell now has two identical sets of chromosomes.

● Can you remember how many chromosomes a human somatic cell usually has, and hence how many it would have at this phase of the cell cycle?

■ The normal chromosome number is 46, so there would be 92 chromosomes after DNA replication has occurred.

As mitosis proceeds, the chromosomes compress even further into short, sausage-shaped structures, which can be clearly distinguished from one another (cell 5). The chromosomes line up in the centre of the cell and then, quite suddenly, one copy of each chromosome migrates to opposite ends of the cell. The two identical sets of chromosomes are separated (cell 8) and a new membrane begins to form across the 'waist' of the cell, dividing it and its contents equally into two. The chromosomes gradually become invisible as the DNA molecules 'stretch out' again and mitosis comes to an end. The result is two daughter cells, each with exactly the same DNA as the original cell, and enough cytosol and organelles for normal cell metabolism to occur (cells 6 and 7; 9 and 10). The new cells go into a 'resting' phase until the time comes for them to divide in their turn: hence the term 'cell *cycle*'.

The part of the cell cycle known as mitosis normally takes between about 30 minutes and three hours, depending on the species of organism. Interestingly, the genes that were switched on or off in the parent cell remain in that state in the daughters: thus, a liver cell divides to produce more liver cells because the pattern of active and silent genes in the parent cell is preserved when the DNA replicates. Cell division involving mitosis enables one cell to become two, and two to become four, and so on; it is the process by which many single-celled organisms reproduce and increase their numbers, and it enables larger organisms composed of many cells to evolve and grow, and to replace worn-out cells.

3.9 Towards larger organisms

We have only a hazy idea from the fossil record of what the evolutionary sequence might have been that resulted in the appearance on Earth of organisms consisting of many cells. The first multicellular organisms may have simply been clusters of cells that did not separate when a single-celled organism divided into two cells, and the daughters in their turn stayed together. Multicellularity provides a number of advantages, such as larger size and mutual protection against a variety of environmental threats. In a comparable way, many large animals live for all or part of their lives clustered together in flocks, herds and colonies, gaining safety in numbers and many other benefits that derive from sociality.

3.9.1 Specialisation of cells

The transition from simple multicellular organisms, that were essentially 'confederations' of identical cells, to more complex organisms such as humans, involved a crucial change in the properties of individual cells. From each cell being entirely self-sufficient and capable of *all* the processes necessary for self-maintenance and reproduction, cells became *specialised*, each carrying out only *some* of the functions required for the survival and reproduction of the whole organism.

Cells on the outside of the body evolved specialised features that formed a protective layer. Within the body, different types of cells formed distinct *tissues* or *organs* with defined functions: some digest food, others collect and excrete waste products, and so on (as we showed early on in this chapter in Figure 3.3b).[10] By analogy, individual members of a human society, or of a bee colony, each perform specialised tasks on behalf of the society or colony as a whole. Specialisation within different cell types occurs because (as mentioned earlier) each cell activates only a part of the full set of genes, and hence produces only those proteins involved in the specialised functions of that type of cell.

As multicellular organisms evolved, they became larger. Above a certain size, cells within a multicellular organism face the problem that they are no longer close enough to the outside world to obtain all the nutrients they need, or to expel their waste, simply by *passive diffusion* across the cell membrane. Nutrients can pass into the body of the multicelled organism, diffusing from one cell to the next, but this is a slow process and above a distance of about 1 millimetre (1 mm) is inefficient.

3.9.2 Transport systems

An early stage in the evolution of multicellular organisms must have been the appearance of channels along which nutrients could be carried to the innermost cells and waste could be carried out. In many kinds of modern-day animals, these channels have evolved into blood vessels and the system includes a pumping organ, such as the human heart, which drives blood around the body. Figure 3.21 shows the basic layout of the human **cardiovascular system** ('cardio' is from the Greek word *kardia*, 'heart', and 'vascular' is from the Latin for vessel). The nutrients transported in the bloodstream are obtained from the breakdown of food by the *digestive system*, but we shall say no more about that here because it is discussed in Chapter 7.

In Chapter 6, we will examine the *lymphatic system*, another transport system in the human body in which many of the cells and molecules of the immune system travel, circulating between the cardiovascular system and back again (you may wish to glance ahead at Figure 6.8). The lymphatic system also replenishes the fluid between cells and transports large molecules such as proteins and fats around the body.

[10] A hierarchy of biological organisation, from atoms and molecules at one end of the spectrum, through increasingly complex levels of organisation (cells, tissues, organs, multicellular organisms), to interactions between species is illustrated in *Studying Health and Disease* (Open University Press, 2nd edn 1994; colour-enhanced 2nd edn 2001), Chapter 9; see particularly Figure 9.1.

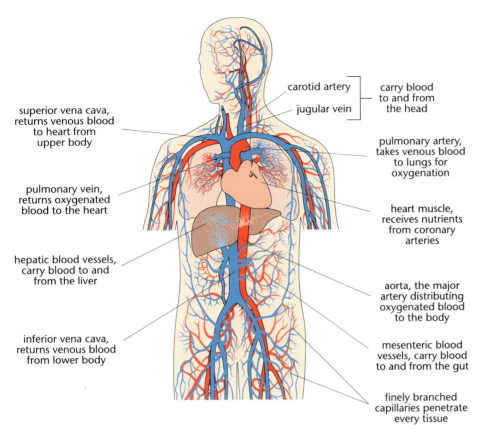

carotid artery
jugular vein
carry blood to and from the head

superior vena cava, returns venous blood to heart from upper body

pulmonary artery, takes venous blood to lungs for oxygenation

pulmonary vein, returns oxygenated blood to the heart

heart muscle, receives nutrients from coronary arteries

hepatic blood vessels, carry blood to and from the liver

aorta, the major artery distributing oxygenated blood to the body

inferior vena cava, returns venous blood from lower body

mesenteric blood vessels, carry blood to and from the gut

finely branched capillaries penetrate every tissue

Figure 3.21   *The main features of the human cardiovascular system. The heart pumps blood to the body in the arteries (shown in red), and it returns to the heart from all parts of the body in the veins (blue). The arteries and veins branch into an extensive network of fine vessels, called capillaries, which penetrate almost all parts of the body. The bloodstream acts as a transporter of oxygen, nutrients and dissolved waste, and of the specialised cells and molecules involved in defending against infection and in regulating growth, development and homeostasis. (You are not expected to memorise the details of this diagram!)*

3.9.3 Communication systems

If large, multicellular organisms, made up of cells of very different types, are to survive and reproduce, it is essential that their activities are coordinated effectively. The *homeostatic* control necessary for cells to function properly becomes a process that must occur, not just at the level of the individual cell as described earlier, but also at the level of the whole organism. Homeostasis at the organism level requires close coordination of the various fluids, cells, tissues and organs of the organism's body. Coordination of activities throughout a complex body requires effective *communication,* so that the requirements of cells in one part of the body can be recognised and responded to appropriately by cells elsewhere. Complex animals have a number of communication and control systems, of which the most important are the nervous system, the hormonal system and the immune system.

The **nervous system** consists of specialised cells, called nerve cells or *neurons*, that are adapted to pass information one to another in the form of electrical impulses and chemical signals (these chemicals are collectively called neurotransmitters). To varying degrees, the nervous systems of animals include a *brain*, which is a large aggregation of neurons that controls the activity of the organism as a whole. An important function of the brain is to receive information about the outside world from sense organs, such as eyes, ears, the nose, etc. and to control the movements of the body through its environment (see Figure 3.22).

The **hormonal system** comprises a number of diverse and scattered groups of cells called *endocrine glands*, together with the hormones they synthesise and secrete into the bloodstream (for example, the pancreas secretes insulin, the ovaries secrete oestrogen). **Hormones** are signalling molecules that are carried around the body in the blood, and which influence the activity of 'target' cells elsewhere in the body.

● From your understanding of membrane structure, how do you expect a hormone to be able to 'select' the correct target cells with which it interacts?

■ By making a lock-and-key interaction with receptor molecules embedded in the surface membrane of the target cells. Cells that do not have the correct receptor cannot interact with that hormone.

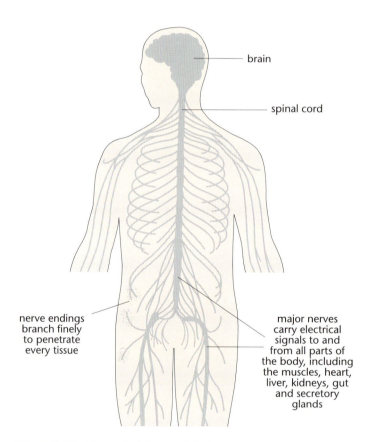

brain

spinal cord

nerve endings branch finely to penetrate every tissue

major nerves carry electrical signals to and from all parts of the body, including the muscles, heart, liver, kidneys, gut and secretory glands

Figure 3.22   *The main features of the human nervous system are conventionally distinguished into the* central nervous system *(the brain and spinal cord) and the* peripheral nervous system *(the nerves that penetrate almost every part of the body). Nerves generally consist of several different nerve fibres, which carry information in the form of electrical signals, either informing the brain and spinal cord about the state of the body, or bringing instructions from the brain and spinal cord to the muscles and organs. (You are not expected to memorise the details of this diagram.)*

Some hormones are chemically related to fats (these are the steroid hormones such as oestrogen and testosterone, involved in sexual development and reproduction); most are short chains of amino acids, some only a few amino acids long, but others (like insulin) are long enough to be called a protein. Certain hormones are intimately linked with the nervous system and some are secreted by the nervous system itself. (For example, the hormone prolactin is secreted by cells in the brain and causes the breasts of female mammals to secrete milk.)

3.9.4 Maintaining the whole

Organisms can only survive if the many processes going on in the body operate within certain narrow limits. This 'whole organism' homeostasis is regulated by the coordinated activity of the nervous system and the hormonal system, together with the processes already described for regulating the internal world of every cell. Precise regulation is essential to life: humans, for example, become very sick and may die if their body temperature deviates by only a few degrees from the 'normal' temperature of around 37 °C.

● Look back at Figure 3.18 to remind yourself of what a negative feedback circuit diagram looks like. What 'response mechanisms' are involved in temperature regulation in humans?

■ You may have thought of sweating to lose heat by evaporation when we get too hot, or shivering to generate heat when we get cold. Other responses involve consciously willed behaviour, such as removing or replacing clothing, and eating or drinking something cold or hot.

Multicellularity has certain drawbacks. Large, multicellular organisms with homeostatically controlled bodies provide wonderful places in which smaller organisms can survive and reproduce. At the very least, these 'passengers' use up precious resources that are needed by their host; at worst, they may be pathogenic and lead to their host's death. A vital aspect of homeostasis involves keeping the organism as free as possible from pathogens; in humans and many other animals, such control is achieved by the *immune system*. It operates in close association with the nervous system and with hormones to ensure, for example, that specialised defensive cells arrive as quickly as possible at places in the body where pathogens have entered. (The immune system is described in detail in Chapter 6.)

3.9.5 Reproduction in multicellular organisms

The evolution of sex was a very important development in the evolution of multicellular organisms. It is a feature that involves certain cells (the *germline* cells) becoming specialised for reproducing the organism, a capacity that is lost by all the other (somatic) cells. Most of the somatic cells in a complex organism can reproduce by mitosis — skin cells can make more skin cells, for example — but they cannot make the special cells (eggs and sperm) from which whole new organisms develop. The production of eggs and sperms involves a quite different form of cell division, called *meiosis*, which is described in Chapter 4.

Whenever cells reproduce by mitosis, whether they be single-celled organisms or cells within multicellular organisms, there is a tendency for small changes, or mutations, to occur in the sequence of bases along their DNA. The rate at which such errors occur is increased by radiation and certain chemicals, as we mentioned earlier in this chapter. In a multicelled organism that lives a long time, and therefore undergoes millions of cell divisions, more of these errors will accumulate than in a short-lived species. This accumulation of mutations is responsible for many of the manifestations of ageing, a topic taken up in Chapter 8.

3.10   Adapting to change

The origin of multicellular organisms and their subsequent evolution into a huge diversity of forms involves the same process of natural selection that was described earlier (for molecules) in our story of life on Earth. Specialisation of cells to form organs with specific functions, the development of homeostatic control, the evolution of an immune system and sexual reproduction are all features that make multicellular organisms better able to survive and reproduce. In the language of evolutionary biology, they are all **adaptations**.

The evolution of the huge diversity of organisms that inhabit the Earth today can be thought of as a series of new adaptations to particular environmental challenges. For example, the ancestors of modern amphibians (frogs, newts and salamanders) evolved a set of adaptations that enabled them to make the transition from the purely aquatic life led by their fish ancestors to one that is lived partly on dry land. Feathers and wings are adaptations in birds that enable them to fly. Chapter 2 described a number of anatomical features, characteristic of humans, that evolved during our evolution as adaptations to our ancestral environment and way of life.

● Can you recall what they were?

■ An upright posture and the ability to walk and run on two legs (bipedality) and a very large brain. These features are described as *adaptive* because they conferred a survival advantage on early humans in the transition to a savannah environment.

3.10.1   Competition for survival

The evolution of organisms by natural selection is a process in which the phenomenon of competition plays a crucial role. The initial stages of the evolutionary process, as discussed earlier, can be regarded as involving competition between different versions of DNA. Those versions that could gather and use chemical compounds from the environment more rapidly would grow and reproduce faster than less effective versions. Competition, both within and between different *species* of living organisms, can be seen essentially as a continuation of the same process, since each individual represents a unique version of DNA, in competition with other versions.

This fundamental element of competition through reproduction raises a problem for any explanation of the evolution of complex organisms from simpler ones. How can one explain the fact that all the somatic cells in complex organisms have *lost* a fundamental property of living things — the ability to reproduce more organisms of that kind? Kidney cells can divide to make more kidney cells, gut cells can make more gut cells, and so on, but only the germline cells can divide to make the sperms and eggs from which all the different cell types of a whole new organism is made.

This problem is resolved when you remember that *all* the cells of an individual contain *the same version of DNA*. Thus all the cells in a complex organism, whatever their specialised functions (skin, kidney, gut, blood, etc.), are more or less directly involved in the survival of the organism and hence the survival of the same version of DNA, and its transmission to the next generation. It is worth noting in passing that cancer cells arise as a result of mutations; their genetic makeup is no longer the same as that of other cells in the body. They reproduce and multiply in a way that, ultimately, threatens the survival of the whole organism in which they grow.

3.10.2 Genotype and phenotype

Before we leave the story of life, it is necessary to make a few final points, and to introduce one more important term. As described above, DNA 'codes for proteins' and thus is responsible for the fact that organisms can produce the molecules that make up their structure, that conduct signals around the body, and which, in the case of enzymes, control the rate of chemical reactions within cells. For an organism to function normally, to be healthy and to be able to reproduce, its DNA must contain all the appropriate genes.

●   Can you remember the collective term given to all the genes that an organism contains? How does it vary between individuals from the same species?

■   The term is *genotype*. In humans, each of us has a slightly different version of DNA and, hence, slightly different genes and a unique genotype (only identical twins have exactly the same genes and hence the same genotype).

Yet, even in identical twins there are distinguishing features, and you can imagine that a person raised under adverse conditions might develop rather differently than they would have done if raised in a healthy environment. The reason is that the *activity* of the genotype (the switching on and off of particular genes) can be influenced by the environment in which the organism grows and develops.

Biologists have a word meaning 'how the organism actually turned out': they describe the 'expressed' characteristics of the organism — its size, shape, metabolism, etc. — as its **phenotype**. Each of us has a unique phenotype, partly because we have a unique genotype, but also because we have undergone a process of development that is particular to each individual. The phenotype of an individual at a given point in its life results from a complex and continuous interaction between its genotype and its environment. You will learn more about the relationship between genotype and phenotype in Chapter 4, particularly in the context of human genetic disease.

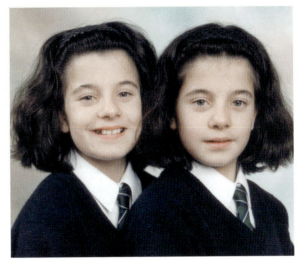

Although the genotype of an individual has to contain the 'correct' genes to produce a viable individual, there is considerable variation between the genotypes of individuals of the same species. Each individual in a species possesses a unique genotype; each of us has some unique *variations* in our genes and some variations that are shared only with the closest members of our family. This fact is exemplified in the technique of *DNA fingerprinting*, a procedure used to determine unequivocally the parentage of individuals, which exploits the fact that specific variations in the genes possessed by an individual's mother or father can be detected in the DNA of their progeny. Genetic variation and inheritance are the subjects of Chapter 4.

Even though they have identical genes, identical twins generally look different enough from each other that close friends and family have no difficulty in telling them apart; different environmental influences as they grow up have affected the way each twin 'turns out', not only in their appearance but also in the metabolic processes within their bodies. (Photo: The Grabowski family)

3.11 Complexity and progress

We end this chapter on a cautious note. The language of evolutionary biology is full of adjectives routinely applied to organisms, which imply various kinds of value judgement. Humans are described as 'complex' and 'advanced', whereas bacteria or molluscs are 'simple' and 'primitive'. The use of such words stems from the fact that biological evolution is typically seen as a process that involves progress, with forms of life that are in some sense 'better' replacing existing forms. There is an important sense in which this view is appropriate and correct. From one generation to the next, those individuals of a given species that survive and reproduce more effectively than others are, by definition, described as being 'fitter'. Thus, over time, natural selection will insure that a species 'improves', in the sense that its individuals become better adapted to their environment.

This scenario assumes, however, that the environment is constant over time, which it is not. The environment is subject to continuous change, both long-term and short-term, and much of the evolutionary change in the form and physiology of organisms that results from natural selection is in response to environmental change. This phenomenon of a constantly shifting environment is central to an evolutionary concept called the Red Queen's hypothesis, after the Red Queen in Lewis Carroll's *Through the Looking Glass* who said

> Now here, you see, it takes all the running you can do, to keep in the same place.

In other words, while natural selection is a process that tends to produce perfectly adapted organisms, a state of perfection is *never achieved*, because a continually changing environment continually alters what 'perfectly adapted' means. This idea is important in the context of disease; as you will see in Chapter 5, organisms such as ourselves have to adapt continually to the rapid changes in pathogenic organisms that occur in our own lifetimes.

Biological evolution involves not only the adaptation of *existing* species to a changing environment, but also the formation of *new* species. Sometimes new species replace existing species but, equally importantly, new species come to coexist alongside already established species. It can thus be misleading to regard all recently evolved species as being in any sense *superior* to their ancestors. The important point is that they are *different*; they have evolved novel characteristics that enable them to exploit the *current* environment in different ways from existing species.

Evolution is not generally, therefore, a process in which new species replace older, less well-adapted ones, but one in which the number and variety of species, the diversity of life, also tends to change over time. From the fossil record, it is clear that during evolution there has been a continual 'turnover' of species; at certain times there have been mass extinctions, when the number of species declined rapidly, and at other times there has been a rapid increase in the diversity of life-forms found on Earth.

At any one time in evolutionary history, as at present, the Earth is inhabited by a large and diverse array of species, some of recent origin, others more ancient, some simple, some complex. The coexistence of complex and simple species is important in the context of disease, because most pathogens, particularly bacteria and viruses, are simple organisms that coexist with complex ones, such as humans. If evolution were a progressive process in which superior forms replaced inferior ones, one might reasonably expect that organisms would arise that are resistant to any kind of disease. That they have *not* is due to the fact that simple organisms hold certain advantages over more complex organisms, notably a very high reproductive rate. The evolutionary interaction between complex and simpler organisms, including pathogenic species, is examined in more detail in Chapter 5 of this book.

OBJECTIVES FOR CHAPTER 3

When you have studied this chapter, you should be able to:

3.1 Define and use, or recognise definitions and applications of, each of the terms printed in **bold** in the text.

3.2 Describe the basic features of a 'typical' animal cell, paying particular attention to the dynamic nature of cell metabolism and the crucial role of the cell membrane as the interface with the external world.

3.3 Give some examples of lock-and-key interactions between biological molecules and comment on their function in cell metabolism.

3.4 Describe the basic features of DNA structure, how it replicates during the cell cycle and is 'shared out' by mitosis; explain the significance of these features for the evolution of life on Earth.

3.5 Describe, in outline, how 'DNA makes RNA makes protein'.

3.6 Explain how a large multicellular organism, such as a human, can be composed of specialised cells of many different types, almost all of which contain exactly the same genes.

3.7 Illustrate the process of maintaining homeostasis by negative feedback, both at the level of a single cell and of a multicellular organism.

3.8 Describe the essential features of natural selection and mutation, and show how they may contribute to the evolution of diverse life-forms.

QUESTIONS FOR CHAPTER 3

1 (*Objectives 3.2 and 3.3*)

Briefly describe the three mechanisms by which substances pass through cell membranes. Which of these mechanisms involves lock-and-key interactions?

2 (*Objectives 3.4 and 3.5*)

How does the sequence of nucleotides in a length of DNA provide the 'genetic code' for the synthesis of a protein?

3 (*Objectives 3.1 and 3.6*)

What is the principal difference between the genetic material of an insulin-producing cell in the pancreas and a pigment cell in the skin of the same individual? Use the following terms in your answer: gene, genotype, gene product.

4 (*Objective 3.7*)

Distinguish between the ways in which a single cell and a multicellular organism maintain homeostasis.

5   (*Objective 3.7*)

Draw a rough sketch of a negative feedback circuit, using Figure 3.18 as a basis, showing how homeostasis of human body temperature is maintained. (A completed diagram appears as Figure 3.23 in the Answers at the end of this book.)

6   (*Objective 3.8*)

The theory of natural selection incorporates the idea of a 'struggle for existence'. Why is there a struggle for existence and why is inheritance of mutations an essential feature of the theory of evolution by natural selection?

CHAPTER 4

Inheritance and variation

Study notes for OU students

This chapter builds on the description in Chapter 3 of the structure of DNA and its replication during the cell cycle in the human body, and the process of nuclear division known as mitosis, which occurs during growth and repair as a body cell divides into two 'daughter' cells. The TV programme 'Bloodlines: A family legacy', which was associated with Chapter 3 and includes an exploration of the structure, function and evolutionary significance of DNA, is also relevant to this chapter. The terms phenotype, genotype and gene were defined in Chapter 3 and are of central importance here. The development of the human organism, from fertilised egg cell to mature adult, is not discussed in this book, but is a major theme in the next book in this series, *Birth to Old Age: Health in Transition* (Open University Press, second edition 1995; colour-enhanced second edition 2001).

4.1 Introduction

This chapter explores three major interacting themes: the way in which genes and environments contribute to the development of the unique *phenotype* of individuals (that is, the sum total of all their characteristics); why individuals tend to resemble their parents; and how the enormous diversity of human phenotypes arises. Some of this variation is shown in Figure 1.1 (the frontispiece to this book). We trace the inheritance from one generation to the next of certain characteristics, including susceptibility to certain diseases, which follow characteristic inheritance patterns. We begin with the individual and then move on to examine the family and finally whole populations. The frequencies of genetic characteristics and diseases in different populations is discussed and we explain how and why these vary within and between populations. We begin by introducing the factors that contribute to the variation between individuals, namely genes and environments.

4.2 Inheritance and the individual

Our first task is to explore the nature of *genetically* determined differences between individuals. Though the focus is on the individual, in order to understand the inheritance of genes it is also necessary to look at events that occur within cells and how these cells interact within the human body; so we jump between focusing on the individual and looking at particular cells, and we explore the relationship between the two.

4.2.1 A family photograph album

Most families have collections of photographs spanning several generations. In these it is possible to follow the growth of individuals from birth, through to the teenage years and into adulthood. Family resemblances are apparent across generations through shared or distinctive *visible* features or characteristics: whether the hair is curly or straight; how tall the family members are, or the colour of their skin. More subtle differences may also be apparent, for example whether the ears are 'unattached', that is with lobes, or 'attached', without lobes (Figure 4.1).

However, what you can *see* is only a very small fraction of a person's phenotype. For example, you cannot 'see' the blood group or the enzymes at work in the digestive system; in fact if you could look within individual cells, at the sequences

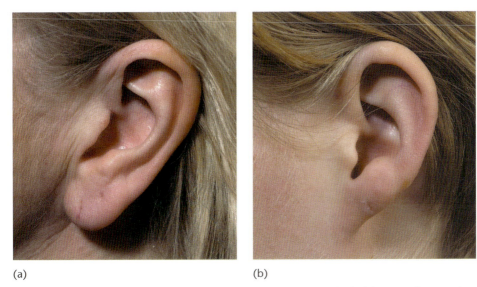

(a)   (b)

Figure 4.1   *Ear-lobes are either (a) free, unattached, or (b) attached. (Photos: Mike Levers)*

of amino acids within the proteins (Chapter 3), you would find that many of them differ very slightly between individuals. A full description of the phenotypes of several (even closely related) individuals, which included all the details of their *morphology* (the shape and structure of their bodies), their *metabolism* (all the biochemical reactions going on in their bodies), their speed of movement and coordination, their temperament, personality and intellectual abilities, would show that — like you — each person is unique. Our uniqueness is a consequence of the enormous amount of phenotypic variation that exists between individuals.

Despite the uniqueness of each individual phenotype, human babies usually resemble their parents, brothers and sisters in particular ways. Why do some members of a family have features in common with most related individuals and yet have strikingly different features which they share with few other relatives? Precisely how this unique combination of features is brought about is a result of a number of factors, as you will see as this chapter unfolds.

In order to understand why an individual develops the particular set of features they have, we need to look at the way in which living organisms reproduce themselves and what is transmitted from parent to offspring. Put another way we need to look at the *genes*, the units of genetic information that children *inherit* from their parents.

4.2.2 Genetic variation between individuals

You will remember from Chapter 3 that genes are composed of a series of DNA components called nucleotides. Whilst all humans share the same *number* of genes arranged in the same *order*, there is some variation between individuals in the exact sequence of DNA nucleotides making up these genes. These variant sequences *within* genes are termed **alleles**, and they have arisen over thousands of years of evolution through *mutation* in the DNA (as described in Section 3.4.5).

The number of different alleles of a gene that exist is highly variable. Some genes show relatively little variation in the human population with perhaps only a few different alleles known to exist. But many genes exist in **multiple alleles** — if the nucleotide sequence of such a gene is compared in a large sample of individuals, several hundred different variants can be found, each containing slightly different sequences of nucleotides in some parts of the gene. And since each of us has around 40 000 genes, each of which can exist in different alleles, the particular alleles that a person inherits is a major source of variation between individuals. Which alleles are inherited primarily depends on a person's ancestors, but new alleles can arise in an individual by mutation, although this is a rare event. Relatives are more likely to have the same alleles in common with each other than are unrelated people, because they have an ancestor in common who has passed down particular variants of their genes. The more closely related two people are to each other, the more alleles they have in common.

● Imagine that two people inherit different alleles of the same gene. What effect might differences in the alleles have upon the protein coded for by the gene?

■ For each allele, the small variations in nucleotide sequence within the gene could lead to instructions for making a protein with a corresponding small variation in its amino acid sequence — such different alleles will code for slightly different proteins; the small structural differences between the proteins could lead to differences in the way the protein functions in the body of these two people. (Look back to Section 3.6.2 if you are unsure why this is the case.)

Most alleles have very little effect upon the function of the protein which the gene encodes. But occasionally a particular allele can result in a significant alteration in the biochemical function of the encoded protein, and this in turn contributes to the variation between one individual and another. In the most extreme of cases, particular alleles of certain genes are the underlying cause of disease.

An important message of this chapter is that individuals are the products of the *combined action* of their genes (the full complement of their genes is called the *genotype*, as defined in Chapter 3) and of their environments. Some characteristics are influenced relatively more by genetic factors than by the environment, and for other characteristics the reverse is true. Later, we will examine examples of each situation, but first we consider how these two aspects — genes and environment — influence the development of the phenotype.

4.3   The process of inheritance

4.3.1 Chromosome pairs

We each begin life as a single cell, which was formed from the combining of two different *gametes* — the collective term for egg cells and sperm cells (Figure 4.2). Each gamete has a *nucleus*, which contains the DNA (the genetic material) and each fertilised egg contains the combined genetic material from sperm and egg.

As you learned in Chapter 3, genes are sequences of DNA that are joined together in a linear order, as long strands called *chromosomes*. Like the gametes, most human somatic (body) cells have a nucleus in which the chromosomes are contained. Laboratory techniques have enabled the preparation and staining of the chromosomes from a single cell, so that they are readily distinguished and can be photographed with the aid of a microscope (Figure 4.3). During *mitosis* (an important stage in somatic cell replication, described in Chapter 3), the chromosomes become visible and their number, size and shape can be most easily studied. Every species has a particular number of chromosomes, each with a characteristic size and shape.

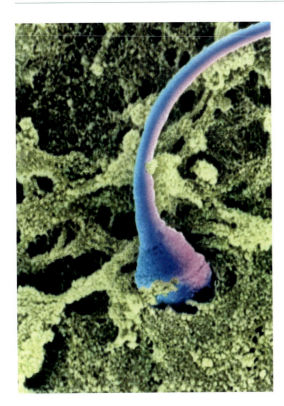

Figure 4.2 *Human gametes: a sperm penetrates an egg ovum, resulting in the combining of genetic material from both gametes. Magnified 6 000 times, photographed with the aid of a scanning electron microscope; the colours have been artificially added. (Source: Dr Yorgos Nikas/Science Photo Library)*

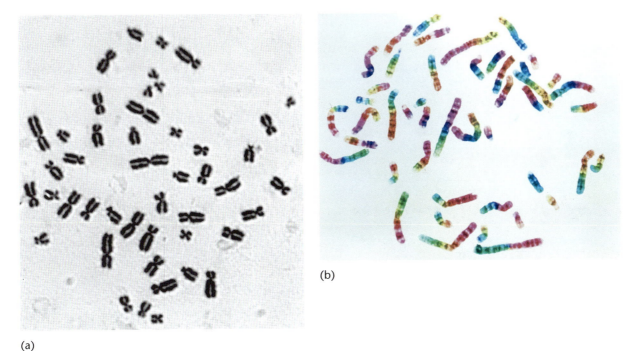

(a)

(b)

Figure 4.3 *(a) Photograph of chromosomes prepared from a single white cell taken from human blood, photographed through a light microscope, magnified approximately 1 000 times. Each chromosome has already replicated, prior to cell division, so it appears 'double'. (Photo: Department of Cancer Studies, The Medical School, University of Birmingham). (b) Here the chromosomes have been chemically treated and coloured using special chromosome-specific 'paints', which reveal distinctive banding patterns on each chromosome. (Photo: L. Willatt, East Anglian Genetics Service/Science Photo Library)*

● Can you remember how many chromosomes are found in the nucleus of most *somatic* cells in humans (i.e. the body cells, excluding the gametes)?

■ There are 46 chromosomes in the nucleus of most somatic cells in the human body. (Mature red blood cells are exceptions; they have no nucleus and no chromosomes.)

If you look more closely at Figure 4.3a you will be able to see that each chromosome in every pair has a 'double image'. This is because the first event at the commencement of mitosis is the replication of each of the 46 DNA molecules in the cell nucleus. So at the stage in the cell cycle when the chromosomes were stained for Figure 4.3a, each chromosome contains *two* DNA molecules, not one. If the cell had been allowed to continue dividing, the two DNA molecules in each chromosome would have separated, one moving to each end of the 'parent cell', thus ensuring that both the new 'daughter' cells have a complete and identical set of 46 chromosomes.

Karyotypes

The chromosomes of a single cell, stained and photographed as in Figure 4.3 to reveal their distinctive features, can then be artificially arranged in a conventional pattern described as a **karyotype**. Figure 4.4 shows the chromosomes of a human female, taken from a cell which has already begun mitosis, arranged in a karyotype — the pattern of chromosomes that is unique to human females. The same term, karyotype, is used for the standard chromosome set of an *individual*, as in 'Mary's karyotype', or of a *species*, as in 'chimpanzee karyotype'.

● What is the most striking feature of the human karyotype shown in Figure 4.4?

■ The chromosomes have been arranged in 23 pairs of varying sizes (numbered from pair 1, the largest, to pair 22, the smallest, plus a pair labelled X); the members of each pair look the same. (Notice that each chromosome in every pair appears as a 'double image' because it consists of two DNA molecules as described above.)

Identifying homologous pairs

Members of the 22 numbered chromosome pairs are said to be *homologous*, which in genetics means 'having a similar structure', thus there are 22 **homologous pairs** of chromosomes in the human karyotype. (You may be interested to know that the chromosomes in our karyotype have a similar genetic organisation to the 48 chromosomes of our closest living relatives, the chimpanzees.) We will return to the 23rd pair — the sex chromosomes — shortly.

Although some homologous pairs have longer or shorter chromosomes than others, it is still difficult to distinguish between several pairs of chromosomes on size alone. For example, look at the pairs of chromosomes numbered 7 to 12 in Figure 4.4: they are all about the same size. This difficulty was overcome in the 1970s by the discovery of special staining techniques, which produce distinctive patterns of bands on chromosomes. More recently, using specially designed chromosome 'paints' as illustrated in Figures 4.3b and 4.4, the technique has improved so much that different chromosome pairs can readily be distinguished on the basis of their different banding patterns (if you know what you are looking for!). Chromosome staining and karyotype analysis has made it possible to look at variants in chromosome structure both between individuals and between cells within the body.

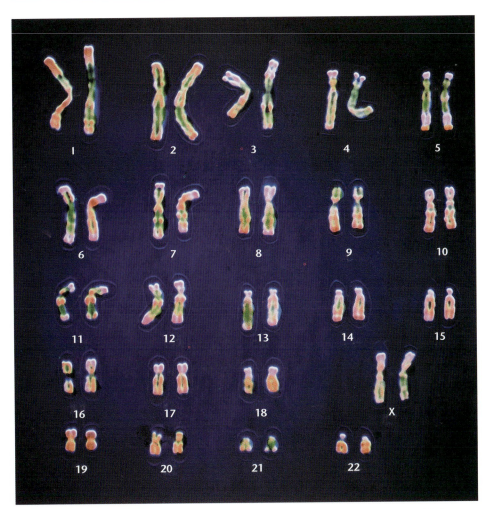

Figure 4.4   *The chromosomes of a human female, arranged as a karyotype, magnified approximately 1 000 times. The chromosomes were first stained and photographed with a digital camera through a light microscope; then the image of each chromosome was manipulated on a computer display to rearrange the chromosomes in a conventional sequence — the karyotype. The pair of X chromosomes has been labelled and the other pairs are numbered 1 to 22. (Photo: CNRI/Science Photo Library)*

● In Figure 4.4, what does the staining reveal about the internal structure of the homologous pairs of chromosomes numbered 7 to 12?

■ If you look closely, you can observe, first, that each chromosome appears to have an identical internal structure as its partner and, second, that each pair can be distinguished from all other pairs.

The two observations that you have just made about chromosomes reveal important information about inheritance. We will look at the implications of each of these observations in turn, but first we must refer to the 23rd chromosome pair.

Sex chromosomes

The human female karyotype (shown in Figure 4.4) contains two chromosomes marked 'X'. In the human male karyotype, one of the X chromosomes is replaced by a much smaller chromosome called the Y chromosome (in fact it is the smallest of all the human chromosomes, even smaller than those in pair 22). The X and Y chromosomes are called the **sex chromosomes** because they play an important role in sex determination: females are often referred to as having the genetic constitution XX, whereas that males are XY. Apart from these sex chromosomes, both males and females contain similar sets of 22 homologous pairs of non-sex chromosomes.

● How many different *kinds* of chromosomes may occur in a human cell?

■ There are 24 different kinds of chromosomes — that is, chromosomes 1 to 22, plus X and Y.

Each unique kind of chromosome carries particular genes arranged in a specific order along its length, and these genes are different from those on other kinds of chromosomes. For example, all human chromosome number 4s, taken from individuals all over the world, carry the *same* genes arranged in the *same* order, and these characteristic 'chromosome 4 genes' are different from the 'chromosome 7 genes', or the 'X chromosome genes', and so on.

As you already know, human cells contain chromosomes in homologous *pairs*, so for example there are two chromosome 7s carrying the *same* genes in the *same* order (Figure 4.5). It follows that every gene on the 22 non-sex chromosomes is present *twice* in the genotype, a feature that has important consequences for inheritance.

The exception to this 'two copies of each gene' rule occurs in males and relates to differences in the two sex chromosomes. The X and Y chromosomes carry different genes and, given the very small size of the Y chromosome, you may not be surprised to learn that it contains very few genes, the most important of which is the gene that carries instructional information for the development of testes rather than ovaries. So males have only *one* copy of the genes carried on their single X chromosome, whereas females have *two* copies since they are XX. Later in this chapter, we will look at the influence of the sex chromosomes on inheritance and, in particular, at the consequences for males of having only a single copy of each of the X chromosome genes.

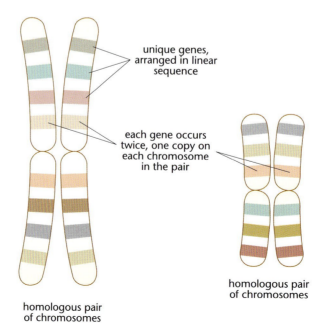

unique genes, arranged in linear sequence

each gene occurs twice, one copy on each chromosome in the pair

homologous pair of chromosomes

homologous pair of chromosomes

Figure 4.5 *Two homologous pairs of chromosomes; each pair has a characteristic set of genes which are different from those found on all the other homologous pairs. Two copies of each gene exist in the cell nucleus, one copy on each chromosome of a pair.*

4.3.2 The formation of eggs and sperm

The presence of homologous pairs of chromosomes is particularly important for understanding reproduction and the passing on or *transmission* of genetic material between generations. Observing the behaviour of chromosome pairs during the production of gametes provides a direct way of obtaining information about the inheritance of genes.

The process of gamete production involves a type of nuclear division, which is different from mitosis and is called **meiosis** (pronounced 'my-oh-sis'). Unlike mitosis, which occurs throughout the organism whenever growth by cell replication occurs, meiosis is confined to the egg-producing and sperm-producing cells in the *gonads*: ovaries in females and testes in males. Meiosis is a much more complex process than mitosis and is remarkably similar in all animal and plant species. The details of the process are not important here, but you should understand how differences between gametes can arise, since this variation has profound consequences for the phenotype of each individual.

Changes in chromosome number

The most striking way in which gametes differ from somatic cells in the body, and from the egg-producing or sperm-producing cells in the gonads from which they arise, is in the *number* of their chromosomes. The changes in chromosome number that take place during meiosis, gamete production and subsequent fertilisation of the egg by a sperm, are summarised in Figure 4.6. As a result of meiosis, each

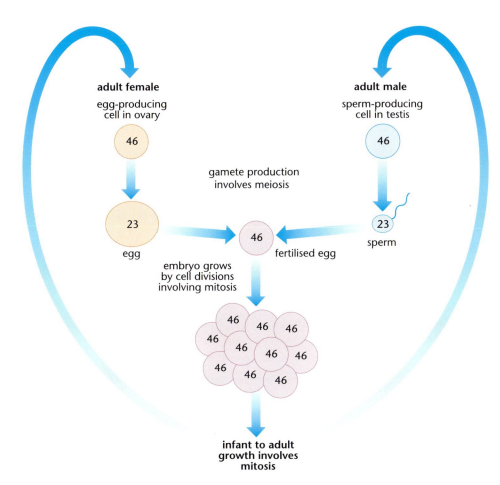

Figure 4.6 *Changes in chromosome number in the human life cycle, beginning with the reduction to 23 chromosomes during gamete production by meiosis (a specialised type of cell division that only occurs when eggs and sperm are produced), the restoration of 46 chromosomes when an egg is fertilised by a sperm, and the production of billions of somatic (body) cells by mitosis (the 'standard' type of cell division), which enables growth and maintenance of the body.*

gamete contains only 23 single chromosomes: one from each of the 22 homologous pairs of non-sex chromosomes, plus either an X or a Y chromosome.

● How many chromosomes will a fertilised egg contain and where did they originate?

■ The fertilised egg has 46 chromosomes in 23 pairs: one member of each pair came from the female parent in the egg and the other member of each pair came from the male parent in the sperm.

Thus fertilisation restores the full chromosome number in the human genotype. It also means that any individual inherits one of each pair of chromosomes from their father and one of each pair from their mother.

● Why is meiosis such an important feature of sexual reproduction?

■ If the chromosome number were not halved in the gametes prior to fertilisation, the fertilised egg would contain 92 chromosomes — twice the normal number in the parents' cells.

Sexual reproduction, which involves the combining of DNA from two different and unrelated individuals, is a powerful source of genetic variation. Growth and development follow, which among other events involve a staggeringly large number of cell divisions involving *mitosis*, in which the normal chromosome number is preserved, to produce a fetus, baby, child and finally an adult.[1] (You, for example, consist of a thousand billion cells.) The mature adult, in turn, produces gametes, some of which are fertilised, and our genetic material continues through this cycle of mitosis and meiosis through the generations, as shown in Figure 4.6.

Sex determination during gamete formation

Now look at Figure 4.7a, which illustrates the production of gametes in each parent with reference to the sex chromosomes only; we have omitted all the other chromosomes to make the sex chromosomes easier to follow. Each of the sperm-producing cells in the testes of the male contain both an X and a Y chromosome, whereas the equivalent cells in the female each contain XX. In the male, the X and Y chromosomes separate from each other during meiosis, the X chromosome going to one sperm and the Y chromosome to another. Similarly, in the female, the two X chromosomes separate from one another, each going into different eggs.

● On the basis of Figure 4.7a, what is the ratio of X gametes to Y gametes produced by the male?

■ It is 1 : 1.

Geneticists frequently use a type of table or matrix, as shown in Figure 4.7b, to determine which combinations of gametes can be produced upon fertilisation and the result of their combination at fertilisation. You can see that it is possible to produce four combinations of X and Y chromosomes.

[1] Biological development from a fertilised human egg to a newborn baby is described in *Birth to Old Age: Health in Transition* (Open University Press, 2nd edn 1995; colour-enhanced 2nd edn 2001), Chapter 3; childhood development and the changes associated with puberty and adolescence are described in Chapters 4–6 of that book; Chapters 7–9 refer to adulthood and midlife and Chapters 10–11 deal with ageing.

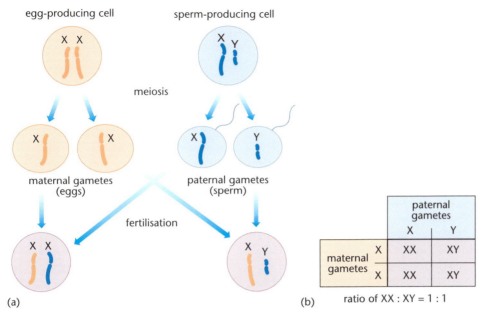

Figure 4.7   *(a) Mating diagram showing the distribution of human sex chromosomes during gamete formation, the consequences for the possible sex of children, and the proportions of children of each sex. (b) Table showing how the combination of maternal and paternal gametes at fertilisation can give rise to four different combinations of X and Y chromosomes in the offspring.*

● Since fertilisation of eggs by sperm is random, what is the expected proportion of female offspring?

■ Half the offspring will be female, since half the sperm contain an X chromosome and so does every egg; therefore, 50 per cent of fertilised eggs will be XX.

Thus, for each conception, there is a 50 per cent chance of the offspring being a girl, and a 50 per cent chance of a boy. The process of meiosis, which governs the separation of X and Y chromosomes during gamete formation, not only accounts for the occurrence of XX (female) and XY (male) individuals, but is also responsible for the production of approximately equal numbers of the two sexes in any population.

4.3.3 Chromosome mixing during meiosis

The behaviour of chromosomes during meiosis is important for understanding how variation arises between gametes and in turn between individuals. Normal cell division involving *mitosis* results in the production of cells that are genetically *identical* to the original cell and to each other (Chapter 3). In contrast, the production of sperm and eggs by cell division involving *meiosis* results in gametes that carry novel mixtures of the original parental chromosomes. This mixing of chromosomes arises through two processes that only occur during meiosis; *crossing over* and *random assortment*. To understand these processes fully, we must first look back at where our genetic material originates.

Crossing over

As we said earlier, each of us inherited one chromosome in each pair from each of our parents, and for each of the genes they passed on to us we inherited a different pattern of *alleles* from our mother and father (since couples are usually completely unrelated individuals). During meiosis, the 'maternal' and 'paternal' chromosomes are mixed together. As a first stage in meiosis, each chromosome pair undergoes a process called **crossing over** to form two new pairs, which are a complementary mixture of the two parental chromosomes. Crossing over is the physical exchange of genetic material between the two chromosomes in an homologous pair, following breakage and rejoining as shown in Figure 4.8a.

Crossing over brings about a considerable rearrangement of genetic material in the original 'parental' chromosomes. Remember that the genetic difference between the parental chromosomes is not in the number or order of genes (which is identical between all people), but in the variants or *alleles* that might lie within each gene. Thus, through the process of crossing over, new combinations of alleles are produced, here represented by the mixing of light and dark shades of blue chromosomes. The points at which this breakage and rejoining occurs is essentially *random* and thus crossing over generates an infinite number of combinations of genetic variants, which end up in the new gametes generated by meiosis (Figure 4.8b).

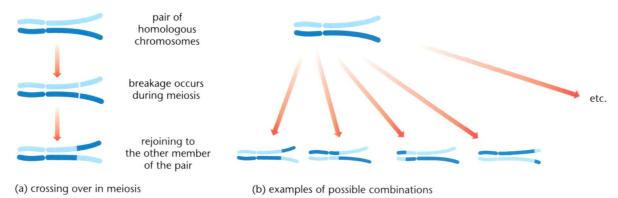

pair of
homologous
chromosomes

breakage occurs
during meiosis

etc.

rejoining to
the other member
of the pair

(a) crossing over in meiosis

(b) examples of possible combinations

Figure 4.8 *(a) The process of crossing over between the two 'parental' chromosomes in an homologous pair, breaks up and rearranges the combination of alleles on individual chromosomes, exchanging alleles between chromosomes inherited from the person's mother (pale blue) and father (dark blue). (b) During each cell division involving meiosis, crossing over in different places along the chromosome generates lots of different combinations of alleles in the chromosomes that end up in each new gamete (egg or sperm). Only one chromosome pair is shown here, but the same process occurs in all 22 homologous pairs.*

Random assortment

Having mixed the parental alleles through chromosome crossing over, the members of each of the 22 homologous pairs of chromosomes in the gamete-producing cells, and the two sex chromosomes, now separate from each other — one member from each chromosome pair entering each gamete (Figure 4.9a and b). It is a matter of chance which chromosome from a given pair enters a particular gamete, so each gamete receives a **random assortment** of the chromosomes, but every new gamete always gets one of each chromosome pair.

With 23 pairs of chromosomes in human cells, random assortment of the individual chromosomes in each pair during meiosis can generate a total of over 8 million different possible combinations! By the time meiosis is complete, one chromosome of each pair is present in each of the resulting gametes, as shown in Figure 4.9b.

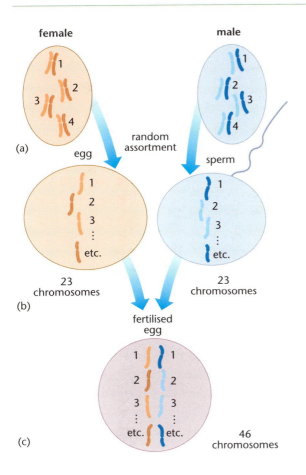

Figure 4.9 *(a) Early in meiosis, chromosomes in gamete-producing cells 'line up' in homologous pairs. (The two shades of orange and blue chromosomes in this diagram represent the two partners in an homologous pair.)*
(b) A random assortment of chromosomes, one from each pair, is donated to each new gamete (only one egg and one sperm are shown here, but the randomisation ensures that every egg and sperm gets a unique assortment of chromosomes). (c) The resulting fertilised egg always contains half maternal and half paternal chromosomes, one in each pair.

The outcome of meiosis

In summary, by the end of meiosis each new gamete contains:

- half the number of chromosomes
- one member of each homologous pair of chromosomes
- one sex chromosome (either X or Y)
- a unique random assortment of chromosomes which have already had their alleles randomly mixed by crossing over.

Upon fertilisation (Figure 4.9c), the 23 chromosomes from the egg and the 23 from the sperm now form a new cell with a *unique* complement of 46 chromosomes. The mixing of genes from two unrelated parents is another major source of genetic variation in a population. The fertilised egg then undergoes billions of cell divisions involving *mitosis* during growth and development into the adult (look back at Figure 4.6). The process by which gametes are produced occurs continuously in males after puberty through the constant production of sperm. In contrast, eggs start to develop much earlier in females, during embryonic life; meiosis begins in gamete-producing cells in the developing ovary in the embryo, but is held in 'suspended animation' until puberty. Upon reaching puberty, the final stages of meiosis occur in a few of the stored eggs during each monthly cycle, culminating with the release of just a single mature egg.[2]

[2] Other changes associated with puberty, in addition to the 'growth spurt' already described in Chapter 2, are discussed in *Birth to Old Age: Health in Transition* (Open University Press, 2nd edn 1995; colour-enhanced 2nd edn 2001), Chapter 6.

4.4   The influence of environment

We turn now to the influence of the environment on the development of the phenotype from the time of fertilisation to adult maturity and into old age. Environmental factors are another very important source of variation between individuals.

You are already familiar with the general meaning of **environment**, but when considering the development of the phenotype, we are using it with a very broad meaning to include (at one end of the spectrum) the cytosol surrounding the nucleus within a cell and a specific biological environment such as the uterus, to contact with pathogens, and (at the other end of the spectrum) the Earth's climate and the whole of human culture. In this context, 'environment' includes any factor *other than the genes* that influences the development of the phenotype. The phenotype, which changes during the lifetime of an individual, is continuously affected by many aspects of that individual's changing environment.

● Given this very broad definition, can you give some examples of environmental factors that affect human physical or mental growth and development?

■ You may have thought of some of the following (there are many others): diet, education and access to books at home, stress, number of children in the family, parental love and attention, level of income in the household, parent's occupation and lifestyle (e.g. whether they smoke), air quality, environmental pollution, exposure to infection, famine, warfare, etc.

Some of these factors may influence the phenotype only at one particular stage of development; for example biological environments are particularly important during fetal development (as discussed briefly below). On the other hand, diet affects the phenotype throughout an individual's lifetime (we return to the subject of human digestion and diet in Chapter 7).

4.4.1   The intra-uterine environment

As discussed in detail elsewhere in this series,[3] the *nutritional* environment inside the uterus has been implicated in possible long-term effects on the susceptibility of adults to a range of diseases in later life, including heart disease and diabetes. The so-called *programming hypothesis* is based on evidence that nutritional deficiencies during fetal life may affect the strength and elasticity of blood vessel walls as they develop, leading to an increased risk of cardiovascular diseases from middle age onwards (O'Brien *et al.*, 1999).

Here we will briefly draw attention to the much faster-acting effects of certain chemical or infectious agents that can enter the intra-uterine environment and cause serious adverse effects on the developing fetus in a matter of weeks or months. Some agents are not harmful to the mother yet can damage the developing fetus. The majority of malformation-producing agents (such as the drug thalidomide, prescribed in the 1960s to combat morning sickness) are especially damaging in

---

[3] Fetal programming is extensively discussed in *Studying Health and Disease* (Open University Press, 2nd edn 1994; colour-enhanced 2nd edn 2001), Chapter 10 and in the associated audiotape for Open University students 'Data interpretation: the programming hypothesis'. David Barker, the leader of the research team that developed the hypothesis, appears in an Open University video 'Status and wealth: the ultimate panacea?' associated with *World Health and Disease* (Open University Press, 3rd edn 2001), Chapter 10.

the early stages of pregnancy, when embryonic limbs and major organs are taking shape. Another example is the rubella virus: if contracted in the first three months of pregnancy this may result in serious eye, ear and cardiovascular (heart and blood vessel) malformations in the fetus, while the mother experiences only the mild symptoms of German measles. In contrast, the harmful effects of excessive alcohol consumption by the mother are not restricted to a sensitive period during pregnancy, but extend through the entire nine months.

4.5   Interactions between genes and environments

The development of the phenotype of an individual is not a simple straightforward process, but rather is the result of the *dynamic interaction* of their genes and their environments. A question that has generated heated debate between biologists and psychologists for the last 50 years or so is 'how much of a person's characteristics are determined by their genes and how much are they influenced by the environment?' Attempts to estimate the relative contribution of the genotype (sometimes referred to as *nature*) and the environment (*nurture*) to the development of characteristics, have been termed the **nature–nurture debate**.

The question is difficult (if not impossible) to answer, because a person's phenotype is a product of growth and development brought about by a certain genotype in a *succession* of environments. The phenotype at a given moment is determined not only by the environment that prevails at that moment, but also by the succession of environments experienced during its lifetime. Every person is the product of their genotype *and* their life experiences.

The nature–nurture debate has gradually given way to a reasonable consensus among scientists that the two are generally inseparable. This *interactionist* view is epitomised by the words of the eminent biologist and expert in animal behaviour, D. O. Hebb who, writing in 1953 about attempts to differentiate between instinct (nature) and learning (nurture) in the development of behaviour, suggested that such attempts are

> … exactly like asking how much of the area of a field is due to its length, and how much to its width. (Hebb, 1953, p. 44)

Nevertheless, many attempts have been made to partition the causes of variation for certain characteristics. The difficulty of this task is illustrated by the example of human birthweight which, although it might be considered a characteristic of the *baby*, is also affected by a number of genetic and environmental factors *outside* the baby.

● Can you suggest some genetic and environmental factors that might affect human birthweight?

■ Among many possibilities are: fetal genotype, maternal genotype, maternal environment including socio-economic factors that might affect maternal diet, smoking, alcohol intake or stress, and contaminants in the intra-uterine environment during fetal development (e.g. infection or toxic chemicals).

This example illustrates the complexity of the interactions between the genotype and environment. Studies on identical twins can shed some light on this interaction. Identical twins are *genetically* identical as they arise from a single fertilised egg which, after a few cell divisions, splits into the two developing fetuses. Twins represent a sort of 'natural' experiment to test whether two individuals who are genetically identical may develop differently in different environments. Clearly, if genes are paramount in determining a characteristic, then that characteristic will be similar in identical twins who are raised *apart*. But suppose, for example, that one identical twin contracts a serious infection such as polio and the other does not; the former may become physically disabled and the latter may not. Clearly, their difference in physical form is then due to environmental factors.

However, it is very rare to find identical twins who were separated early in life, so the information on humans is limited; we will consider some examples later in this chapter. It is much easier to carry out studies of how the same genotype may react to different environments in plants. In the case of grasses, for example, it is possible to split one individual into a number of genetically identical pieces, grow them in different environments and observe the phenotypic differences between them. The results of one such experiment are shown in Figure 4.10. You can see from this drawing how wide the range of phenotypes, all with the same genotype, can be. Experiments such as this show that the phenotype is the result of the *interaction* between gene action and the particular environment.

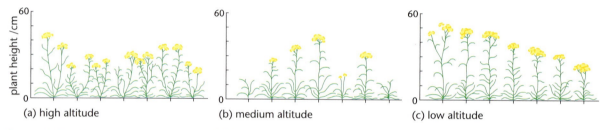

Figure 4.10 *Responses of seven different* Achillea *(yarrow) plants to environments of different altitude. Cuttings from each of the seven plants were grown at (a) high altitude, 3 040 metres above sea-level, (b) medium altitude, 1 400 metres, and (c) low altitude, 30 metres. Plants from the same parent have been planted in the same order, from left to right. (Redrawn from Suzuki, P. T., Griffiths, A. J. F. and Lewontin, R. C., 1981,* An Introduction to Genetic Analysis, *2dn edn, W. H. Freeman, San Francisco, p. 18)*

This interaction is as important in humans as it is in other organisms. *The genotype sets the boundaries within which the phenotype develops in different environments.* For example, however perfect the diet that promotes the growth of a particular individual, there is a maximum height above which he or she cannot grow that is determined by the genotype. On the other hand, the potential height may never be reached because of an inadequate diet and/or the extent of childhood diseases the individual has suffered.[4] We can put these ideas into a broader context by considering a different example — tuberculosis (TB).

● If every individual in a family of two parents and four children has a similar characteristic, such as TB, would you conclude that the condition was bound to be genetic in origin (that is, a result of family members sharing similar genes)?

■ No. If a condition is *familial*, which means that it runs in families, one may *suspect* a genetic origin, but there could be something about the environment that they all share which leads them all to succumb to the same disease.

[4] The relationship between nutrition and infection during childhood and the effects on growth and development, including final adult height, are discussed in *World Health and Disease* (Open University Press, 2nd edn 1993; 3rd edn 2001), Chapter 11.

To be sure that a characteristic is inherited, it is necessary to look at the occurrence of the characteristic in more distant relatives, including grandparents. This is our next task: to explore the patterns of inheritance and the extent to which different characteristics recur in different members of the same family.

4.6   The family

We now turn to an examination of specific characteristics, or phenotypes, in order to explore patterns of inheritance in family members and examine how these patterns contribute to the production of variation between individuals. The word phenotype, as well as meaning the sum total of all characteristics, has another more-restricted meaning; it is used by geneticists as a 'shorthand' way of referring to the expression of a *particular* characteristic. So instead of talking of the 'characteristic of brown hair', geneticists frequently talk of the 'brown hair phenotype', as in 'all the members of a brown-haired family share the brown hair phenotype'.

If we return to our family photograph album, we can ask why any one individual has a particular characteristic, such as curly hair or a certain blood group. To understand the reasons, we need to broaden our interest to look at other family members. By examining the family as a whole, we can determine if a particular phenotype is genetically influenced and, if so, show why some children in a family share some characteristics, but differ from each other in many ways.

Another word of warning about the terminology sometimes used to describe the *relationship* between genes and the phenotype is appropriate here. Biologists often use a shorthand such as 'the gene for brown hair' or 'the brown hair gene' (and we shall do this in this book). This expression suggests a direct causal relationship between a particular gene and the production of brown hair. But this may be an over-simplification because the gene involved in making hair brown may *primarily* be involved in pigment formation throughout the body, not just hair colour.

4.6.1   Tracing the inheritance of single genes

You have seen that each single human chromosome carries many genes, each with its own function and each with its own specific location on that chromosome. Here we focus on the behaviour of *single* genes during gamete production and fertilisation, by tracing the patterns of **single-gene inheritance**. As we have already discussed, many variants or alleles can exist within the DNA that encodes a gene. If these alleles actually cause a difference in the biological activity of the gene, they can often also influence what we see as the phenotype of the individual who carries that gene in their genotype. Across a whole population therefore, the presence of multiple alleles for a single gene coding for any one characteristic (such as hair colour) give rise to what we see as *normal variation* between individuals.

However, the phenotypes associated with some alleles are seen in the form of human disease. As the inheritance pattern of our genes determines who carries these alleles, these conditions are referred to as **genetic diseases**. As human disease is so apparent within a healthy population, we know much more about disease-causing alleles than alleles (the great majority) that do not result in disease. The examples used in this chapter, and in all human genetic texts, reflect this emphasis on disease-causing alleles, but you must not lose sight of the fact that much of the *normal* variation between individuals is genetically influenced and is due to the inheritance of different combinations of alleles in each of our 40 000 genes.

Now that we have introduced the term allele to mean 'alternative forms of a gene', we can re-state in a more precise genetic language that in any individual, as they have two of each chromosome, there are two *alleles* of each gene present. For each gene, an individual inherits a *paternal allele* (from the father) and a *maternal allele* (from the mother). Whilst there may be many hundreds of alleles of any single gene within the human population, we each inherit only *two*.

4.6.2 Tracing disease alleles: multiple lipoma

We will illustrate the vital importance of alternative alleles for the pattern of single-gene inheritance by considering a specific example, the inheritance of alleles within a gene which is known to cause a disease called *multiple lipoma*. Multiple lipoma is probably the most common form of tumour in adults and is not normally harmful to health; individuals develop benign (non-cancerous) fatty tumours, usually occurring beneath the skin. In the whole of the human population, there are only two alleles of the gene concerned in this condition: one that causes the tumours and one that does not.

Before proceeding, we must first explain some conventions in genetic nomenclature. It is conventional in genetics to represent each allele by a letter (either capital or lower case), printed in *italics*. In this example, we will use the letter *L* for the allele associated with tumours, and *l* for the allele associated with their absence. You already know that in any individual, there are *two* copies of each gene present in every somatic cell, one inherited from the mother and one from the father, each on one chromosome of a homologous pair (if you are unsure, look back at Figure 4.5). Therefore, any one individual could have two copies of the tumour-associated allele (*L L*), two copies of the allele not associated with tumours (*l l*) or have one of each (*L l*). An individual with two copies of the *L* allele is said to have the *L L* genotype; such individuals will develop multiple lipomas. A person with two copies of the *l* allele has the *l l* genotype and will be free of tumours. (Note that here we are using 'genotype' in its restricted sense to mean the inherited alleles of a *particular* gene, rather than in the comprehensive sense used up to now to refer to the sum total of all the genes of an individual.)

In Figure 4.11, you can follow what happens to the *L L* and *l l* alleles, first during meiosis when gametes are produced, and at fertilisation when gametes combine. The two alleles of the multiple-lipoma gene are located on a pair of homologous chromosomes, one allele on each, as shown in the egg-producing and sperm-producing cells at the top of the figure. Remember that during meiosis, each member of this pair will separate during gamete formation (as shown earlier in Figure 4.9), and hence the alleles they contain *also* separate.

● How many alleles of the multiple-lipoma gene are present in each gamete?

■ Only one allele in each gamete. Remember that the total number of chromosomes is reduced to half (i.e. 23) with just one copy of each present (look back at Figure 4.6 if you are unsure).

● What alleles do the gametes contain in this example?

■ The female's gametes all contain *L*, whereas the male's gametes all contain *l*.

● What are the possible genotypes of the children of this couple with respect to the multiple-lipoma gene?

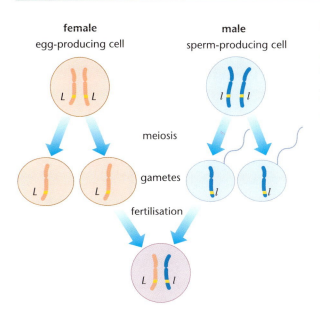

Figure 4.11 *Mating diagram between a female with the genotype L L and a male with the genotype l l, illustrating the behaviour of these alleles during gamete formation and fertilisation. (Only the chromosomes containing the multiple-lipoma gene are shown here.)*

■ Each child must receive one allele from each parent and therefore they must all be *L l*.

Notice that not only do *all* the progeny have the *same* genotype, *L l*, but that it is also a different genotype from either of the parents. We need some way to distinguish between situations in which the two inherited alleles of a particular gene are the *same* and where the two alleles are *different*. Geneticists use the following terms, which will recur many times in this chapter and elsewhere in this book. Where the two alleles are the *same*, the alleles are said to be **homozygous** (pronounced 'hom-oh-zy-gus') and the individuals are referred to as **homozygotes** ('hom-oh-zy-goats') for that particular gene; where the two alleles are *different* they are said to be **heterozygous** ('het-er-oh-zy-gus') and the individuals are referred to as **heterozygotes** for that particular gene.

In our example, the offspring shown in Figure 4.11 are heterozygotes (they have two different alleles) with respect to the multiple-lipoma gene, whereas their parents are both homozygotes for different alleles (the mother is *L L* and the father is *l l*).

4.6.3 Dominant and recessive characteristics

Now we know the genotypes of the individuals in Figure 4.11 with respect to the multiple-lipoma gene, but what is the *phenotype* of offspring with the heterozygous genotype *L l*? One of their alleles (*L*) is associated with the presence of tumours, but the other (*l*) is not, so how do the offspring 'turn out'? (Or to put it in more precise genetic language, how is the (*L l*) genotype 'expressed' in the phenotype?) In fact, the offspring all have multiple lipoma like their mother. The characteristic that we see in the phenotype of a heterozygote individual is said to be the **dominant characteristic**, because it masks the effect of the other allele. The characteristic that is *not* expressed is said to be the **recessive characteristic**.

In this example, 'absence of lipomas' is *recessive to* (or masked by) the dominant characteristic, which is 'presence of lipomas'. Another way of putting it is to say that the *L* allele is dominant and the *l* allele is recessive. (Note the convention in genetics to signify dominance by using a capital letter, whereas recessive alleles are given lower case letters.) Alleles are therefore frequently classified by their effects upon the phenotype; an allele that gives rise to a dominant characteristic in the phenotype (such as the presence of lipomas) is termed a dominant allele. Conversely, the recessive phenotype results from a recessive allele. In the shorthand of genetics, multiple lipoma is often referred to as a **dominant disorder**, because it appears in the phenotype as a consequence of the expression of a single dominant allele. (You will learn about *recessive disorders* later in the chapter.)

The patterns of inheritance of alternative phenotypes (such as presence or absence of lipomas) associated with single-gene inheritance, are found not only in humans but in all organisms with sexual reproduction. It is noteworthy in the example of multiple lipoma that there is no 'blending' of the two different alleles in the heterozygote to produce an intermediate condition, and the children (*L l*) have the same phenotype (presence of tumours) as one of the homozygous parents (*L L*). As you will see in the following section, there are cases when blending of two different alleles does occur and these alleles are called **co-dominant**.

Understanding the patterns of inheritance for recessive, dominant and co-dominant alleles helps us to learn more about *normal variation* between individuals and why particular characteristics tend to run in families. These patterns are even more important when the inheritance of genetic diseases is considered. We return to this theme later in the chapter.

4.6.4 Several alleles: ABO blood groups

So far in this section, characteristics with just two alternative phenotypes have been described because the gene involved exists in only two alternative alleles. However, many genes have multiple alleles. A well-known example is that of the **ABO blood groups**, where at least three alternative alleles (*A, B* and *O*) of the *ABO* gene exist. A person's blood group partly depends on which of these alleles he or she inherits. This information is vital for blood transfusion. Blood cannot be transfused between one person and another without first checking the blood groups of both the recipient and the donor. It is safe to transfuse blood from an individual of one group into another individual of the *same* group; but when blood is transfused between individuals with *different* blood groups, strict rules of compatibility must be followed. Breaking these rules may result in serious harm or even the death of the person receiving the transfusion.

● Three alternative alleles of the *ABO* gene exist, but how many of them are present in any one individual?

■ Only two, one on each member of a pair of homologous chromosomes.

An individual may be *homozygous* for any one of the three possible alleles (that is, *A A* or *B B* or *O O*) or *heterozygous* for any possible combination (*A B* or *A O* or *B O*). To determine the phenotype (that is, the blood group) arising from these genotypes, you need to know that both the alleles *A* and *B* are *dominant* to *O* (or put another way, *O* is recessive to both *A* and *B*).

● What is the blood group of individuals with the following genotypes: *A O, B O*, and *O O*?

■ Blood group A, B and O, respectively.

When an *A* and a *B* allele is inherited by an individual, the blood cells carry *both* an A and a B phenotype and the blood type is referred to as AB. In such cases, the A and B alleles are said to be *co-dominant*.

The existence of multiple alleles of the same gene is quite common; a great variety of characteristics are known to be associated with multiple alleles and others are sure to be found in the future. Although the pattern of inheritance seems more complicated for multiple alleles than for those with just two alternatives, the same rules are obeyed: only *two* of the many possible alleles of a gene are present in each individual, these are separated and reduced to one during gamete production, and two are restored when the egg is fertilised by a sperm.

4.6.5 Multiple alleles: haemoglobin

As we noted several times in earlier discussions, multiple alleles of a gene represent an important source of variation within the human population. To emphasise the amount of variation that exists within the human species consider the blood protein **haemoglobin**, the most widely studied of all our body constituents.[5] Haemoglobin, which is present in red blood cells, transfers oxygen from the lungs to all the cells in the body. This complex protein is made up of a sequence of amino acids which is the same in most people. However, nearly 500 variant forms of haemoglobin have been found, each coded for by a gene containing a different allele. These multiple alleles have arisen due to rare mutations in the DNA nucleotide sequence within the haemoglobin gene.

If you consider that humans have an estimated 40 000 genes coding for proteins, many with multiple alleles, you will begin to get a measure of the variation that exists within our species. We shall return to this theme later in the chapter, but now we explore how families can reveal the genetic nature of normal and disease characteristics in their family trees.

4.7 Patterns of inheritance in families

Recognising the patterns of inheritance is one of the first stages in genetic counselling for families affected by a disease which appears to have a genetic contribution.[6] Knowing this pattern and being able to follow the inheritance through family members allows predictions to be made about future generations. Whilst this might not be as important for characteristics such as non-malignant tumours, it is crucially important when a debilitating or potentially fatal disease is involved (a topic we return to in Chapter 9). Here we will describe how particular patterns of inheritance appear within families when the phenotype is either dominant or recessive, or when the pattern is dependent upon the chromosomal location of the gene. We will be looking at *disease phenotypes*, i.e. those that are considered to be outside the usual range, but the rules or laws of inheritance described in earlier sections apply to all our genes.

[5] Mutations in the haemoglobin gene leading to altered forms of the haemoglobin protein, with different outcomes including the blood disorder 'thalassaemia', are explored in the TV programme 'Bloodlines: A family legacy' for Open University students, which is associated with this chapter (and with Chapter 3).

[6] An article, entitled 'Beyond the disorder: one parent's reflections on genetic counselling', by Ruth McGowan describing her family's experiences, appears in *Health and Disease: A Reader* (Open University Press, 3rd edn 2001); it is set reading for Open University students studying this book during Chapter 9, but you could also read it now if you have time.

Human diseases can be classified in a number of ways, from those caused by nutritional factors (such as rickets), those caused by infectious agents (such as polio or tuberculosis), and those that are genetically determined. In the case of genetic diseases, individuals are ill because they are born with a defective gene. Over 5 000 genetic diseases have been shown to be due to defective genes, many of them rare, but a few are surprisingly common. About 1 in 30 children born in the UK has a genetic disorder and these account for about one-third of all hospital admissions of young children.

4.7.1   Sex-linked inheritance: colour-blindness

The X chromosome carries many genes which have a pattern of inheritance described as **sex-linked inheritance** (sometimes referred to as *X-linked inheritance* because it refers specifically to the genes 'linked together' on the X chromosome). If you look back to Figure 4.7, you will remember that females have two X chromosomes and males one X and one Y chromosome. Therefore, males have only *one* copy of each of the X-chromosome genes. In this special case, *all* the alleles on the inherited X chromosome are seen in the phenotype in males.

●   Can you explain why males differ from females in this respect?

■   Since males have only one copy of each gene on their single X chromosome, there is no 'alternative' dominant allele to mask the X-linked genes the male has inherited, so they are all expressed. Females have two X chromosomes, which may carry different alleles of the same gene; the dominant allele will be seen in the phenotype, regardless of which X chromosome it is carried on.

The different patterns of sex-linked inheritance in males and females can be illustrated by examining the X-chromosome gene associated with red colour vision, for which two alleles exist; one for normal colour vision and one that gives rise to red colour blindness. The normal colour vision allele is dominant and red colour-blindness is therefore a *recessive* characteristic. If we represent the normal colour vision allele as (*C*), and the recessive colour-blindness allele by (*c*), we can examine what happens in a mating between a *heterozygous* female (*Cc*) who has normal colour vision, and a male with normal colour vision (Figure 4.12). In Figure 4.12a you can see that two types of female gamete are produced, half with the normal allele, (*C*), and half with the colour-blindness allele (*c*). In the male, there are also two types of gametes — one bearing the X chromosome with the (*C*) allele and the other carrying the Y chromosome, which does not have the red colour-vision gene at all (remember, the Y chromosome is the smallest in the human cell and has very few genes). Using the matrix in Figure 4.12b you can determine the possible combinations that could arise at fertilisation.

●   What are the possible phenotypes of the children of the couple in Figure 4.12a, for both sex and red colour-blindness? (You might want to look back to Figure 4.7 to refresh your memory about inheritance of sex chromosomes.)

■   Half the children would be female and half would be male. The daughters' genotypes would be either (*CC*) or (*Cc*) and therefore they would all have *normal* colour vision, since the (*C*) allele is dominant. *All* the sons inherit the Y chromosome from their father. *Half* the sons would inherit the (*C*) allele from their mother and have normal vision, whilst *half* would inherit a single recessive (*c*) allele and so would be red colour-blind.

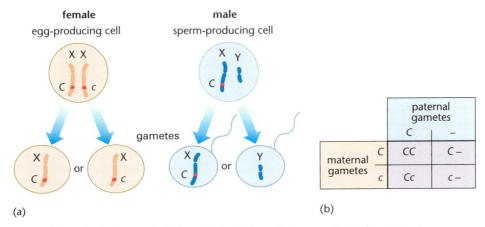

(a)   (b)

Figure 4.12 *(a) Diagram illustrating the behaviour of alleles on the X chromosome associated with normal colour vision (C) and with red colour-blindness (c) during gamete formation. The red colour-vision gene does not occur on the Y chromosome. (b) Table showing how the combination of maternal and paternal gametes at fertilisation gives rise to four possible genotypes with respect to colour vision in the offspring.*

●   What genotype would you expect to find in colour-blind females?

■   Females always inherit two copies of every X-linked gene because they have two X chromosomes; if either of these chromosomes carries the dominant (*C*) allele, the person will have normal colour vision, so colour-blind females must inherit *two* copies of the recessive red colour-blindness allele (*c c*) — one from each parent. A colour-blind female will therefore always have a colour-blind father.

Colour-blindness in females is an example of a **recessive disorder**, i.e. a genetic condition expressed in the phenotype of individuals who have *two* copies of a faulty recessive allele. The probability of inheriting two faulty alleles of the same X-linked gene is much lower than the chance of a male inheriting just one, so red colour-blindness — like *all* sex-linked characteristics — is more common in males than in females. (You may be interested to know that the bright orange colour of the bold terms in the index of this book was chosen as the most visible option by men with red colour-blindness.)

●   Sex-linked characteristics are never passed from father to son. Why is this?

■   Sex-linked characteristics are encoded in genes on the X chromosome. In order for an individual to be male, he must inherit a Y chromosome from his father. As you can see in Figure 4.12a, a man's gametes either contain an X or a Y chromosome, but *never both*. Therefore a father cannot pass on any X-linked genes to his *sons* (only to his daughters).

4.7.2 Family trees

Red colour-blindness is an example of a **single-gene disorder**, i.e. a genetic disease arising from the inheritance of a single gene. (Multiple lipoma, described earlier, is another example.) To learn more about the inheritance of single-gene disorders, genetic pedigree charts or **family trees** can be drawn describing the incidence of a particular characteristic within the family over several generations. The degree to which the characteristic recurs in different members of the same generation, and between generations, provides the first clue as to the mode of its genetic transmission.

In drawing up genetic pedigrees or family trees, certain conventions are used. Each generation is numbered, starting at the oldest, as I, II, III, IV, etc. Then, within each generation, individuals are numbered so that each can be identified. Individuals are also usually drawn with the oldest from left to right within a family, and different symbols are used for males and females. Where the purpose of the family tree is to trace the patterns of inheritance of a genetic disease, affected individuals are usually shaded.

● Most people know at least some details of their family of origin, or their adoptive family, across two or three generations. You may like to try and draw a family tree using the conventions described above. Try and think of each person, their parents, brothers and sisters and then move onto the next.

■ You probably found that it was quite hard and you had to keep going back and adding people you had forgotten, or moving them around. This illustrates why genetic counselling usually starts by drawing up a family tree: it collects together and organises all the information required in order to assess fully an individual family.

Below we consider two examples of family trees, which have been drawn up to reveal patterns of inheritance of genetic disorders within families. The first is *Huntington's disease*, a rare dominant disorder, and the second is a relatively common recessive disorder, *cystic fibrosis*, which commences in early childhood. (Remember that when we refer to a condition as a 'dominant or recessive disorder', it is a shorthand way of saying that it is caused by a faulty dominant or *two* faulty recessive alleles of a single gene.)

4.7.3 Inheritance of a dominant disorder: Huntington's disease

Huntington's disease is a degenerative neurological disorder, which is progressive and causes increasing motor (movement), cognitive (thought) and psychiatric disturbances. The disease starts in adult life, usually between 35 and 45 years, and affected people survive with progressive degeneration for between 10 and 15 years. There is no known cure for this disease, only treatment for the various symptoms.

The family tree in Figure 4.13 is a typical representation of a family in which Huntington's disease is present. The family members affected by the disorder (numbers 2, 3, 8, 9 and 13) are shaded green. You can see that in generation I, couple 1 and 2 had three children (numbers 3, 5 and 6), of which their only daughter (3) has the disorder; she had three children with an unrelated male (4), but neither of her brothers (5 and 6) had offspring.

● What is the most obvious feature of this family tree?

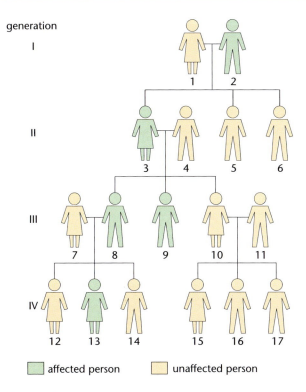

Figure 4.13   *A typical pattern of inheritance through four generations in a family affected by a dominant disorder, in this case Huntington's disease.*

■ The most striking feature is that there is at least one affected family member in each generation and that every affected person has an affected parent.

● Why is this inheritance pattern typical for a dominant genetic disorder?

■ In the case of a dominant disorder, the person only needs to inherit *one* copy of the disease-causing allele from one of their parents in order to develop the disease phenotype. The offspring of each affected parent has a 50 per cent risk of inheriting the parental chromosome carrying the disease allele. Note also that one branch of the family (arising from couple 10 and 11) do not have any affected offspring; these individuals have inherited the normal allele and therefore cannot pass the disease to their own children.

As we will discuss later in this chapter, Huntington's disease is caused by an unusual change to the DNA within a single gene; a direct DNA test is now available to detect whether a person in an affected family has inherited this disease-causing allele. We will also return to this disease in Chapter 9 when we discuss the impact of a diagnosis of Huntington's disease within just such a family and the range of issues it highlights.

4.7.4 Inheritance of a recessive disorder: cystic fibrosis

We now move on to a family tree with a very different appearance from that in which Huntington's disease is present. Figure 4.14 overleaf shows a typical pattern of inheritance for a recessive disorder such as **cystic fibrosis (CF)**. This disease is relatively common in northern Europe and the USA, affecting 1 in 2 000 children.

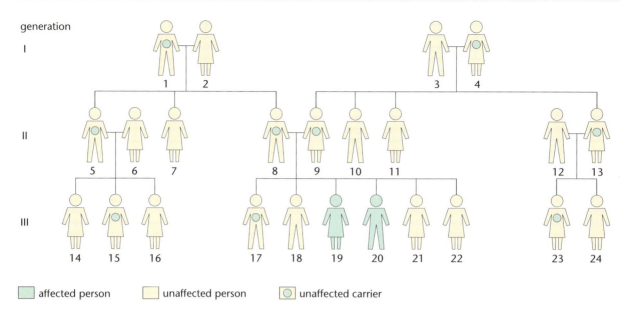

generation

I

II

III

▢ affected person   ▢ unaffected person   ◉ unaffected carrier

Figure 4.14   *A typical pattern of inheritance through three generations in a family affected by a recessive disorder, in this case cystic fibrosis.*

The inheritance of the faulty *CF* alleles causes the body to produce thick, sticky mucus that clogs the lungs, leading to infection, and blocks the pancreas, leading to problems in the intestines. Affected individuals develop symptoms in early childhood and, even with intensive physiotherapy, the average life expectancy is currently only until the mid to late 20s (though some people with CF have survived longer and life expectancy is slowly improving). If you contrast the family tree in Figure 4.14 with that represented in Figure 4.13, you can see that of the 24 individuals depicted only two have the disorder.

The low prevalence of cystic fibrosis in an affected family is because it is a *recessive* disorder, so affected individuals must inherit *two* faulty alleles, one from each parent.

● Explain why the parents of affected individuals 19 and 20 do not have the disease phenotype, even though they have each passed on the disease allele.

■ The parents do not have cystic fibrosis themselves because they each carry one recessive disease allele masked by a dominant normal allele (i.e. they are heterozygotes with respect to this gene — a state often described as being a 'carrier' of the faulty gene; other carriers are indicated in Figure 4.14).

The sudden appearance of the disease in a previously unaffected family is the usual way in which cystic fibrosis comes to light clinically; over 85 per cent of cases have no apparent family history of the disease. (In the family in Figure 4.14 it appeared 'out of the blue' in generation III, but there had been carriers in at least the two previous generations; notice that every carrier has at least one parent who is either affected by the disease or is also a carrier.) This situation is typical of a recessive disorder, whose incidence is dependent upon the frequency of carriers within the population. In the case of CF, approximately 1 in 20 people in the UK is a carrier for a disease-causing *CF* allele (there are several different *CF* alleles, each causing slightly different manifestations of the disease).

The chances of two carriers meeting and having children is therefore one major determinant of whether a recessive disease comes to light. Take a look at the family

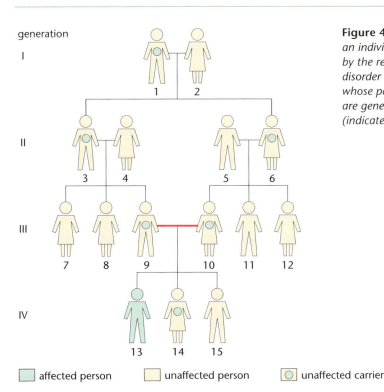

Figure 4.15 *Family tree of an individual (13) affected by the recessive genetic disorder cystic fibrosis (CF), whose parents (9 and 10) are genetically related (indicated by a red bar).*

generation

I

II

III

IV

☐ affected person   ☐ unaffected person   ☐ unaffected carrier

in Figure 4.15. You can see that the parents (9 and 10) of the affected child (13) are related via their grandparents (1 and 2); they are in fact first cousins. In this example, the grandfather (1) in generation I was a carrier of cystic fibrosis; he transmitted that allele to both his children (3 and 6), each of whom passed it on to one of their offspring (9 and 10) in generation III. When this couple had children, they are in fact transmitting the *same* allele that they *both* inherited from their grandfather through their own parents. Thus, two copies of the same recessive *CF* allele were transmitted to the affected individual (13). The tendency of recessive disorders to appear with a high frequency in the offspring of inter-cousin marriages was recognised long before the genetic principle was understood, and it led to the prohibition of cousin marriages in many societies.

In recessive disorders such as CF, where the presence of the disease alleles in a family only becomes apparent after the birth of an affected child, ethical issues arise, for example about informing other family members (some of whom will be carriers) and making decisions about future children. These issues will be discussed in Chapter 9.

4.8   Multifactorial characteristics: growth in childhood

4.8.1   Continuous variation

So far in this chapter, we have only considered patterns of *single-gene* inheritance associated with the *presence* or *absence* of a characteristic (e.g. the presence or absence of multiple lipoma or Huntington's disease or cystic fibrosis, or the inheritance of a particular ABO blood group). But the inheritance of many phenotypic characteristics does not follow this pattern: characteristics such as height, blood pressure, susceptibility to infectious diseases, rate of growth, or skin pigmentation, do not fall into two or three clearly defined alternative phenotypes (for example, height does not occur as either 'tall' or 'short'). Instead they show *continuous variation*, each category of which differs from the next in the range by only a small measurable amount. ('Continuous' in this context means that there are no 'gaps' in the distribution, for example, there are no heights within the normal range for humans that have no individuals in the population reaching that height.) Such phenotypic characteristics are usually described as **continuously variable characteristics** because they are distributed continuously in the population, in the manner shown in Figure 4.16. They are *quantitative* traits (i.e. 'how much' of the characteristic is expressed in the phenotype, for example 'how tall are you'?), rather than *qualitative* (present or absent).

The pattern shown in Figure 4.16 is called a **normal distribution** curve: the majority of individuals fall within the middle of the range, with few people at the two extremes. If this diagram represented, for example, the range and distribution of the height of adult Englishmen, then the majority of individuals fall around the national average height, with few very tall or very short men.

Figure 4.16 *A normal distribution curve.*

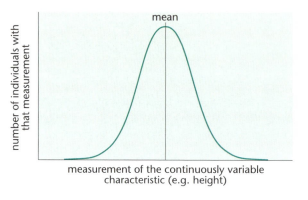

Height is a continuously variable characteristic. (left) Ugandan John Ofwono, aged 40, eight feet two inches (249 cm) tall, with his parents; (right) Jordanian Younis al-Edwan, aged 24, 65 cm tall, being measured by his brother. (Photos: (left) Reuters/ Popperfoto; (right) Ali Jarekji/Reuters/ Popperfoto)

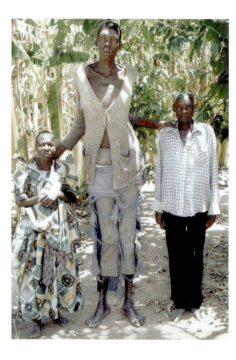
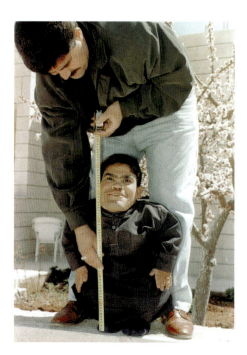

Continuously variable characteristics, such as height, are thought to reflect the *cumulative* effect of *several different* genes, each of which has a small individual impact on the phenotype. These *multiple* genes are scattered throughout the DNA, on several different chromosomes, in sharp contrast to the *single-gene* effects we discussed earlier, which are due to alternative forms (alleles) of the *same* gene occurring on a single homologous chromosome pair.

In addition, environmental factors play a particularly large part in the development of continuously variable characteristics, which is why they are also often referred to as **multifactorial characteristics**, since many interacting genetic and environmental factors are involved in determining how the phenotype turns out. Blood pressure is a good example of a continuously variable characteristic, which is multifactorial in its origin, being influenced by variations in several different genes interacting with environmental factors such as weight, diet, history of smoking and stress.

4.8.2 Studying growth in twins

As we pointed out earlier in this chapter, studying identical twins is one way of estimating the *relative influence* of environmental and genetic factors on variations between individuals for multifactorial characteristics such as height. Identical twins raised together are compared with those in which members of each twin-pair are separated at birth and raised in different households. Each twin-pair is genetically identical since both individuals are formed from a single fertilised egg, which splits early in development to form two distinct embryos with identical genes.

Table 4.1 presents a quantitative comparison of four multifactorial characteristics in three groups of twins. In the far right-hand column, you can see that for non-identical twins raised together, on average, there was a difference of 4.4 cm in their height, 4.5 kg difference in their weight and so on. Now look at the first two data columns relating to genetically identical twins raised together or raised apart, and consider the data on height. Regardless of whether they were raised together or apart, the difference in height between the two members of an identical twin-pair is very small, between 1.7 cm and 1.8 cm, (compared to a height difference of 4.4 cm for non-identical twins raised in the same environment).

● 　What do the results in Table 4.1 suggest about the genetic influence on weight compared with that on height, head width and head length?

Table 4.1   Average intra-pair difference for four multifactorial characteristics between the two individuals in pairs of identical and non-identical twins, raised in similar and in different environments.

Multifactorial characteristics	Average intra-pair difference		
	Identical twins raised together	Identical twins raised apart	Non-identical twins raised together
height/cm	1.7	1.8	4.4
weight/kg	1.9	4.5	4.5
head length/mm	2.9	2.2	6.2
head width/mm	2.8	2.9	4.2

Source: Newman, H. H., Freeman, F. N. and Holzinger, K. J., (1937), *Twins: a Study of Heredity and Environment*, University of Chicago Press, Chicago, p. 369).

■ The results indicate that a greater genetic influence exists for height and head dimensions than for weight; the latter is more subject to environmental influences. (If you are unsure about this, notice that height and head dimensions are similar for identical twins, regardless of whether they were raised together or apart, and the difference between identical twin-pairs is much less than it is between non-identical twins. In contrast, the weight difference between identical twins raised apart is much larger (4.5 kg) than the difference when they were raised together (1.9 kg), suggesting that weight is strongly affected by the child's environment.)

This example illustrates an important general point: there is considerable variation between multifactorial characteristics in the amount of influence exerted by the environment or by the genes.

4.8.3 Studying growth in different populations

More can be learnt about genetic and environmental influences on multifactorial characteristics by broadening the view to compare populations who live in different parts of the world. There are enormous differences in both the rate of growth and the ultimate height of children belonging to different countries of the world. Are these differences related (at least partly) to differences in their genes? To answer this question we can, for example, estimate the growth rate between the age of onset of puberty and achievement of ultimate adult height, and compare people in the Far East with those in Western Europe. Studies reported by J. M. Tanner (1992), have shown that people with good nourishment in the Far East, such as the Japanese, have puberty about a year earlier than Western Europeans and end up about 6 cm shorter.

● Assuming that environmental conditions were ideal in both populations, what do these data suggest about genetic influences on growth rate and ultimate height?

■ They suggest that there are genetic differences between different populations for these characteristics.

Thus, even among children who are well nourished, there are clear indications that genes influence growth and height differently in different countries. But there are a number of environmental factors that can lead to enormous differences in the size of children within and between populations.[7]

● What environmental factors might contribute to these differences?

■ Among many such factors are relative wealth or poverty within the child's family, affecting the quality and sufficiency of their diet, domestic hygiene, crowding, damp, etc.; urban or rural environments with different levels of pollution; stress, access to education, health and social services; repeated exposure to infection, abuse or neglect.

---

[7] *World Health and Disease* (Open University Press, 2nd edn 1993; 3rd edn 2001), Chapter 11, contrasts the height and weight of individuals from 'traditional' hunter–gatherer societies, a present-day Asian country such as Bangladesh, and an industrialised country such as the UK.

As living conditions improve, the growth of children speeds up and adult height increases. In the industrialised nations, these trends towards taller individuals reaching their adult height at earlier ages are now slowing down and in some cases height and growth rate have almost stabilised, at least in the children of the well-off. Differences in growth between rich and poor are still present in practically all countries; only in Norway and Sweden have they been eliminated (these trends are reviewed in Brundtland *et al.*, 1980, and Lindgren, 1976). Because similar environmental factors affect growth and health, one of the best monitors of the health of a nation is the growth of its children. Continuous surveillance of childhood growth is carried out in a number of countries, including the UK; this has practical value in monitoring the health of individuals and *indirectly* surveying the living conditions of populations.

You saw above that in the case of characteristics caused by an allele of a *single* gene (such as the allele that causes multiple lipoma), inheritance of the characteristic follows a distinctive pattern from generation to generation. But for multifactorial characteristics, such as height, there is no distinctive pattern of inheritance. Since many disorders are multifactorial, this information is crucially significant when trying to make predictions about the likelihood of genetic relatives inheriting or manifesting such disorders, as discussed later in this chapter.

4.9   The biochemical and cellular basis of disease

The primary aim for medical science in trying to understand any disease is to determine the link between the cause of the disease and its symptoms. In this section, we will explore the mechanisms by which an abnormal gene gives rise to a disease phenotype (i.e. to the signs and symptoms of the disease). In some disorders, such as cystic fibrosis, the link between the faulty allele and the manifestations of the disease is quite clear (as you will see), but in other disorders it is less so. In most cases, a disease-associated allele has a direct effect upon the gene product, or protein. We will investigate how a knowledge of the protein's function can be used in both diagnosis and in understanding and possibly in curing the disease.

Salt transport in cystic fibrosis

In cystic fibrosis, let us first consider what the *normal* protein coded for by the normal allele does in the body. You should recall from Chapter 3 that every gene is made of a chain of DNA bases which serve as a code for the synthesis of a protein. The gene that is defective in cystic fibrosis is called *CFTR* (the Cystic Fibrosis Transmembrane Regulator gene). The normal CFTR protein encoded by the normal *CFTR* gene lies within the surface membrane of cells lining the lungs and intestines and plays an important role in pumping salt across the membrane.

● The cystic fibrosis disease allele has an altered sequence of DNA bases, which in turn alters the CFTR protein structure (in fact there are several such alleles, but this point need not concern us here). What effect is this structural change likely to have on the transport of salt across membranes?

■ The protein has an altered shape (conformation), which reduces its capacity to transport salt (Figure 4.17a overleaf).

In people affected by CF, the complete absence of any functional CFTR protein results in the failure to transport salt effectively and leads to the secretion of thick mucus within the lungs. There is, therefore, in this case, a very obvious link between

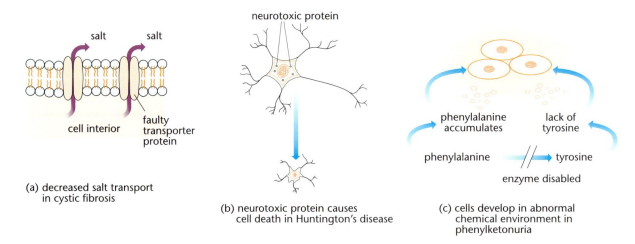

Figure 4.17 *(a) Reduced salt transport across cell membranes in cystic fibrosis is a consequence of the altered shape of the transporter protein, encoded by the faulty allele. (b) The altered protein in Huntington's disease is toxic to nerve cells. (c) In phenylketonuria (PKU), the faulty allele fails to instruct the production of a protein enzyme that converts one amino acid into another, so phenylalanine accumulates to toxic levels and levels of tyrosine become very low.*

the disease-causing allele, the protein and the cellular phenotype seen in the lungs. Furthermore, it also highlights why the disease is recessive; carrier individuals have one functional copy of the gene and can produce enough CFTR protein to pump salt across the lung's surface. You will see in Chapter 9 how attempts are being made to reintroduce the normal CFTR protein into the lung cells of people with CF by using gene therapy. In most genetic diseases, the link between the disease gene, the protein it encodes and cell function is not so clear.

Neurotoxicity in Huntington's disease

In the case of Huntington's disease, the disease-causing allele results in additional amino acids being added to the protein encoded by the affected gene (you will learn how this happens later). This structural change results in the protein becoming toxic to nerve cells, causing them to die and eventually leading to neurodegeneration. The level of neurotoxic protein produced is sufficient to kill nerve cells even in the presence of the normal allele of the gene; hence the disease allele acts in a dominant fashion and Huntington's disease is a dominant disorder (Figure 4.17b).

Amino acid imbalance in PKU

Phenylketonuria (PKU) was the first disease for which treatment in the form of dietary restriction was successfully used. The first insights came in 1934 when a Norwegian physician showed that babies who failed to make a certain enzyme developed mental retardation. This enzyme breaks down the amino acid phenylalanine into another amino acid, tyrosine. The absence of the enzyme results in both an accumulation of phenylalanine and a deficiency of tyrosine in the body (Figure 4.17c). The effect of too much phenylalanine disrupts the synthesis of another protein called myelin, which is an important protective fatty sheath that surrounds nerves and is essential for their proper function. The situation can be redressed through the diet by strictly controlling the intake of phenylalanine and by ensuring that enough tyrosine is present. Affected children who are managed in this way from soon after birth develop healthily. The 'treatment' can be thought of as modifying the effects of the faulty allele by changing one aspect of the body's environment (diet).

PKU is a recessive disorder and therefore two disease alleles must be present for the individual to develop the disease. The disease phenotype in PKU can actually vary considerably between individuals. At least part of this variability is due to the existence of multiple alleles, each with different nucleotide base changes to the DNA within the PKU gene. All of these alleles can cause the disease if a person inherits any two of them; they all disable the protein involved in the amino acid conversion described above, but to differing degrees. However, even in patients carrying two copies of the *same* allele, there is often a difference in the manifestations of the disease between one such person and another. Variability probably exists in other genes which affect the rate of removal of phenylalanine, or the cell's sensitivity to it. These differences highlight that what is seen in the phenotype is actually the result of many interactions within the cell, the body and with the environment.

Thus, the effect of a single allele cannot be considered in isolation from the rest of the genotype. What a person inherits is not a set of independent characteristics but a vast number of genes, the products of which interact with both other gene products and the environment. Variability amongst these genes will add to the range of phenotypes, but how does this variability arise? It is time to complete the discussion of mutation we began in Chapter 3.

4.10   The process of genetic change: mutation

As you already know, allelic differences between genes are caused by *mutation*, the introduction of permanent changes in the nucleotides that make up DNA. Mutation is the raw material of evolutionary change and the accumulation of genetic changes over time has contributed to the evolution of different species, including humans, and their separation from other primates.

4.10.1   Different mutations, different outcomes

●   Different kinds of mutation can occur in the DNA. Can you remember from Chapter 3 what some of these changes can be?

■   We discussed the addition or loss of nucleotides, ranging from the alteration of single nucleotides to more gross rearrangements of larger quantities of genetic material.

Other changes that also occur relatively frequently in humans, as you will see later, result in the deletion or duplication of entire chromosomes.

Changes in the DNA strand can arise spontaneously as errors during the process of DNA replication in any cell. However, as less than 5 per cent of our DNA codes for proteins, most DNA changes are likely to be irrelevant as they will occur in the non-coding portions of our chromosomes (Figure 4.18).

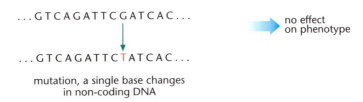

...GTCAGATTCGATCAC...

...GTCAGATTCTATCAC...

mutation, a single base changes
in non-coding DNA

no effect
on phenotype

Figure 4.18   *Hypothetical example of a single base change from G to T, with no effect on the phenotype since it occurs within a non-coding region of the DNA and so is not 'translated' into a protein.*

Figure 4.19a shows the hypothetical nucleotide sequence of part of a gene coding for the most frequently found protein in people with the normal phenotype. Figure 4.19b illustrates that some mutations in coding regions of the DNA (i.e. within genes) might have no, or very little effect on the phenotype because the structural alterations to the encoded protein do not alter its function significantly; some mutations might even have a beneficial effect upon an individual's phenotype because the new variant protein functions better than the most common version. Figure 4.19c shows one example of a mutation that results in a disease allele,

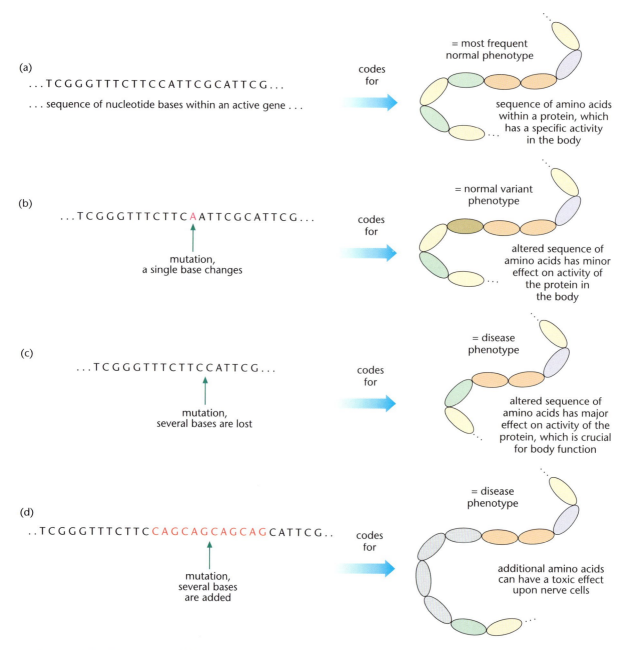

Figure 4.19 *Mutations in DNA sequences and their effects upon proteins and disease phenotypes. (a) The normal DNA base sequence for a gene encoding the normal protein. (b) A single base change from C to A has little effect on the resulting protein. (c) Loss of AATTCG from the gene results in an altered protein responsible for a disease phenotype. (d) Insertion of several repeated CAG sequences of nucleotides can lead to the construction of a protein that is toxic to nerve cells.*

coding for an altered protein which is responsible for causing a disease phenotype. In Figure 4.19d, the gene acquires several additional repeated base sequences, with serious consequences, which we discuss in more detail in the next section.

These types of mutation events occur in many genes and are essentially random occurrences. They will only be passed on to succeeding generations, if they occur within the cells from which gametes are produced, and if they do not cause disorders serious enough to prevent the individual from reproducing.

4.10.2   Mutation and the origin of genetic disease

We will now examine two types of mutation involved in human disease — those that cause cystic fibrosis and Huntington's disease.

Although the majority of DNA changes are minor, affecting only one or a few nucleotides, they can have profound effects. For example, consider the *CFTR* gene which is mutated in cystic fibrosis. The messenger RNA carrying the coded instructions from which the protein is synthesised is over 5 000 nucleotides in length; the most common mutation in families with cystic fibrosis involves the loss of just *three* of these nucleotides, leading to the loss of just *one* amino acid in the CFTR protein. This is an incredibly small change when you consider that the human genome contains three billion (three thousand million) nucleotides.

● Is the origin of alleles that cause a genetic disease such as cystic fibrosis different to the process that produces alternative normal alleles?

■ No, mutation underlies both (for example, see Figure 4.19b and c).

In the early 1990s, a novel form of DNA mutation was described which occurs in several human neurological diseases, including Huntington's disease. It occurs within areas of a gene in which the same series of nucleotides is repeated many times over (as shown earlier in Figure 4.19d). In this example, the stretch of repeated DNA consists of the three nucleotides CAG (called a *triplet*); this triplet instructs the inclusion of the amino acid glutamine at the corresponding location in the encoded protein (remember from Chapter 3 that every amino acid is specified by a code consisting of three nucleotides). In individuals with over 35 copies of the CAG triplet, an unusual event occurs during the copying of DNA prior to cell division; additional copies of the CAG triplet repeat are added to the gene. This mutation happens during the generation of gametes and, as a result, successive generations within a family inherit more and more CAG triplets within the affected gene.

● What is the result in the protein of adding additional CAG triplets to the gene?

■ As CAG codes for the amino acid glutamine, the protein will contain additional glutamines.

The presence of the additional glutamines makes the protein toxic to the nerve cells in which it is synthesised, causing them to die and leading to neuro-degeneration. In fact, the degree of cellular toxicity is directly related to the number of 'excess' glutamines in the protein, so alleles that contain longer stretches of CAG triplet repeats result in earlier neuro-degeneration and death. In the case of Huntington's disease, the direct measurement of the length of CAG triplet repeats at a specific location in the person's DNA forms the basis of a DNA test for the disease allele.

It is important to remember that only mutations that occur within gametes can be passed from one generation to the next. If you were to examine your own DNA, many of the variant alleles you are carrying will have accumulated over preceding generations and have been copied and passed down to you. In addition, there are almost certainly new mutations, which arose in your parents as new gametes were formed. Most of these mutations will remain hidden as the alleles they produce are either recessive or have no biological effect. Since mutation occurs during the process of DNA copying, it is more likely to occur in cells that are continually dividing — like the gamete-producing cells. A high proportion of the cases of some genetic diseases are known to arise by *new* mutations, which have occurred spontaneously during gamete formation.

4.10.3   Chromosomal mutations

In addition to small changes at the DNA level, mutations can also occur at a chromosomal level, that is they involve such a large portion of DNA that a change is visible on a karyotype. This can involve the loss or rearrangement of portions of a chromosome or can be the loss or gain of complete chromosomes. In all cases, these mutations often involve large chains of DNA and therefore multiple genes.

A **chromosomal mutation** underlies the development of Down's syndrome, in which the affected individual has received an additional complete copy of chromosome 21. This can clearly be seen in Figure 4.20. As many as 120 characteristic features have been described in Down's syndrome. With the exception of some degree of learning disability, there is no feature of Down's syndrome that is present in all individuals with the condition. Some features such as eyes that slant slightly upwards, a flat profile, a slightly flattened back of the head, a single crease across the palms of the hands, short stature and 'stubby' hands and feet are more common than others. (It is a myth that children with Down's syndrome always have a loving nature; they are as much products of their environment as any other human beings.) How the additional chromosome produces these phenotypic features is unknown.

The incidence of Down's syndrome increases with maternal age (Figure 4.21) and in order to explain this we must go back to the process of meiosis discussed earlier in this chapter. During meiosis remember that each chromosome of a pair is usually separated into different gametes. In the case of Down's syndrome, this process fails to happen and two copies of chromosome 21 end up in the same egg.

The effects of Down's syndrome vary between individuals, particularly in the degree of learning disability. (Photo: John Birdsall Photography)

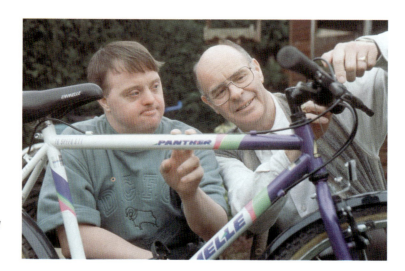

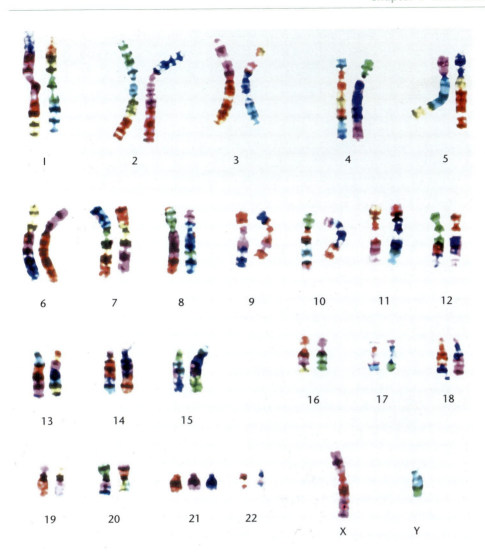

Figure 4.20   *The karyotype of a person with Down's syndrome, showing the characteristic pattern of three chromosome 21s. (Photo: L. Willatt, East Anglian Regional Genetics Service/Science Photo Library)*

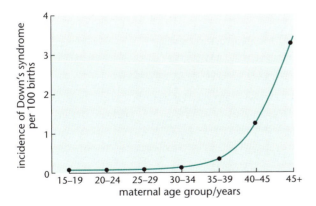

Figure 4.21   *The incidence of Down's syndrome births and maternal age. (Source: Jones, S. et al. (eds) (1992) The Cambridge Encyclopedia of Human Evolution, Cambridge University Press, Cambridge, un-numbered Figure, p. 275, acknowledged 'after Penrose, L. S. and Smith, G. F. (1966) Down's Syndrome, Churchill Livingstone)*

● Can you think why the risk of producing an egg with an extra chromosome rises with maternal age? (You might want to go back and read through Section 4.3.2 to remind yourself of how mature eggs are produced.)

■ The age-dependency arises from the fact that meiosis in the female actually occurs over a long period of time. During development, cells in the newly formed ovary undergo the initial stages of meiosis but stop just before the point at which chromosomes are separated. Only after puberty are eggs activated (once per month) to finish this process. It appears that as the length of time over which the process of meiosis increases, so the chance of a chromosome separation going wrong also increases.

Chromosomal mutations are rarely perpetuated, either because the affected individual has a short lifespan, or because he or she is infertile. In about half of all miscarriages occurring in the first 3 months of pregnancy, the developing baby has an altered number of chromosomes. However, the average life expectancy of live born children with Down's syndrome is now between 50 and 60 years. Although it is a rare occurrence, a woman with Down's syndrome can have children and men with Down's syndrome have been known to father children.

Before we leave the subject of mutation, it is important to stress that an important concept of medical genetics is that genetic diseases are only the most extreme manifestations of genetic change superimposed upon a background of normal variation, all generated through the random process of mutation. The question of where we draw the line between 'normal' and 'abnormal' is a complex issue to which we return in Chapter 9.

4.11   Genes, populations and environments

We have confined ourselves so far to a discussion of the inheritance of genes within individuals and within families, but in order to understand more about the distribution of genetic diseases around the world we must turn to look at wider groups within countries and continents. This is because the genotype of individuals, including those with a genetic disease, is a reflection of the population to which they belong. The genotype of an individual is affected not only by his or her immediate kin (blood relatives), but by the genotype of the population that has married into that family. Why is it, for example, that cystic fibrosis affects mainly people of northern European ancestry, whereas sickle-cell disease (as you will see later) affects those from more tropical regions of the world?

The focus of this section of the chapter is on *population genetics*, the study of factors influencing the distribution and frequencies of genes in populations. Here we are using the term **population** in a biological sense, to mean a group of individuals among whom mating occurs more often than with members of other populations.

4.11.1   Differences between populations

In order to understand the present-day genetic structure of human populations we need to look at our evolutionary history (as described in Chapter 2). About 10 000 years ago the number of humans on Earth was at least 1 500 times smaller than it is today. At this low population density, breeding populations were relatively isolated from each other and evidence suggests that major genetic differences between populations must have occurred *before* population growth increased the contact between previously isolated groups.

There are some striking geographical patterns for genes that influence visible characteristics. For example, body form and proportions are in the main due to the influence of a person's genes (as you have already seen in the discussion of twin studies and Table 4.1). Most tropical peoples have slim bodies and long limbs (which help them to lose body heat through increased surface area), in contrast to the shorter, stocky, heat-conserving shape of the Inuit (Eskimo) and other arctic peoples.

However, these striking physical differences have often led to the assumption that humans can be divided into genetically different 'races'. Colloquially, race usually refers to a set of physical characteristics such as skin colour, hair texture, body shape and cultural features associated with people whose ancestors come from a particular part of the world. To a geneticist, **race** means a group with certain frequencies of alleles which differ significantly from the patterns found in other groups. In fact, *no such differences* are present between what we colloquially term 'races'.

The large amount of DNA sequence information now available as a result of the Human Genome Project and the extent to which genes vary between human populations has been extensively studied. The extent of DNA nucleotide differences that exist globally *within* human populations is at a level of approximately 0.1 per cent. This means that if you compared two people at random from the same population (say two Masai, or two Inuit), they would differ by roughly 1 nucleotide in every 1 000, which means that any two people have approximately 3 million differences in their DNA sequences!

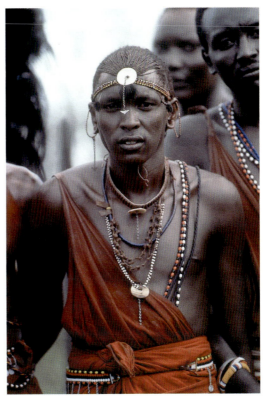

Masai tribesmen from Kenya have slim bodies and long limbs, which increases the rate of heat loss, but there are no significant differences in the frequency of alleles between these tribesmen and (say) Inuit, or white-skinned Europeans, or any other culturally defined 'race' of people. (Photo: Muriel Nicolotti/Still Pictures)

Most of the variation that exists in the whole of the human species presently on Earth can actually be found within a very small regional population of several million people, such as the inhabitants of a large city. If you look at differences between 'racial' groups, only 5 to 10 per cent of these differences distinguish one 'racial' group from another. Put another way, the differences that exist between a white European and a black African are not significantly different to those that exist between two Europeans or two Africans.

Each population (interbreeding group) is said to have a **gene pool** — a term which encompasses all the alleles ever found in this population; in other words, the gene pool represents the total genetic diversity existing in that group. Many populations will, of course overlap and interbreeding between populations does occur, particularly on its territorial margins or when transportation of people between populations occurs. Even within some populations, however, variations in the frequency of certain alleles exists; for example, people living in a remote region may have a higher frequency of a particular allele than their countrymen or women living some miles away, yet the two populations are indistinguishable in terms of their appearance and culture.

In order to address the question as to why such variations within populations arise, studies have focused on the frequencies and distribution of disease-causing alleles because these can easily be scored or detected, but the same principles apply to any allele. Several processes have been identified, which together explain why frequencies of alleles vary in different parts of the world. These are the mutation rate, chance or random processes and natural selection. We consider each of these in turn, and in passing also consider some sociocultural factors.

4.11.2   Mutation rate

Mutation is a constant process and continues to occur within our bodies as we age. Depending upon the nature of the mutation, its location in the DNA, and the tissue affected by the gene product, the accumulation of mutations might contribute to our ageing or possibly lead to cancer (we shall discuss this further in Chapter 8).

Although mutations occur at random, the **mutation rate** (the frequency with which mutations occur or, put another way, the chance of a change happening in the DNA), falls within a range between 1 and 12 mutations per gene in every 100 000 gametes. The rate can be increased by external agents such as ultraviolet light, X-rays and chemicals, which can all interfere with DNA within our cells — particularly those that are rapidly dividing.

● Explain why the gonads are protected by a lead apron when an X-ray is being taken.

■ The gonads are the site of rapidly dividing gamete-producing cells, so they are particularly vulnerable to mutations caused by exposure to X-rays. Once a mutation has occurred in a gamete, then it is transmitted to all the cells in the individual formed from that gamete (after fertilisation), because the mutant allele is *copied* when DNA replicates before each cell division, in just the same way as the normal alleles are copied.

The incidence of certain genetic diseases depends *solely* on the mutation rate because, in such diseases, the mutation results in such a severe genetic abnormality that it prevents the person from having children. Mutations that produce a *dominant* disease allele often prevent reproduction and so are not transmitted to the next generation. Since the disease allele is not transmitted, it can only occur in a population as a newly arisen mutation. Thus, the incidence of the disease reflects the rate at which new mutations of the affected gene arise. This also applies to chromosomal mutations. For example, the incidence of chromosomal mutations involving a whole chromosome (as in Down's syndrome) is about 6 per 1 000 newborn babies and about 250 per 1 000 miscarriages. As we noted earlier, these chromosomal mutations are rarely passed on since children who survive are usually infertile.

● Why is the mutation rate less significant for *recessive* diseases?

■ Recall that recessive alleles can be transmitted invisibly from generation to generation by carriers, their presence being masked by the normal dominant allele. Therefore, mutant recessive alleles accumulate in the population without causing disease until, by chance, two carriers produce an affected offspring.

In the case of recessive alleles, the risk that any carrier will have an affected child depends partly on the *carrier frequency* (proportion of heterozygotes) in the general population; the higher the frequency, the greater the chance that a carrier will mate with another carrier and produce an affected child. Consider the following data for PKU, which can be determined from the known incidence of the disease in the white population of the USA, estimated to be 200 million people in 1976 when these figures were quoted by Lerner and Libby (p. 238):

- number of carriers of newly arisen PKU mutations in 10 million gametes = 400
- number of carriers with inherited PKU mutations = 2 500 000

These data clearly demonstrate the importance of carriers of mutations descended from previous generations, relative to the number of newly arisen mutant alleles, in determining the frequency of the disease.

4.11.3   Chance or random processes

Human populations that are geographically close to each other, or who have recently evolved from a common ancestor, usually share some of the same alleles. There is, however, an important exception to this, which occurs when a population lives in relative *isolation* from other populations. A rare genetic mutation may arise in such an isolated population as a chance event, but can be absent in a related but geographically separate population. The inhabitants of the island of New Guinea provide a remarkable example of this. Until relatively recently, isolated populations lived in separate valleys unaware of each others' existence. These populations had their own distinctive genetic abnormalities, such as premature ageing in one valley, delayed puberty in another, and one population had the highest known incidence of profoundly deaf individuals in the world. Such effects suggest that a different ancestral disease mutation became prevalent in each isolated population.

Groups may be isolated not only for geographic reasons, but because they hold strong religious beliefs, as in the case of the Old Order Amish, an American religious sect which split into three isolated communities in Pennsylvania, Ohio and Indiana. Even today, rare recessive diseases exist with an increased frequency, each one in a different community, clearly illustrating the strong interrelationship of social structure and genetic structure. The Amish in Pennsylvania is a small genetically isolated population with large families and with a high frequency of marriages between relatives, leading to unusually high frequencies of some genetic diseases. A form of dwarfism (Ellis–van Creveld disorder) is present at a high frequency in the Pennsylvania Amish, but is absent in the Amish in Ohio and Indiana.

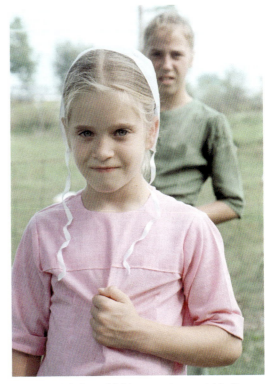

- Can you deduce when in time the mutation leading to this disorder arose?

- It must have arisen after the three groups of Amish separated from each other, or have been present in one of the founders of the Pennsylvanian group.

There is one important systematic difference in the incidence of recessive diseases between industrialised countries and more traditional populations in other parts of the world. In general, in the populations of industrialised countries, recessive diseases are much rarer than in parts of the developing world because the proportion of marriages between genetic relatives (for example, first cousins) went

Religious beliefs prohibiting marriage outside the faith sustain the genetic isolation of small populations around the world, for example the Old Order Amish in the USA. (Photo: David Turnley/ Corbis Images)

down sharply during the twentieth century. Cousin-marriages were previously quite common, and indeed encouraged among people with land and other property, because intermarriage kept ownership 'within the family'. For this reason, they still occur more frequently in the populations of developing countries.[8]

4.11.4   Natural selection in action

The process of natural selection (described in Chapter 3) is one of the driving forces by which the frequencies and patterns of certain gene variants (alleles) change over time. Harmful mutations are 'weeded out' because they reduce the affected individual's fitness and reproductive success, so are less frequently passed on to offspring; conversely, mutations that increase the ability of individuals to survive and reproduce are favoured by natural selection. Variations in environmental conditions interact with variations in the genotypes of organisms in those environments, ensuring that evolution never stands still. We shall discuss later an attempt to identify the environmental selection pressure that has led to the high prevalence of the cystic fibrosis mutation in northern European populations. But first we shall examine by far the best understood case of natural selection acting on gene frequencies in populations — that of sickle-cell disease and the haemoglobin gene.

Sickle-cell disease and malaria

As you learnt earlier, more is known about haemoglobin and its variants than any other human protein. Remember that haemoglobin is present in red blood cells and has the crucial function of carrying oxygen from the lungs to all the cells of the body. One of the variants of this molecule, called *haemoglobin S* or sickle-cell haemoglobin, is common only in regions of the world where there is (or once was) a high prevalence of malaria.

Haemoglobin S is the protein product of an allele conventionally represented by the letters Hb^S. Individuals with two copies of this allele ($Hb^S Hb^S$) have *sickle-cell disease*, a severe recessive disorder in which the red blood cells take on a sickled shape instead of being round.[9] The sickle cells block capillaries and produce a variety of symptoms from anaemia to heart failure. In the absence of medical care, many individuals with this genotype die before they can reproduce and so do not pass on the mutant allele. Despite this, the mutant allele persists in certain parts of the world at a high frequency. For example, in Africa south of the Sahara and north of the Zambezi river, Hb^S is so common that in some groups 5 per cent of newborn babies are homozygous and thus suffer from **sickle-cell disease**.

Why then is the Hb^S allele so common in Africa and also in parts of Asia? You might have expected that natural selection would lead to its gradual disappearance, since it clearly reduces the reproductive potential of people with sickle-cell disease. The answer lies in the remarkable advantage gained by *heterozygotes*, who carry one copy of Hb^S and one normal haemoglobin allele, Hb^A. They have some resistance to the organism that causes malaria. Let us look at the evidence for this explanation. Figure 4.22a shows the distribution of malaria in Africa and southern Asia. Compare this with Figure 4.22b, which shows the distribution of the Hb^S allele in the same part of the world.

[8] *World Health and Disease* (Open University Press, 2nd edn 1993; 3rd edn 2001), Chapter 4, discusses the problem of land title disputes in a rural village in Bangladesh arising from division of land and property following marriage.

[9] Sickle-cell disease is introduced in *World Health and Disease* (Open University Press, 2nd edn 1993; 3rd edn 2001), Chapter 3; Figure 3.4 is a photograph of sickle-shaped red blood cells.

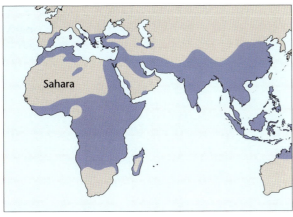
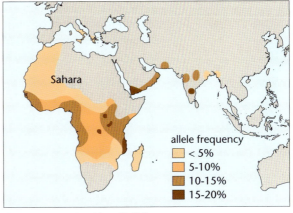

(a) distribution of malaria

(b) frequency of sickle-cell allele

allele frequency
- < 5%
- 5-10%
- 10-15%
- 15-20%

Figure 4.22   *Distribution (a) of malaria and (b) of the sickle-cell allele; shading denotes the percentage of the population that has this allele. (Source: Jones, S. et al. (eds) (1992)* The Cambridge Encyclopedia of Human Evolution, *Cambridge University Press, un-numbered Figure, p. 16, based on Strickberger, M. W. (1990)* Evolution, *Jones and Bartlett, Figures 21–23)*

● What relationship is there between the two distributions?

■ They overlap. The regions with a high frequency of the *Hb*^{S} allele, and hence of sickle-cell disease, coincide with areas of the world where malaria is rife. In areas where malaria is less common, such as the Sahara and southern Africa, the *Hb*^{S} allele is also less common.

The parasite responsible for **malaria** (a single-celled organism called *Plasmodium*, of which there are four main species) spends part of its life cycle in the red blood cells of mammals, including humans, where it multiplies.[10] The red blood cells of normal homozygotes (*Hb*^{A} *Hb*^{A}) are susceptible to this parasite and consequently they, like sickle-cell homozygotes (*Hb*^{S} *Hb*^{S}), produce fewer children than heterozygotes

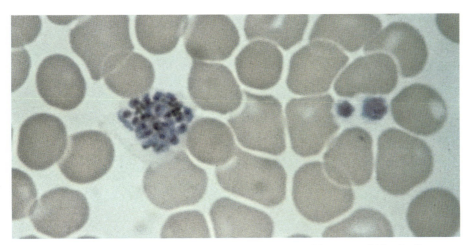

*A malarial parasite (*Plasmodium vivax*) living inside a normal human red blood cell. Carriers of a single copy of the sickle-cell gene have red cells which are less able to sustain the parasite's life cycle, so they have greater resistance to malaria. (Photo: Wellcome Trust Photo Library)*

[10] The life cycle of the malarial parasite is represented in Figure 3.3 of *World Health and Disease* (Open University Press, 2nd edn 1993; 3rd edn 2001), Chapter 3.

($Hb^A Hb^S$), who have some resistance to malaria. People who are heterozygotes with only one Hb^S allele have *sickle-cell trait*, an intermediate phenotype with respect to the red blood cells since some are the normal round shape and some are sickle-shaped. The sickled shape confers some protection against the debilitating effects of malaria since the parasite is killed inside the collapsed sickle cells.

Thus, heterozygotes tend to have more surviving children than either of the two homozygote genotypes and some of these children will inherit the Hb^S allele. Another way of saying this is that natural selection acts to retain the Hb^S allele in the population because it confers some advantage in areas of the world where malaria is rife. A summary of the phenotypes associated with each genotype of the Hb^A and Hb^S alleles is given in Table 4.2.

Table 4.2   Genotypes and phenotypes of the Hb^A and Hb^S alleles.

Genotype	Phenotype
$Hb^A Hb^A$	normal homozygotes: at risk of dying from malaria
$Hb^S Hb^S$	sickle-cell homozygotes: at risk of dying from sickle-cell disease
$Hb^A Hb^S$	sickle-cell trait heterozygotes: some resistance to malaria, some symptoms of anaemia

For a final piece of evidence that the Hb^S allele confers some resistance to malaria, we can look at a population genetically related to those shown in Figure 4.22a, which became geographically separate in a part of the world where malaria is absent. 15 million black Africans were transported to the Americas as slaves in the eighteenth century, taking the sickle-cell disease allele with them.

● If sickle-cell disease confers an advantage only in those regions of the world where malaria is rife, would you expect the frequency of the mutant Hb^S allele to have decreased, increased or stayed the same in the present-day black population of the USA?

■ Since sickle-cell homozygotes ($Hb^S Hb^S$) rarely leave descendants and heterozygotes ($Hb^A Hb^S$) would no longer be at an advantage compared with normal homozygotes ($Hb^A Hb^A$), the frequency of the mutant Hb^S allele would be expected to decrease in the population.

In fact, the frequency of heterozygotes in US blacks has decreased to 1 in 500 of the population, compared with 1 in 25 in parts of present-day equatorial Africa.

The example of sickle-cell disease shows clearly how the environment affects the distribution of a genetic disease. The transmission of the malarial parasite to human hosts depends in part on a suitable climate and habitats for mosquitoes to breed. It also illustrates the influence of culture on the change of gene frequency, since the introduction of agricultural practices to Africa involved the clearing of forests, which improved the environment for the mosquito. So the increased probability of malarial infection depends in part on agricultural practices among different African populations.[11]

[11] Malaria persists in various regions of the world for complex social and cultural (as well as biological) reasons, outlined in *World Health and Disease* (Open University Press, 2nd edn 1993; 3rd edn 2001), Chapter 3. The difficulties encountered in eradication campaigns aimed at either the malarial parasite or its mosquito vector are discussed in *Caring for Health: Dilemmas and Prospects* (Open University Press, 2nd edn 1993; 3rd edn 2001), Chapter 8.

The case of malaria and sickle-cell disease has been established over many decades of study. It is not always clear, however, how selection can act upon the frequency of a gene and its alleles. In the case of cystic fibrosis, it has proved difficult to identify the selection pressure.

Cystic fibrosis and cholera?

Mutations that cause cystic fibrosis are found in all populations around the world but their frequency in the USA and northern European populations (and their descendants) is remarkably high, at approximately 1 in 20 individuals. At first sight it is hard to imagine why the prevalence of *CF* alleles is so high, when individuals with CF will not, in the main, survive to pass on their alleles. As you have seen in the case of the sickle-cell trait, the most likely answer lies in the process of natural selection. To understand what this effect might be, we need to return to the function of the CFTR protein as a salt transporter across cell surfaces. When the protein is completely defective (as in people who are homozygotes carrying two defective *CF* alleles), the failure of salt transportation leads to the development of the disease. So, does carrying a *single CF* allele confer any advantage?

Cholera is a bacterial infection of the gut, which leads to such severe diarrhoea that untreated individuals can die in a few days from dehydration and salt imbalance. The toxin produced by the cholera bacteria acts by 'jamming open' various molecular channels in the cells of the gut wall, leading to severe salt and fluid loss. Studies of mice infected with the cholera bacterium have found that animals with a defective CFTR protein (similar to that in CF individuals) have lower than expected loss of salt and fluid from the small intestine, compared to normal mice (Gabriel *et al.*, 1994).

●   The reduction in the amount of salt and fluid lost by infected mice was greater in *homo*zygotes than in *hetero*zygotes. What does this suggest about the mechanism of protection?

■   The degree of protection from cholera seems to be directly related to the amount of defective CFTR protein present; homozygotes have two copies of the defective gene, so produce more of the protein than heterozygotes.

If a similar mechanism operates in humans, then even a small advantage in a heterozygote *CF* carrier might alter the frequency of the allele within a population as a result of natural selection 'favouring' the persistence of this allele. *CF* carriers might be more likely to survive in a cholera epidemic and so pass on their *CF* alleles.

While this model is attractive because it suggests a direct link between the function of the CFTR protein and an important infectious disease, it is still speculation as to whether cholera has anything to do with the persistence of *CF* alleles in human populations. Cholera epidemics were not known in Europe until the early 1800s — it seems implausible that in just 200 years natural selection could account for the unusually high allele frequencies found today. However, it is possible that other infections have played their part in promoting the spread of *CF* alleles, because many other diarrhoeal infections (such as that due to *E. coli*) operate through a similar mechanism to that of cholera.

Although natural selection is responsible for many geographical changes in gene frequency, it is important to remember that such patterns can also arise at random. Differences in gene frequencies between populations and ethnic groups means that, in order to determine the *current* risk of being affected by a disease allele, it often matters whether a family has its origins in, for example, the UK, Italy or

Japan. Given the changes in movement of people round the world, particularly in the last 5 000 years, how are gene frequencies being affected? This is the topic with which we conclude this chapter.

4.12   Present trends and future prospects

With the advent of global travel and in the process of global environmental conquest, human populations have undergone a basic change in their relations with one another. Our long heritage of cultural diversity is being blurred, leading to the gradual 'homogenisation' of language and culture. What might the effect of these cultural changes be on the genes carried within and between populations? The genes found in most present-day populations show evidence of their origins in the relatively isolated populations of the past. For example, Welsh-speaking Welsh have a higher frequency of certain alleles than English-speaking Welsh, and vice versa, but as the two cultures mix, so will their genes.

● How do you think the exchange of people between formerly separate populations might affect the frequency of recessive genetic disorders?

■ They will decline in incidence, because the chance of a carrier of the recessive allele mating with another carrier will go down.

Recessive genetic disorders are usually associated with particular populations (for example, cystic fibrosis is highest in white Americans and Europeans, but rare in black African peoples, whereas sickle-cell disease shows the opposite distribution). Increasing rates of intermarriage between people from different population groups will tend to reduce the incidence of any recessive genetic disorders that either population experiences.

Conversely, improvements in social, economic and medical provision tend to *reduce* the impact of natural selection on disadvantageous genes. In the past, natural selection acted against the passing on of genes that increased a young person's susceptibility to infectious disease, or contributed (at least in part) to certain congenital abnormalities, low birthweight and so forth. By the end of the twentieth century, an increasing proportion of human babies were surviving to reproduce in their turn, passing on to future generations genes which might not, in the past, have been passed on. However, disease-causing organisms themselves evolve in unpredictable ways, and it is difficult to determine whether new infectious diseases might influence the selection of particular alleles in human populations in the future.

This point is emphasised by the evolution of one relatively new disease, Acquired Immune Deficiency Syndrome (AIDS). A few individuals appear to be resistant to infection by the causal agent of AIDS, the Human Immunodeficiency Virus (HIV).[12] These individuals carry a genetic difference which affects the structure of a protein on their cell surface to which the virus attaches; without this 'anchor' HIV cannot infect human cells. People with this *CCR5-32* allele are resistant to HIV infection.

● In areas of high HIV infection, such as parts of East and Southern Africa, what do you predict would happen to the frequency in the population of this allele over time?

[12] HIV and AIDS are the subject of a case study in *Experiencing and Explaining Disease* (Open University Press, 2nd edn 1996; colour-enhanced 2nd edn 2001), Chapter 4.

■ An allele that confers resistance to HIV infection would be expected to *increase* in the population as more children would be born to people who had that allele, and more of the children who inherited it would survive to reproduce in their turn. (This is the opposite case to that described earlier for the Hb^S allele, which is *decreasing* in the USA as selection pressure favouring its transmission declines in the absence of malaria.)

In Chapter 6, we will return to the subject of infectious diseases and genetic resistance to infection and, at various points later in this book, we will continue to speculate about the future course of human evolution. It may be closely bound up with the evolution of other species; in Chapter 5 we turn to the relationship between humans and other organisms and examine their impact on our health and disease.

OBJECTIVES FOR CHAPTER 4

When you have studied this chapter, you should be able to:

4.1 Define and use, or recognise definitions and applications of, each of the terms printed in **bold** in the text.

4.2 Use examples to illustrate the difference between: genotype and phenotype; dominant and recessive characteristics; homozygotes and heterozygotes; and sex-linked and non-sex-linked characteristics.

4.3 Explain why each individual is phenotypically unique, with reference to: the behaviour of chromosomes during meiosis and at fertilisation; single-gene inheritance and multifactorial characteristics; the contribution of mutations, and the influence of the environment.

4.4 Using phenylketonuria (PKU) as an example, explain (a) how the diverse clinical features of an affected individual are related to a single deficient gene product, and (b) how the overall genotype and the environment can influence the expression of this disorder.

4.5 Describe the mechanisms that influence the distribution and frequencies of genes in populations, and discuss how this knowledge explains the patterns of genetic diseases (with reference to particular examples) in the world today.

QUESTIONS FOR CHAPTER 4

1   (*Objectives 4.2 and 4.3*)

Match one of the *situations* described in (a) to (e) with one of the *explanations* 1–5 given in the list below.

Situations

(a) Parents of normal stature have a child with the dominant disorder *achondroplasia* (short-limbed dwarfism).

(b) A study was conducted on twins in which at least one member of each twin-pair had club-foot at birth. All these twin-pairs had a similar home environment. In 32 per cent of the *identical* twins in the study, *both* twins in the pair had club-foot; of the remaining 68 per cent of identical twins, only one twin in each pair was affected. In 3 per cent of the *non-identical* twins in the study, *both* had club-foot; of the remaining 97 per cent of non-identical twins, only one twin in each pair was affected.

(c) A child is born with the recessive disorder *atrophy of the retina,* in which the back of the eye degenerates, but neither parent has the disease.

(d) A woman is heterozygous for two genes, one associated with PKU, which is on chromosome pair number 12, and the other gene associated with cystic fibrosis which is on chromosome pair 7. She transmits the defective allele for PKU and the normal allele for cystic fibrosis to her daughter.

(e) A woman has two sons, both of whom have *haemophilia*, a disease in which the blood fails to clot, and four unaffected daughters. Neither she nor the children's father have the disease, but *her* father had haemophilia.

Explanations

1   A new mutation occurred during gamete formation in one parent.

2   Assortment of chromosomes during meiosis accounts for this situation.

3   This situation is best understood as a multifactorial characteristic with both genetic and environmental influences.

4   The affected individual is homozygous for two recessive alleles of the gene.

5   This situation is characteristic of a sex-linked recessive disorder.

2   (*Objective 4.2*)

What is the sex of the person whose karyotype is shown in Figure 4.20?

3   (*Objective 4.3*)

Normal individuals have an enzyme that repairs damage in the DNA of skin cells brought about by exposure to ultraviolet light. Individuals with *xeroderma pigmentosa* are unable to repair such damage because of a defective enzyme and consequently they develop skin cancers. How could the development of skin cancers be prevented?

4   (*Objective 4.3*)

What are the possible genotypes of the gametes of a person who is heterozygous for the gene that causes cystic fibrosis?

5   (*Objective 4.4*)

Using PKU as an example, describe the diverse clinical features of this disease and explain how these are related to a deficiency in the product of the defective gene.

6 (*Objective 4.5*)

Explain the distribution of each of the following diseases: (a) porphyria, (b) thalassaemia, and (c) neurofibromatosis, each of which is described below.

(a) The dominant genetic disorder *porphyria* is rare in most parts of the world but is relatively common in South Africa. The gene normally has little effect, but its carriers have a severe, and sometimes fatal, reaction to barbiturate drugs. About 30 000 Afrikaners carry the disease allele today, which we know they all inherited from a couple from Holland who arrived in South Africa in the 1690s.

(b) *Thalassaemia* (featured in the Open University TV programme 'Bloodlines: A family legacy') is a recessive genetic disease, prevalent in Mediterranean countries, the Indian sub-continent, Malaysia and the Far East and in parts of Central and West Africa. Affected individuals have anaemia and other associated blood problems. The disease is associated with loss of part of the haemoglobin molecule. Its distribution overlaps part of the area where malaria is currently or was once prevalent.

(c) The dominant disorder *neurofibromatosis* affects the nervous system and is associated with the risk of malignant tumours. It occurs at high frequency in certain families, but these families have no known previous history of the disease.

CHAPTER 5

Living with other species

Study notes for OU students

This chapter discusses the relationship between humans and those organisms, collectively referred to as pathogens, that cause communicable human diseases. It builds on an understanding of the story of human evolution presented in Chapter 2, and of the theory of biological evolution by natural selection, which was discussed in Chapter 3. From Chapter 2, we assume a knowledge of the origin of a number of infectious diseases caused by pathogenic organisms that humans have acquired from other animals; from Chapter 3 we assume some understanding of the concepts of natural selection, adaptation and fitness.

5.1 Introduction

In the 1990s, the global burden of **communicable diseases** — the collective term for infectious and parasitic diseases — increased rapidly due to the epidemic of AIDS (acquired immune deficiency syndrome) caused by the human immuno–deficiency virus (HIV), closely associated with a sharp rise in cases of tuberculosis in the developed as well as the developing world. New, often fatal, infections emerged, for example Ebola fever, *E. coli* 0157 food poisoning and Hanta virus pneumonia. In 2000, the World Health Organisation (WHO) announced that 17 million people were dying every year from communicable diseases — 50 000 people every day — most of them children under five (WHO, 2000b). The growing resistance of pathogenic bacteria to commonly used antibiotics was another cause of concern, prompting newspaper headlines on the 'threat from superbugs'. The fear was widely expressed by organisations such as the WHO that rates of infection had returned to levels not seen since the nineteenth century.

This chapter is about relationships between pathogenic organisms and their human hosts. *Pathogen* is the term we are using in this book to refer to any organism, large or small, that causes disease by infecting or infesting another organism. When you fall ill with an infectious disease caused by a pathogen, such as the measles virus, you probably regard it as an unfortunate, random event, like falling off a ladder. In fact, your misfortune is part of a pattern, and a manifestation of a complex relationship that exists between us, as members of the human species, and whichever organism has caused the disease that has afflicted you. This relationship has a history and an origin, as outlined in Chapter 2. The pathogenic organism may have been affecting humans for many thousands of years or may be comparatively new. Infectious diseases can kill and, if we are to survive and reproduce, we must respond to every infection by inactivating the organism that causes it, or by becoming less adversely affected by it.

The history of *host–pathogen relationships* is like a very prolonged war, made up of countless, often-repeated battles fought out within individuals in the form of illnesses that end in the incapacitation or death either of the pathogen or of the host. The outcome of each little battle changes, by an infinitesimal amount, the relationship between pathogen and host *at the species level* and determines whether, over evolutionary time, the disease becomes more or less common and harmful to humans. (Note the use of 'military metaphors' in this account, a common form of expression in discussions of infectious disease, which is considered further in Chapter 6.)

The phrase 'at the species level' defines what this chapter is about. Here we are concerned with the ways in which species (rather than individuals) are affected by communicable diseases and how, over evolutionary time, the host species and the pathogen species respond to one another.

The chapter begins by describing in very general terms the ways in which species interact with one another in nature. We discuss the biological importance of pathogenic organisms, their diversity, classification and effects on their hosts, giving most attention to those pathogens that affect humans. In the middle of the chapter, we examine the interaction between infectious diseases and the life history of the host. The life of humans, and of other hosts, consists of a series of stages, in which birth, reproduction and death are the three crucial biological events. What impact does infectious disease have on the normal progression from one stage to the next?

The chapter then looks in more detail at the idea that hosts are engaged in a protracted, evolutionary 'war' with their pathogens; we expose the limitations of this militaristic analogy and describe some of the different outcomes that can result during host–pathogen evolution. Host–pathogen relationships change over evolutionary time but rarely come to a definite, stable conclusion; we consider the intrinsic instability of this relationship and how it is influenced by environmental changes.

A brief overview of how diseases are thought to have influenced the course of evolution of humans and of other species brings the chapter almost to a close, as we consider how pathogens are implicated in some fundamental aspects of human biology, such as the fact that we reproduce sexually, that we choose our mating partners and that we live socially. Finally, we emphasise the importance of micro-organisms in maintaining the survival of life-forms on Earth.

5.2   Interactions between species: a general framework

● Can you recall the definition of a species from Chapter 2?

■ A species is a group of organisms that most closely resemble one another and that, typically, can mate with one another in their natural habitat and produce fertile offspring.

The current concern for the future of the Earth and its living inhabitants has given a sharp emphasis to the question 'How many species are there?'. It is estimated that the Earth currently contains some 30 million species, of which only about 1.5 million have been named and described by biologists. It may well surprise you that, despite all their efforts, biologists are apparently so woefully ignorant. A major problem is that biological knowledge is very fragmentary and biased. Most of the Earth's approximately 4 000 mammal and 9 000 bird species have been described, but much less is known about the majority of insects, which account for more than half of the world's species. Knowing about the Earth's species is not simply an academic exercise. The Oxford evolutionary biologist, Robert M. May wrote in 1992:

> More immediately, utilitarian reasons for counting and cataloguing species are also noteworthy. A considerable fraction of modern medicines has been developed from biological compounds found in plants. Society would be well advised to keep looking at other shelves in the larder rather than destroying them. Many nutritious fruits and root crops remain largely unexploited; cultivating them could expand and improve the global food supply. (May, 1992, p. 19)

Species of organisms are not only very numerous; they are also very diverse. They exist in a vast range of sizes and have a rich variety of life styles. To cope with this diversity, biologists need to classify organisms, to arrange them in sensible groupings of manageable size. There are many ways to classify organisms, just as there are several ways of organising books in a library. They could be categorised, for example, by size, by colour, by method of movement, by habitat, and so on (we shall attempt to classify pathogens in some of these ways in a moment). At this early stage in the chapter, however, we shall classify organisms according to the major ways in which they *interact* with one another.

Two simple examples can help to clarify important differences in types of interaction. When a cow browses on a plant, it destroys much of the plant's previous growth and perhaps its flowers, preventing it from reproducing. In this interaction, between a *herbivore* (plant-eating animal) and its food, the cow gains food that it needs to sustain its own survival, growth and reproduction, while the plant loses tissue and reproductive potential; this relationship is one of *exploitation*. When a bee visits the flowers of a plant, it gains food in the form of nectar. This modest loss to the plant is greatly offset, however, by the fact that the bee takes pollen from the flowers and pollinates other plants elsewhere, promoting the plant's reproduction; the relationship is one of *reciprocal benefit*. Table 5.1 lists a number of kinds of relationship between organisms according to whether the participants appear to gain (+) or lose (−) from the relationship or whether it has a neutral effect (0) on their survival and reproduction.

● In which of the categories of interaction in Table 5.1 would you place the association between humans and the bacteria that live in our guts and which help us to digest our food?

■ Because both species benefit from the association, it is an example of *mutualism*.

Table 5.1   A classification of interactions between species.

Interaction		Consequences for species A and B		Comments
		A	**B**	
competition		0	−	competition for one or more essential resources (e.g. food, space) in which A excludes B: *competitive exclusion*
		or		
		−	−	competition in which A and B compete for resource(s) but neither excludes the other: *coexistence*
predation		+	−	carnivorous animals: A typically kills B
		+	−	herbivorous animals: A typically browses on but does not kill B
symbiosis	parasitism	+	−	A is a parasite on or in B, its host; A derives benefit at a cost to B
	commensalism	+	0	A derives benefit by living on or with B, but at no cost to B
	mutualism	+	+	A and B live in close association and both derive a benefit
	neutralism	0	0	A and B live in close association but neither derives a benefit or incurs a cost

While much of the emphasis of this chapter is on organisms that cause human disease, it is important to remember that humans have other kinds of relationship, sometimes positively beneficial, with other organisms. Many help us to lead healthy, disease-free lives. The last four interactions in Table 5.1 can be grouped under the single heading **symbiosis**, meaning 'living together' in intimate and prolonged association. (Note that in some older biology texts symbiosis is used in the same sense as 'mutualism' in Table 5.1, but in modern biology it is used, as here, in a more general sense.)

In the context of health and disease, however, the type of interaction described as **parasitism** in Table 5.1 is of the greatest relevance, because it covers the various relationships that exist between large animals, including humans and their livestock, and simpler pathogenic organisms that actually or potentially cause disease.

5.3   The nature of human pathogens

To a biologist, all pathogenic species, from microscopic bacteria and viruses to large tapeworms, are properly described as **parasites**, a term defined in Table 5.1 as any organism that derives benefit from living in or on another organism (the host), at a cost to the host. The cost may be anything from using small amounts of the host's food supply to causing a fatal illness. However, in everyday language, the word 'parasite' tends to refer only to multicellular *animals* and the single-celled *protoctists* that cause significant irritation or illness (for example, the parasite that causes malaria is a protoctist); the common meaning of parasite generally *excludes* pathogenic bacteria, viruses and fungi. To avoid confusion, we shall make it plain whenever we use the term parasite exactly what kinds of organisms we are referring to.

5.3.1 Parasitic animals and protoctists

● Compile a short list of parasitic animals or protoctists that you have directly encountered or heard about (some were mentioned in Chapters 2 and 3).

■ The list is potentially enormous. If you own a cat or a dog, you have probably had to treat it for worms in its gut, or for fleas, ticks and lice in its fur. Many of us have had to comb head lice out of children's hair, or combat them with special shampoo. At some time in your life, a small amount of your blood has surely been sucked out of your body by a midge or a mosquito. Protoctists cause malaria, sleeping sickness, some diarrhoeal diseases (e.g. amoebic dysentry) and some genital tract infections (e.g. *Chlamydia, Trichomonas*).

Figure 5.1 overleaf summarises the type and location of the principal animal and protoctist (single-celled) parasites that can be found in and on a human host. These range from tiny organisms resembling an amoeba to quite large, complex creatures like tapeworms and ticks. (Note that the larger parasites and those living on the *outside* of the host are often referred to as 'infesting' rather than 'infecting' their host — a term which is usually reserved for microscopic parasites, bacteria, viruses and other pathogenic micro-organisms. But for simplicity, we will use 'infection' here.)

One important general distinction is between **endoparasites**, those that live within the body of their host, usually within a specific organ, and **ectoparasites**, those that live attached to the outer surface of the host, like leeches, fleas and lice. As well as animals and protoctists that live inside cells and organs, the term

Figure 5.1 *Some examples of animal and protoctist (single-celled) parasites that infect humans. (Photographs of* Trypanosomes *and* Trichomonas *appeared in Figure 3.17.)*

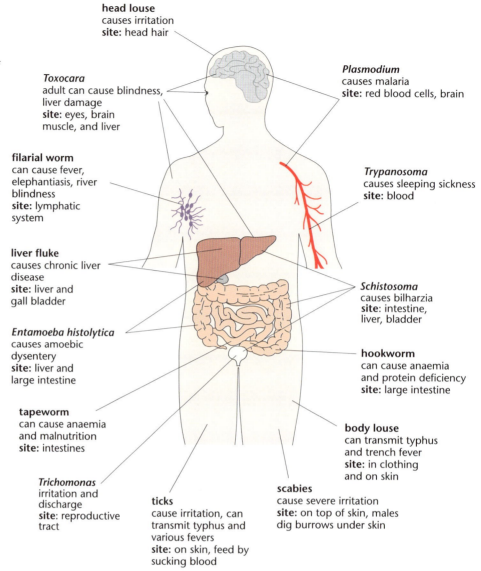

head louse
causes irritation
site: head hair

Toxocara
adult can cause blindness, liver damage
site: eyes, brain muscle, and liver

filarial worm
can cause fever, elephantiasis, river blindness
site: lymphatic system

liver fluke
causes chronic liver disease
site: liver and gall bladder

Entamoeba histolytica
causes amoebic dysentery
site: liver and large intestine

tapeworm
can cause anaemia and malnutrition
site: intestines

Trichomonas
irritation and discharge
site: reproductive tract

ticks
cause irritation, can transmit typhus and various fevers
site: on skin, feed by sucking blood

Plasmodium
causes malaria
site: red blood cells, brain

Trypanosoma
causes sleeping sickness
site: blood

Schistosoma
causes bilharzia
site: intestine, liver, bladder

hookworm
can cause anaemia and protein deficiency
site: large intestine

body louse
can transmit typhus and trench fever
site: in clothing and on skin

scabies
cause severe irritation
site: on top of skin, males dig burrows under skin

'endoparasites' includes a huge variety of bacteria and viruses. Ectoparasites commonly suck blood from their host and, in themselves, are often little more than an irritant. In some instances, however, they carry endoparasites and provide the means of transmission (they are the *vectors*) by which endoparasites get from one host to another. For example, the malarial parasite (*Plasmodium* species) is transmitted by several species of mosquitoes. A feature of many endo- and ectoparasites is that they are, to a greater or lesser degree, highly specific to particular species of host. For example, as described in Chapter 2, species of *Toxocara* are nematode worms, which are specific parasites of dogs and cats.

It follows from the great number and diversity of parasites of all kinds (in the widest biological sense of the term), and from their specificity in certain hosts, that there must be many more species of parasite in the world than there are of hosts. It is estimated that 25 per cent of all insect species (which account for more than half the world's species) are parasites of *other insects*, laying their eggs inside the eggs or juvenile stages of other insect species.

So, naturalists observe, a flea
Hath smaller fleas that on him prey;
And these have smaller fleas to bite 'em,
And so proceed *ad infinitum.*
(Jonathan Swift: 'On poetry', 1733)

This maxim is most clearly demonstrated by a group of viruses known as *bacteriophages,* which infect bacteria.

Parasitic animals and protoctists are at the larger end of the scale of pathogens that cause disease in humans; they range from metre-long tapeworms to viruses that are only visible with the electron microscope (Figure 5.2). Size is another way of classifying the enormous diversity of human pathogens; put simply, the big ones are termed *macroparasites* and the tiny ones are termed *microparasites.*

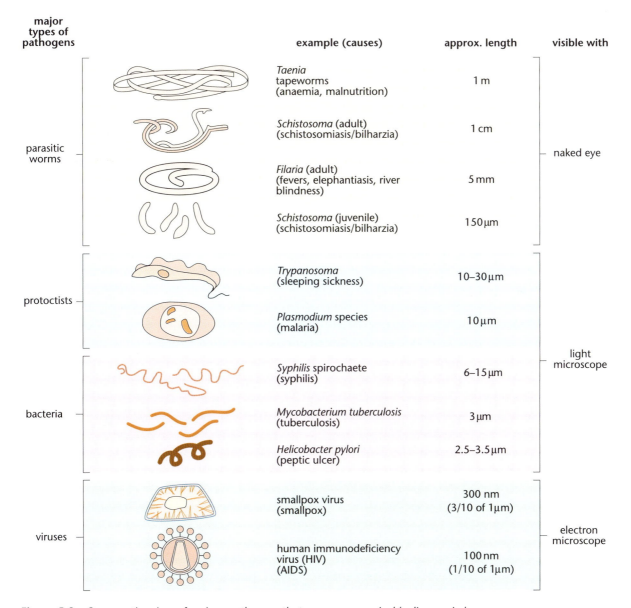

Figure 5.2   *Comparative sizes of various pathogens that cause communicable diseases in humans.*
(1 μm or 1 micrometre = one-millionth of a metre; 1 nm or 1 nanometre = one-thousand-millionth of a metre.)

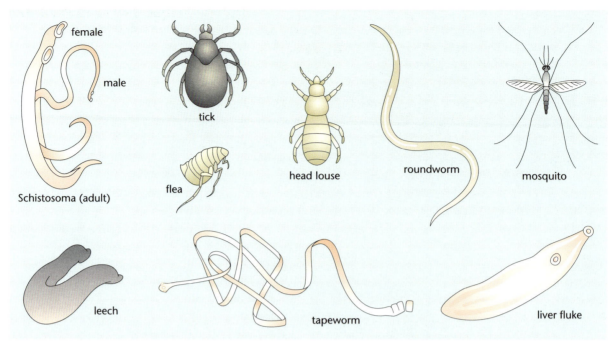

Figure 5.3   *The huge variation among the macroparasites that infect humans is illustrated in these drawings (by Tim Halliday, one of the editors of this book). The mosquito is also a vector of other smaller parasites that cause human disease. These animals have not been drawn to scale; simply admire their diversity!*

Macroparasites are relatively large, multicelled *invertebrate* animals ('invertebrate' means without a backbone), which mainly belong to two groups: the *flatworms*, which include flukes, tapeworms and nematode worms; and the *arthropods* (a large group of jointed-limbed invertebrates), which include lice, fleas, mosquitos and ticks (Figure 5.3).

Some macroparasites have complex life cycles involving two or more host species; this complexity prolongs the time it takes to produce the next generation. Typically the eggs are laid in one host, but they mature in another. Tapeworms (Figure 5.4), for example, reproduce sexually in the human gut; their eggs are passed out in the host's faeces and are later eaten by, and develop in, other large mammals, such as pigs or cattle (described in Chapter 2).

5.3.2 Parasitic diseases

Humans who live in an affluent modern society generally fail to appreciate the biological importance of parasites because they are so rarely encountered in everyday life. In fact, on a worldwide scale, the **parasitic diseases** are a major cause of human sickness, as Table 5.2 (opposite) shows.

● According to Table 5.2, approximately how many cases of parasitic diseases did the WHO estimate occurred in the years shown?

■ Between 3.7 and 3.9 billion cases. Even allowing for the fact that a high proportion of cases can be attributed to individuals who were infected with several different parasites at the same time (each parasitic infection counting as a 'case'), the prevalence of diseases caused by these organisms is immediately apparent.

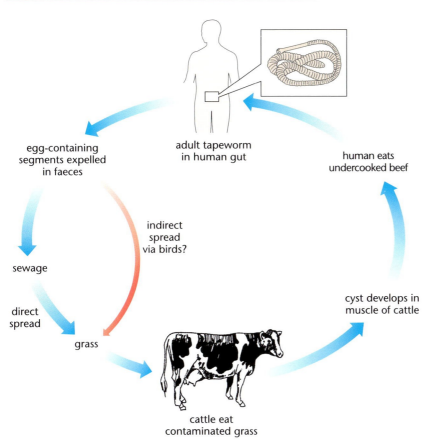

Figure 5.4 *The life cycle of the tapeworm* Taenia saginata.

Table 5.2 Estimated numbers of people infected worldwide with the commonest diseases caused by parasitic animals and protoctists (various years).

Medical name of disease	Common name of disease	Infected people (millions)
dracunculiasis (1997)	guinea worm	0.08
Intestinal parasites (1989)		
amoebiasis	amoebic dysentery	400
ancylostomiasis	hookworm	900
ascariasis	roundworm	1 000
giardiasis	giardia	200
strongyloidiasis	threadworm	30
trichuriasis	whipworm	500
leishmaniasis (2000)	kala azar	12
lymphatic filariasis (2000)	elephantiasis	120
malaria (1998)	malaria	300–500
onchocerciasis (2000)	river blindness	18
schistosomiasis (1996)	bilharzia	200
trypanosomiasis (African) (1998)	sleeping sickness	0.04
(South American) (1997)	Chagas disease	16–18

Source: World Health Organisation (WHO) estimates for 1989, quoted in Dobson, A. (1992) Chapter 10.4 in Jones, S. *et al.* (eds) *The Cambridge Encyclopedia of Human Evolution*, Cambridge University Press, pp. 418–9. More recent data from WHO Fact Sheets (from http://www.who.int/inf/) [accessed 26 February 2001]

The emphasis on parasites that infect humans should not obscure the fact that parasitic animals and protoctists are also a major cause of mortality and of reduced reproductive success among non-human animals and plants; a major preoccupation of agriculture is to control parasites that can wipe out crops and livestock.

Macroparasites present a major problem in many parts of the world because they infect very large numbers of people (as Table 5.2 shows).[1] They have particular properties that make them very difficult to eradicate; immune responses against them are not fully effective (as you will see in Chapter 6), so parasitic diseases are typically chronic in form, flaring up episodically or progressing slowly over many years, causing long-term morbidity rather than mortality. Macroparasites are persistent; individuals can become re-infected and, consequently, people tend to carry such parasites for the greater part of their lives. In many countries in Sub-Saharan Africa, over 90 per cent of the children are infected with parasitic worms.

5.3.3 Microparasites and infectious diseases

Microparasites, as their name implies, are very small organisms visible only through a microscope. They are generally endoparasitic, that is, they live in their host's cells and organs, and typically the entire life cycle is completed in a single host. They include all the pathogenic viruses, bacteria, protoctists and a few fungi (for example *Candida*, growing as white fungal spots in the reproductive tract or in the mouth, causes the intense inflammation known as 'thrush'). These pathogenic micro-organisms are responsible for the **infectious diseases**, which are the largest cause of mortality worldwide — causing 6 or 7 times as many deaths as the macroparasites. Table 5.3 shows the major categories of infectious diseases, with annual mortality in millions of deaths annually. The toll on children under five is immediately apparent.

● Which of the infectious disease categories in Table 5.3 will make the greatest economic impact on countries where prevalence is high?

■ The categories where the majority of deaths are among young adults are AIDS and tuberculosis.

In some parts of the world (e.g. South Africa) more than 10 per cent of the labour force is already infected with HIV.[2] By 2000, the global death rate from TB had risen to 2 million.

The disease categories represented in Table 5.3 illustrate the importance of all three of the major types of microparasites: protoctists, bacteria and viruses. Fungal infections do not generally contribute to fatalities, except in people whose immune system has collapsed (for example, due to AIDS), so we will say no more about them here. The protoctists are the largest of the microparasites, and their diversity was described earlier, so we will focus here on bacteria and viruses, and briefly mention prions.

---

[1] The proportion of deaths caused by communicable diseases in developed and developing countries are compared, and their underlying causes are discussed, in *World Health and Disease* (Open University Press, 2nd edn 1993; 3rd edn 2001), Chapters 2 and 3.

[2] HIV/AIDS is a major case study in *Experiencing and Explaining Disease* (Open University Press, 2nd edn 1996; colour-enhanced 2nd edn 2001), Chapter 4. The impact of AIDS on South Africa is examined in a video for Open University students, 'South Africa: Health at the crossroads'.

Table 5.3 The leading categories of infectious disease and annual mortality rates, millions of deaths worldwide, all ages, 1998.

Infectious disease category	Total number of deaths (millions)	Deaths under age five (% of total)
acute respiratory infections	3.5	55
AIDS	2.3	18
diarrhoeal diseases	2.2	80
tuberculosis	1.5	10
malaria	1.1	73
measles	0.9	100
total (millions)	**11.5**	**6.0**

Data derived from World Health Organisation (1999) *Removing Obstacles to Healthy Development*, Graph 5 (from http://www.who.int/infectious-disease-report/pages/graph5.html) [accessed 28 February 2001]

Bacteria

Bacteria are among the most ancient organisms in terms of life on Earth. They are true cells and so are capable of independent life; their basic cellular structure has already been described in Chapter 3. The great majority have a tough cell wall outside the cell membrane, which gives them additional protection from drying out and other hazards during transmission from host to host. This cell wall also betrays their presence to the human immune system, since it contains molecules unique to bacteria (discussed further in Chapter 6). Differences in the chemical structure of this outer layer are also responsible for an important distinction in bacterial classification into Gram-positive and Gram-negative bacteria, depending on their reaction to a stain named after its nineteenth-century Danish inventor, Christian Gram.

Several groups of bacteria can form *spores*, which have such resistant coats that they can survive for many years in a dormant condition and be re-activated when environmental conditions are favourable. Some bacterial spores are so tough they can survive boiling!

● Can you suggest some major bacterial diseases affecting humans?

■ They include bacterial pneumonia, bronchitis and meningitis; diphtheria and many ear, nose and throat infections; tuberculosis, leprosy, plague, cholera, salmonella poisoning and several other diarrhoeal diseases; syphilis, gonorrhoea and several other sexually transmitted infections; typhoid and tetanus.

Consider two examples. The WHO estimates that there are around 4 billion cases of **diarrhoeal diseases** annually — most of them caused by bacteria — resulting in the deaths of 2.2 million people, mainly children under five. The bacterium that causes **tuberculosis**, TB (*Mycobacterium tuberculosis*) kills around 2 million people every year, including 200 000 children. One-third of the world's population is already infected with TB, and it is 'active' in about 10 million of these people. After the successes in treating and preventing TB in the first half of the twentieth century, it began increasing rapidly in the mid-1980s.[3] Later in this chapter (Section 5.7.1) we will consider the reasons for this new epidemic of an 'old' infectious disease.

[3] The history of tuberculosis is described in *Medical Knowledge: Doubt and Certainty* (Open University Press, 2nd edn 1994; colour-enhanced 2nd edn 2001), Chapter 4.

Viruses

Viruses are so small they cannot be seen with a light microscope. They are not living 'cells' but consist of a small strand of genetic material (either DNA or RNA) encoding at most a few tens of genes (compare this with around 40 000 in the human genome), enclosed in a protein coat assembled from pre-formed components. An individual virus is termed a *virion*, or more simply a virus particle. The regular building blocks from which the coat is made, give viruses the appearance of geometrical models when viewed under the electron microscope. Some viruses also surround the coat with a membrane acquired from the host cell in which the virus was assembled, so the outer surface of the virus is partly 'disguised' from the host's immune system (we return to this point in Chapter 6).

Viruses have no means of generating energy for metabolic processes inside the virus particle itself; they have no cytosol and none of the organelles described in Chapter 3. They cannot grow, and they cannot reproduce without first 'hijacking' the biochemical stores of the host cell they have infected, by instructing that cell to make components of new virus particles instead of carrying out its normal functions. The small number of genes in each virus particle is just enough to convert the host cell into a virus production factory.

More than 3 600 different types of viruses have been identified, infecting hosts as diverse as humans and other animals, plants of all kinds, protoctists, fungi and even bacteria (we mentioned the bacteriophage viruses earlier, which specialise in infecting bacteria). The range of infectious diseases caused by viruses is very large.

● Can you name some viral diseases of humans, other than HIV/AIDS?

■ Several of the common childhood infections are caused by viruses, e.g. measles, mumps, chickenpox and rubella (German measles); also the common cold, influenza and many other respiratory infections; the herpes viruses cause 'cold

Human papilloma virus particles photographed at a magnification of 70 000 with an electron microscope (the colours have been artificially added); this virus causes genital warts and is implicated in the causation of cancers of the cervix and penis. (Photo: EM Unit, VLA/ Science Photo Library)

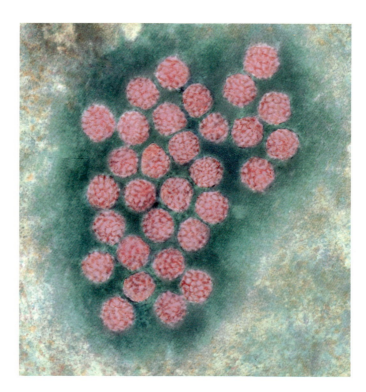

sores', genital herpes and 'shingles' (as well as chickenpox); hepatitis viruses cause liver disease; other significant viral diseases in developing countries include rabies, tick-borne encephalitis, Ebola fever, Dengue haemorrhagic fever and Lassa fever; and several viruses are implicated in the causation of certain cancers.

But there have been some notable triumphs in reducing some viral diseases. In the past, smallpox was a major killer but was eradicated worldwide in 1980. Another success story is the decline of polio, reduced to just 1 500 cases in 1999, with large areas of the world (including the Americas, Europe and China) declared 'polio free'.

Prions

We cannot leave the discussion of microparasites without briefly mentioning another 'non-living' source of infectious disease — **prions**, which we introduced in Chapter 2.

● Why did prions achieve worldwide prominence in the 1990s?

■ Mutant prions were shown to be the causative agents of *bovine spongiform encephalopathy* (BSE) in cattle and of its human form *variant Creutzfeld–Jakob disease* (vCJD).

Prions are composed of small proteins (only 253 amino acids in length — most proteins have well over 1 000) which have no known function, but everyone has them in their bodies. Infective prions are mutants, i.e. they have a slightly altered amino acid order in the protein, which results in the formation of solid masses of protein in the brain of animals that they infect. Areas of brain degeneration appear around the protein masses, with increasing destruction of tissue and progressively greater loss of muscle coordination, speech and cognitive function. Prion infections are common in sheep, where they cause a disease termed scrapie. As noted in Chapter 2, by 2000 over 70 people — most of them young — had died of vCJD in the UK and it was beginning to appear in Europe and other parts of the world, including the USA. The likely route by which vCJD entered the human population is by eating beef containing the mutant prions.

The extraordinary variety of the organisms that infect people around the world helps to explain their great importance for human survival and for the structure of human populations, the economic output of different nations and, ultimately, the survival of the human species.

5.4 Impact of pathogens on human survival

Some infectious diseases are relatively trivial and self-limiting (e.g. the common cold), but others reduce the survival chances of their human hosts, either by killing people directly, or by debilitating them so that they become more susceptible to other infections, or by limiting their capacity to work and hence acquire the means of subsistence. In this section, we look at the impact of communicable diseases on the general shape of **survival curves** for humans living in a prosperous, industrial society and in a poor, developing country in recent times (Figure 5.5 overleaf). The difference between the two is largely attributable to the impact of infection, exacerbated by malnutrition, in the developing world.

● What aspects of survival are similar in the two populations shown in Figure 5.5, and what aspects are different?

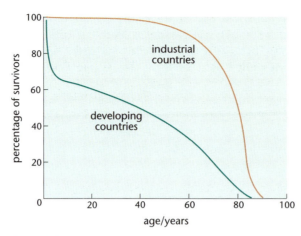

Figure 5.5   *Survival curves showing the percentage of individuals living to a given age in a prosperous industrial country and in a poor developing country. (Source: Begon, M., Harper, J. L. and Townsend, C. R., 1990,* Ecology: Individuals, Populations and Communities, *2nd edn, Blackwell Scientific Publications, Oxford, Figure 12.19(b), p. 418; adapted from Bradley, D. J., 1977, in* Origins of Pest, Parasite, Disease and Weed Problems, *edited by Cherrett, J. M. and Sagar, G. P., Blackwell Scientific Publications, Oxford)*

■   The maximum survival in the two populations is very similar, at 90 and 85 years. The main difference lies in the survival rate during the first five years of life. This is much lower in the developing country's population, with the result that a much smaller proportion of those born survive to reproductive age.

Differences such as these between developed and developing countries have become *more* apparent since the mid-1980s. Although life expectancy has improved throughout the world, it has been rising so much faster in developed countries that the gap between 'rich' and 'poor' nations has grown wider over time. And in some parts of the world, particularly in Sub-Saharan Africa and in the Russian Federation since the break-up of the Soviet Union, life expectancy has been *falling* quite sharply since the 1990s.[4]

●   What are the principal reasons for the decline?

■   In Sub-Saharan Africa, by far the most important cause is rapidly increasing infection with HIV, leading to AIDS and greatly increased susceptibility to other infections, particularly TB. In the Russian Federation, the largest contributory factor is thought to be alcohol abuse, but close behind are large rises in the rates of respiratory infections (influenza, pneumonia) and HIV.

The general shape of the curves in Figure 5.5 shows that, from one part of the world to another, or from one period of human history to another, infectious diseases can have a varying effect on the *age structure* of the human population.[5]

[4] The falling life expectancy in Sub-Saharan Africa is discussed in *World Health and Disease* (Open University Press, 2nd edn 1993; 3rd edn 2001), Chapter 8 and also in the video for OU students 'South Africa: Health at the Crossroads'; falling life expectancy in the Russian Federation is discussed in Chapter 7.

[5] Population age structure is discussed in *Studying Health and Disease* (Open University Press, 2nd edn 1994; colour-enhanced 2nd edn 2001), Chapter 7; and also in *World Health and Disease* (Open University Press, 2nd edn 1993; 3rd edn 2001), Chapter 2, which includes a comparison of remaining life expectancy at different ages in the UK and in Bangladesh.

Parasites may adversely affect the reproductive success of their host in a variety of ways. Some kill their host before it reaches reproductive age, while others allow the host to survive but cause infertility; some reduce the host's life expectancy or cause reproduction to be delayed to later in the host's life, so that it produces fewer offspring. However, the survival of the pathogen species depends on an adequate population of hosts surviving long enough for the pathogen to reproduce and be transmitted to new hosts. This brings us to the central aspects of existence!

5.5 Life, sex, death and disease

Viewed from an evolutionary perspective, in the life of an individual organism there are two fundamental events, reproduction and death. These reflect the two components of biological *fitness*, survival and reproductive success, survival being (in essence) the delaying of death.

● Can you recall, from Chapter 3, what the word 'fitness' means in a biological context?

■ It is a measure of the lifetime reproductive success of an individual, usually expressed in relative terms. For example, an individual that leaves six surviving offspring who themselves survive to reproduce has twice the fitness of one that produces and raises three.

5.5.1 Life histories

The pattern and timing of reproduction and death during the lifespan of an organism are called its **life history**, and *life-history theory* seeks to explain how the very different life histories of different species have evolved by natural selection. It examines such questions as why individuals of some species are short-lived, while those of others are long-lived; why some species reproduce only once in their lives and others do it several times. In answering such questions, life-history theory seeks to address the general hypothesis that different kinds of life history are *adaptations* to particular features of the environment of the species under consideration.

Of major concern in the study of life histories is the reproductive 'schedule' which is characteristic of a species. Some species breed early in life, others delay breeding until they are relatively old. Some produce several young at each breeding episode, others a few or only one. In comparison with other animals, humans are late breeders, breed several times and produce a small number of young at each breeding episode.

Most animals and plants die soon after breeding or, put another way, continue to breed until they die. The timing of death in a given species depends a lot on whether or not there is parental care of the young. Some species of salmon, which do not care for their young, die immediately after spawning, but in many other fishes and in most mammals and birds a protracted period of postnatal feeding and care is essential for the survival of the young. Death of the parents does not occur, except by disease or predation, until the rearing of their offspring has been completed. A very unusual feature of the human life cycle is that women have a protracted period of post-reproductive life that continues long after all the children have become independent (a point we return to in Chapter 8 when we consider human ageing). In this chapter, we are concerned with the question of why organisms die when they do; indeed, why do they die at all?

A superficial interpretation of the theory of natural selection suggests that the fittest organisms would be those with the highest *fecundity*, i.e. those that produce the greatest number of surviving progeny in the shortest possible time; in the words of Oscar Wilde, 'nothing succeeds like excess'. We might expect evolution, therefore, to have produced a 'super-organism' that shows all the life-history features that confer high fitness.

● What might these features be?

■ Such an organism would reproduce soon after birth, producing large numbers of progeny, and would continue to do so throughout an extremely long life. It would out-compete any competitor, would be highly efficient at finding food, would ward off all predators, and be resistant to all diseases.

Such super-organisms do not exist, and nor could they, for a number of reasons, of which we shall consider two.

5.5.2 Why do organisms die?

Consider, first, the specific question 'Why do organisms die?'. The evolution of death is an interesting problem, about which there are several theories. One such theory argues that natural selection cannot prevent death because it cannot eliminate certain kinds of *genes*. Genes that cause death *before* an individual has reproduced are, obviously, not passed on to progeny and so are eliminated by natural selection whenever they arise by mutation. However, genes that cause death *after* reproduction has begun are passed on to the progeny and thus persist in the gene pool of the species. (The term 'gene pool' refers to all the genes carried by all the individuals of a population or a species, as defined in Chapter 4.)

Put another way, the capacity of natural selection to eliminate harmful genes becomes weaker as an organism progresses through the reproductive phase of its life. According to this argument, death is an inevitable *consequence* of natural selection, but it is not an *adaptation*, that is, a characteristic that has been favoured by natural selection.

5.5.3 Trade-offs between competing activities

The second, more general, reason why super-organisms cannot evolve invokes the concept of **trade-offs** between one component of a life history and another. Trade-offs arise because the resources organisms need in order to survive and reproduce, such as food, water and energy, are often in limited supply, at least for part of an organism's life cycle. This shortage arises largely because individuals, of the same and of different species, are sometimes in competition with one another for such resources. Given a finite supply of resources that they have managed to acquire, organisms have to make what amount to life-history 'decisions'. A major decision is how much of their available resources should be allocated to bodily survival and growth (*somatic* effort) and how much to reproduction (*reproductive* effort). An individual that puts everything it has into reproduction may not have enough left to survive to another breeding episode, whereas one that limits its reproductive output at its first breeding episode may have enough left to survive and then breed again.

● Humans typically have one child at a time, though twins and triplets occur occasionally. What trade-offs do you think might be involved that prevent twins becoming the norm for humans?

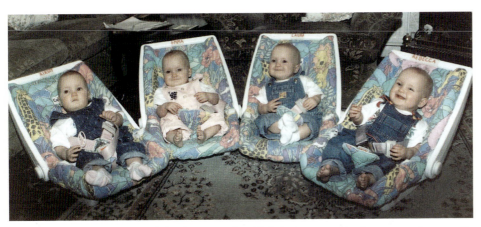

In a species where growth and development after birth is slow, reproductive success is generally greater when one baby at a time is produced at short intervals, than when a larger number are born from a single pregnancy. But in industrialised countries, the survival advantage of single births is small. (Photo: Courtesy of The Multiple Births Foundation)

■ There are at least two possible trade-offs to be considered. First, space in the womb and nutritive resources for the developing fetus or fetuses are limited, leading to twins typically being born prematurely and each being smaller than single babies. The apparent twofold advantage of producing twins may be offset by their postnatal survival chances being reduced as a result of their smaller size. Second, babies have to be fed by their mother. The effort of feeding twins may cause a delay before the next breeding episode can be undertaken. Thus, the reproductive success of a woman having one baby at a time at short intervals may be greater than that of a woman having pairs of twins at longer intervals.

As a result of many trade-offs such as these, various aspects of the life history of organisms tend to be associated with one another. So, for example, animals that breed only once tend to have a large number of young during their single breeding episode and to be short-lived, whereas those (like ourselves) that breed several times tend to produce a small number of progeny per breeding episode and to be long-lived.

Small animals usually breed early in life and die young; large animals are older when they first breed and tend to live long, although there are exceptions to these general rules. As a general rule, small, short-lived, fast-breeding animals and plants, pursue what is often called a 'boom and bust' life history, and are found in environments that are unpredictable or unstable, and in those habitats where there are a large number of competing species. Large, long-lived, slow-breeding species are more typical of environments that are stable over long periods and in which the level of competition between species is relatively low. Like all generalisations in biology, however, there are many exceptions to this general rule.

5.5.4 Vulnerable stages in the life history

Many diseases and other causes of death typically occur most often at particular stages in the life history of a certain species. For example, young individuals are particularly vulnerable to infectious disease; hence the low survival of humans up to five years in developing countries (as shown in the survival curve in Figure 5.5). There are two major reasons for this pattern.

First, young individuals have not had the opportunity to develop **immunity** to common pathogens. Many infectious diseases, such as measles and whooping cough, can affect individuals at any age but, typically, are 'diseases of childhood'. This is because once an individual has recovered from the first episode of infection, he or she is *immune*, i.e. never susceptible to that pathogen again (the mechanisms by which this occurs are discussed in Chapter 6). Some young individuals who have not yet developed immunity succumb to an infection and die. Second, early life is a period of rapid growth requiring abundant food that, in a harsh, unpredictable environment, may not be available. In many species, including our own, high mortality early in life is due partly to malnutrition leading to increased vulnerability to infection.

Once the early growth stage is completed, the survival curve for most species declines much less rapidly. The next vulnerable stage in the life history is during reproduction. This exposes animals to disease risks peculiar to reproduction, in the form of **sexually transmitted diseases** (STDs). An interesting feature of STDs such as syphilis and gonorrhoea is that individuals do not develop immunity to them and can be reinfected again and again. STDs typically do not kill their hosts immediately but may have a debilitating effect leading to premature death. Very little is known about STDs in other animals and so it is not clear whether the effects that they have on humans are typical of animals generally. STDs are known for some plants; they are carried from flower to flower by pollinating insects.

Reproduction is also typically very stressful for animals, particularly for females, though often also for males. In red deer (*Cervus elephas*), for example, the autumnal mating period, or rut, involves intense fighting among stags which leaves some of them injured or so weakened that they are unable to survive the winter. Females may be so weakened by feeding their calves that they are unable to breed in the following year.

●   Patterns such as these have echoes in human lives. Can you suggest some parallels?

■   As described in Chapter 2, birth in humans is more stressful than it is in the majority of primates. Some male violence against other males is undoubtedly linked to sexual competition.

Finally, old age is a period of increasing susceptibility to infectious disease and therefore reduced expectation of survival. As we age, the immune system generally becomes less and less capable of coping with infections, as you will see in Chapter 6.

We turn now to the question of how these life-history relationships between humans and their pathogens may have evolved.

5.6   The evolution of host–pathogen relationships

5.6.1 Generation times

We can speculate that when the first bacterial cells evolved on Earth they lived suspended in a slurry of mud and water containing a variety of chemical compounds, which provided the raw materials to support their survival, growth and reproduction. Much later in evolution, a few of the descendants of these early life-forms had new environments to invade, which offered a much more hospitable habitat than the 'primeval soup'. This new environment was inside the cells and organs of multicelled animals and plants, a protected place, full of nutrients. In such a favourable environment, micro-parasites are able to reproduce at a very high rate.

A bacterium that infects a human may generate several dozen generations within a single day. For example, the time that it takes for a common inhabitant of the large intestines of mammals, the bacterium *Escherichia coli* (known as *E. coli* for short), to complete the process of reproduction is 20 minutes under optimal conditions. Put another way, the **generation time** of *E. coli* is just 20 minutes. Many pathogenic bacteria can reproduce just as quickly. *E. coli* sometimes occurs in pathogenic forms and can cause severe outbreaks of diarrhoea and may even lead to death in vulnerable groups such as older people, as has happened frequently with the consumption of meat products contaminated with the strain *E. coli* 0157. Viruses can also replicate at an astonishing rate. Someone infected with HIV is attempting to defend against the production of 10 billion new virus particles a day!

The difference between the very short generation time of a microscopic pathogen and the relatively long generation time of its host has profound implications for the evolution of the relationship between them. During the course of its host's life, a pathogen living within it can complete many hundreds or thousands of generations and may therefore actually *evolve*, becoming better and better adapted to life in its host and acquiring ever-improving counter-defences against the defences of its host.

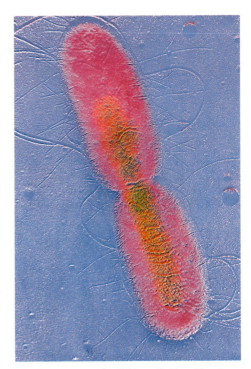

The bacterium Escherichia coli (E. coli) *takes only about 20 minutes to grow and divide into two bacterial cells. (The photograph was taken at a magnification of 9 400 with an electron microscope; the colours have been artificially added.) (Photo: CNRI/Science Photo Library)*

● What are the main processes underlying the ability of a population to evolve and adapt (become fitter) in a given environment (described in Chapters 3 and 4)?

■ They are *mutation*, random changes in the sequence of nucleotides in an organism's DNA, which are passed on to its offspring in the gametes; *crossing over* and *random assortment* creating new combinations of genes during gamete formation; *sexual reproduction* combining genes from unrelated individuals; and *natural selection*, which ensures that advantageous genes gradually spread throughout a population over many generations.

Under pressure from the reproductive advantage of micro-organisms, the immune systems of larger animals have evolved enormous flexibility, which gives the host some chance to counter any new varieties of pathogen that evolve. These immune defences are the subject of Chapter 6. In recent times, 'natural' defences have been reinforced by artificially produced chemicals, which (in some cases) have changed the balance of survival in favour of the host species. For example, in the middle years of the twentieth century, the incidence of malaria worldwide was greatly reduced through the use of drugs to combat the malarial parasite itself and of insecticides that killed the mosquitoes which transmitted it to humans. However, both the rapidly reproducing parasite and its mosquito vector have evolved resistance to these compounds; this is one reason why malaria is returning to areas until recently declared free of infection.

5.6.2 Coevolution

The consequences of the great difference between pathogen and host reproductive rates are of great concern to an evolutionary biologist. Viewed from this perspective, there are three important features of **host–pathogen relationships** (Box 5.1).

Box 5.1   Important features of host–pathogen relationships

1   The association is often very intimate. Pathogens typically possess a number of adaptations that enable them to maintain a position in or on their host and to resist all the host's efforts to remove them. For example, different species of mammals have fleas and lice with grasping limbs specifically adapted to clasp the hair of their host species (Chapter 2). Thus cat fleas cannot maintain a secure grip on human hair. Pathogenic organisms of all kinds are adapted to resist the defensive responses of their host's immune system (as you will see in Chapter 6).

2   The pathogen is largely or wholly dependent on its host for the resources that it requires for survival, growth and reproduction. A major problem for pathogens is that, to reproduce, they, at some stage in their life cycle, must get to a new host before their current host dies. In many macroparasites, dispersal is effected by means of one or more vector species.

3   The activities of the pathogen, to varying degrees, reduce the fitness of the host by reducing its survival and/or reducing its reproductive success. In extreme instances a pathogen may kill its host.

Such is the specificity and intimacy of the relationship between pathogens and their hosts, that it is clear that each has become *adapted* in many ways to the other — an example of what is called **coevolution**. Coevolution refers to specific, reciprocal adaptations between two or a few species, which have evolved through prolonged, intricate interaction between those species. Coevolution between hosts and pathogens, one or both of which has a harmful effect on the other, is often likened to the human arms race because any adaptation by one side that increases its effectiveness tends to lead to counter-adaptations by the other side. This analogy is a poor one, however, because, in the natural world, coevolution commonly leads to adaptations by each organism that *reduce*, rather than increase, its harmful effects on the other.

5.6.3 Virulence

The harm caused by the same species of pathogen within the same species of host is very variable. Within a host species, for example humans, there are typically individuals who are totally unaffected by a particular pathogen, others who have mild infections that cause little or no impact on their fitness, and some who are seriously debilitated or even killed. The same sort of variation also occurs within the pathogen population — some individuals are more effective at surviving their host's defences than others — and consequently they vary in the degree to which they harm their hosts, a property called **virulence**.

The virulence of a particular pathogen is measured as the percentage of infections that lead to death. Among human pathogens, the bacteria that cause cholera can have a virulence of 15 per cent (i.e. 15 per cent of infected people die), whereas pathogens causing other diarrhoeal infections typically have a virulence closer to 5 or 6 per cent. Cholera was among the most virulent of human pathogens until the advent of HIV, which currently has a virulence of over 90 per cent (though this is falling in countries where the newest combination drugs can be afforded).

Any new mutation arising in the host, which causes it to be more resistant to a pathogen, or mutations in the pathogen causing it to be more virulent, has the effect of altering the relationship between them. This leads to evolutionary changes in the other 'partner' in that relationship. If the pathogen becomes more virulent, the host must evolve greater resistance or die out; if the host evolves a more effective immune response, the pathogen evolves counter-measures. For this reason, host–pathogen relationships are evolutionarily *unstable* and are subject to change over time, favouring one partner or the other at different times. This instability becomes particularly apparent when a disease is passed from its usual host to a new host. For example, plague, which has devastated human populations many times during recorded history, is contracted from rats and other rodents, in some of which it is a far less lethal disease.

● What is the term that is used for such diseases?

■ They are called zoonoses (Chapter 2).

Other examples of diseases that are more harmful to humans than to their natural hosts are rabies (which originated in foxes), yellow fever (which originated in monkeys) and brucellosis (which originated in cattle). These and other examples suggest that host–pathogen relationships tend to evolve towards a situation in which *both* organisms can coexist without the host being affected as severely as it once was. Is this due to evolutionary changes in the host, the parasite or both?

5.6.4 Coevolution in action: myxomatosis

The history of myxomatosis provides some answers to this question. The *Myxoma* virus is indigenous to South America and rabbits there are prone to the disease, which produces fibrous lesions on the skin, but do not usually die from it. The virus was unknown in other parts of the world until it was deliberately introduced into Australia in 1950 in an attempt to control the rabbit population, which threatened the livelihood of sheep farmers. Rabbits had themselves been introduced to Australia from Europe in the late nineteenth century and had undergone a population explosion.

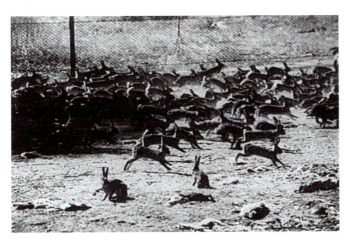

Faced with abundant food and few natural predators, rabbits introduced into Australia from Europe in the late nineteenth century underwent a population explosion which, by the mid-twentieth century, was devastating farm land. (Photo courtesy of Dr Roger Trout)

Carried by mosquitoes, the newly introduced *Myxoma* virus caused an epidemic that killed 99.8 per cent of all rabbits; a second epidemic killed 90 per cent of the generation that resulted from those that survived the first. A third epidemic, however, killed only 50 per cent of the remaining rabbits. This rapid decline in the virulence of myxomatosis was due both to the rabbits evolving resistance to the virus, and to the virus evolving reduced virulence.

● Why do you suppose that reduced virulence might be *adaptive* for the *Myxoma* virus (i.e. improve its chances of surviving long enough to reproduce)?

■ A pathogen that does not kill its host has greater opportunity itself to survive, reproduce and infect new hosts than one that kills its host quickly. At the point when it had reduced the host population by 99.8 per cent, the *Myxoma* virus must itself have been at some risk of becoming extinct.

We would like to add a word of caution here, to dispel a common misconception about the coevolution of host–pathogen relationships. It is all too easy, having seen examples of how coevolution has occurred in specific examples (such as rabbits and *Myxoma*), to be left with the feeling that the pathogen and host somehow 'know' in advance what the other will do and so direct their own evolution to counteract this. Or that pathogens 'know' it is not in their best interests to kill their hosts too soon. This is not the case. The DNA mutations which drive evolution are completely random events — what we see as 'successful' adaptations in pathogens or in hosts are simply those that survived natural selection. Billions of other less-successful mutants were also created by random changes in DNA, but were lost in the competition for survival. Just as lottery winners do not know in advance what the winning combination of numbers will be, so organisms cannot predict what DNA sequences will be the best adapted to survival in the ever-changing environment they will meet.

5.6.5 Transmission routes and the evolution of virulence

It appears to be a feature of some host–pathogen relationships that, during evolution, they have changed from being one of true parasitism towards one of commensalism (recall Table 5.1). It has been widely assumed that there is a general trend during evolution for pathogens to become less virulent, but this view is erroneous. There are other directions in which pathogens may evolve.

An alternative adaptive solution to the pathogen's problem of getting from one host to another is to evolve the ability to survive for a long period outside the host. For example, the bacillus (a rod-shaped bacterium) that causes anthrax, a highly virulent disease, can survive in soil, in a dormant state, for many years. The small island of Gruinard off the coast of Scotland was uninhabitable for more than 40 years after it was used for testing the anthrax bacillus as a biological weapon in World War II. A pathogen with the ability to survive outside its host, and which can thus survive if its host has become rare, does not need to adapt to the problem posed by a reduced host population by evolving decreased virulence. By contrast, a pathogen that cannot survive independently for long (like *Myxoma*) can adapt to a shortage of hosts by evolving reduced virulence.

The mode of transmission between hosts may be a key factor in the evolution of virulence. Transmission from host to host may be through a variety of mechanisms (Box 5.2).

Box 5.2 Modes of transmission of pathogens to new hosts

1   Simple transmission from host to host through the external environment, for example, in airborne water droplets, e.g. the viruses that cause the common cold can be transmitted by sneezing.

2   Transmission from host to host through intimate contact involving exchange of body fluids, e.g. HIV which can be transmitted sexually or through blood transfusions.

3   No direct transmission between hosts, but infection occurs by contact of a new host with intermediate stages of the parasite in the external environment, e.g. the anthrax bacteria can be transmitted in soil.

4   Transmission by vectors or intermediate hosts in which development and reproduction of the microparasite may or may not occur, e.g. typhus is transmitted by lice, and the worms that cause schistosomiasis (bilharzia) are transmitted by snails.

Parasites that are carried by vectors tend to be more virulent than those that are passed directly from host to host; if their hosts become rare, they can survive for some time within the vector. Where evolution *does* appear to have led to decreased virulence is in pathogens that are passed directly from host to host, by direct contact or through the air, such as the rhinoviruses that cause the common cold (Chapter 2). If such pathogens were to make their hosts very ill so that they had to 'go to bed' and thus engage in much less social contact, the transmission of the pathogen to new hosts would be greatly reduced. Rhinoviruses and other pathogens that are transmitted directly tend to have low virulence. There are exceptions, however, to this generalisation, for example, HIV.

● HIV remains dormant in the body for several years without causing any symptoms. How might this be an adaptive feature of this virus?

■ The long period of dormancy allows more opportunities for it to be passed from person to person than would be the case for a pathogen that debilitates or kills its host soon after infection.

Medical and social intervention can influence the evolution of a pathogen's virulence, in either direction. For example, the increasing availability of purified water in parts of India in the 1950s and 1960s led to an evolutionary change in the water-borne cholera pathogen, *Vibrio cholerae*. This bacterium exists in two forms: the original form has a virulence of up to 15 per cent, but there is a less virulent 'El Tor' form of the bacterium, with a virulence of 2 per cent. As the water purification schemes progressed, the proportion of El Tor forms of cholera in India rose, but the original, more virulent form still persists in Bangladesh where water purification schemes have been delayed by natural disasters such as flooding, and lack of finance.

● Can you explain this phenomenon?

■ Water purification tilted the balance of survival against the more virulent bacteria, but the El Tor form increased in the population because its lower virulence allowed more opportunities for transmission between infectious individuals who (usually) did not die.

Conversely, there is evidence that attempts in hospitals in the USA to counter outbreaks of pathogenic *E. coli* with disinfectants have led to the evolution of more virulent strains. The virulence of *E. coli* ranges from 0 to 25 per cent (Ewald, 1993 includes this and other examples). In the UK, the 1990s saw increasing concern about *hospital acquired infections*, including multiple-drug resistant strains of *Staphylococcus aureus* (the 'flesh-eating' bacteria of tabloid headlines), which were reported in official statistics as affecting 100 000 people a year in England alone (National Audit Office, 2000).

5.6.6 Host–pathogen dynamics

Another common feature of host–pathogen interactions is that pathogens are distributed in the population such that the number of pathogens per host individual does not show a *normal distribution*, that is, one in which a majority of host individuals carry an average number of pathogens. This is difficult to demonstrate with bacteria and viruses, but can be easily shown with ectoparasites such as the head louse.

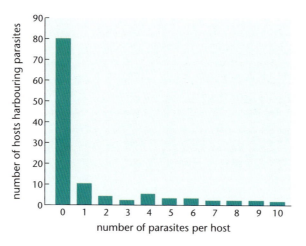

Figure 5.6 *The distribution across a population of people of the head louse* Pediculus humanis capitis. *(Adapted from Begon, M., Harper, L. J. and Townsend, C. R., 1990,* Ecology, *2nd edn, Blackwell Scientific Publications, Oxford, p. 407, Figure 12.13(b))*

● Look at Figure 5.6. How are head lice distributed among individual people?

■ Their distribution is highly 'clumped', such that most individuals carry no lice, some carry a few, and only a small proportion are heavily infested.

There are a number of possible reasons for this distribution pattern, each of which may apply more or less in different cases. It may, for example, reflect the fact that it is difficult for pathogens to disperse from one host to another, with the result that infections only affect a restricted number of individuals living in a confined area. Another common factor is that pathogens may reproduce prolifically only in individual hosts that are already weakened by other factors such as starvation or another kind of infection. A third possibility is that a large proportion of the host population is resistant to the pathogen.

The dynamic properties of an infection by a pathogen, that is, the way the impact of the infection on the host changes over time, can be described and analysed by reference to certain properties of the host population. Every individual in the host population must belong to one of four categories (numbered i to iv), which are represented in Box 5.3 and in Figure 5.7.

Box 5.3   Categories of infection status in a host population

(i) *Susceptibles*: individuals who are capable of being infected, but have not been infected by the pathogen.

(ii) *Latents*: individuals who are currently infected with the pathogen, but do not show symptoms of infection. Individuals with latent infections may or may not be *infectious*, i.e. capable of passing the pathogen on to susceptibles. Some latents are not infectious because the pathogen has not yet produced infective stages; others are infectious even though symptom-less. The length of time between a host becoming infected and the first symptoms appearing is called the **latent period**; it is highly variable between pathogens (we return to this point in Section 5.6.7).

(iii) *Symptomatic infected*: individuals who are currently infected with the pathogen, show symptoms of infection and are usually capable of passing the pathogen on to susceptibles.

(iv) *Immunes*: individuals that have previously been infected with the pathogen, have recovered from their symptoms and are now immune to that pathogen. Immunes may or may not still be carriers of an infection; if they are they can pass it on to susceptibles, as in the celebrated case of Typhoid Mary. She was a domestic cook named Mary Mallon, who worked in the USA at the turn of the twentieth century. In a ten-year period she is believed to have infected 54 people with typhoid, three of whom died. She always denied that she was the source of the infection.

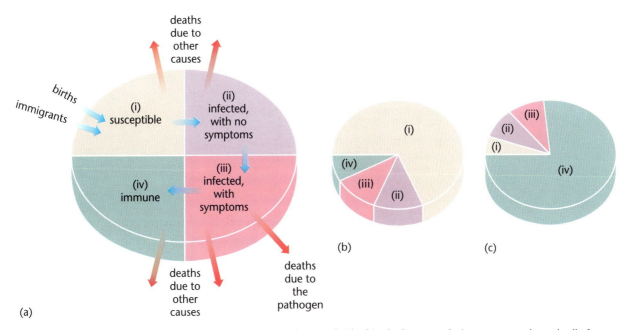

Figure 5.7   *(a) During the course of an infectious outbreak, an individual in the host population may pass through all of categories (i) to (iv), which are defined in Box 5.3. For most infectious diseases, the relative proportions of the four categories in the population of a host species are different in (b) an early stage of an epidemic, compared with (c) a late stage.*

Any one host individual may pass through all of categories (i) to (iv) during the course of its life, or may die at any stage (Figure 5.7a). If the individuals in the host population are adult, all can reproduce and replace members of the population that die. Deaths occur in all four categories, but only those in category (iii) can be the direct result of the disease caused by the pathogen. As discussed above, it is generally not adaptive for pathogens to kill their hosts early in the course of an infection.

● If you were to draw a diagram like Figure 5.7 for HIV, a relatively new infection in the UK with a very high fatality rate, what would the relative proportions of the various segments look like, and why?

■ It should look something like Figure 5.8. HIV is of relatively recent origin, so in most Western populations the susceptibles segment is still very large; however, in some cities in the developing world it is much smaller than shown here, because a high proportion of the population are infected with HIV. The majority of infected individuals are in category (ii), the latents, who show no symptoms of HIV-related illness (the long period of dormancy of this virus was mentioned earlier), but *all* of these are believed to be infectious. The proportion of infected people who belong to category (iii), symptomatic infected, is small because of the high rate of fatality within a short time of symptoms developing. Virtually no one falls into category (iv) because, to date, only a very few individuals have developed immunity to HIV.

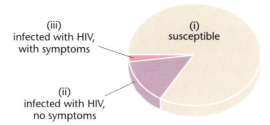

Figure 5.8 *The relative proportions of susceptible, latent (those who show no symptoms) and symptomatic individuals in a theoretical population, with respect to HIV. The proportions shown here vary enormously from one population to another, but the rarity of immunes is common to all. Everyone with a latent HIV infection is believed to be infectious to susceptible individuals.*

The rate at which the number of hosts infected by a given pathogen increases depends upon a number of features of the pathogen itself and on certain properties of the host population. For example, if the host population contains a high proportion of immunes and a low proportion of susceptibles, then the rate at which the pathogen spreads is likely to fall. If the rate falls below that at which each pathogen produces one surviving offspring in each generation, the diseases will become extinct.

● Under what circumstances do you suppose that these conditions would arise?

■ In the late stages of an epidemic, when most members of the host population have been infected by the pathogen and, if they have not died, have become immune to it.

Thus, diseases to which humans can develop immunity tend to occur erratically, with epidemics separated by periods in which their impact is slight or negligible. By contrast, sexually transmitted diseases, to which hosts do not generally become immune, persist in human populations at a more constant frequency. Immunisation programmes, by increasing the proportion of immune individuals in a population, greatly reduce the impact of a pathogen and can sometimes eliminate it altogether; as in the case of smallpox.

5.6.7 Latency, infectious periods and host density

If a pathogen has a long *latent period* and/or *infectious period*, as in the case of HIV, the transmission of the pathogen to relatively few new hosts in a widely dispersed population will adequately maintain its survival in the population.

● Can you explain why this is so?

■ The longer a pathogen has a hold on an individual, the more time there is to come into contact with potential new hosts, even if these are few and far between, so the greater is its chance of being transmitted to susceptibles.

In contrast, measles is a disease with a relatively short latent period (6–9 days) and an even shorter infectious period (6–7 days). Host density becomes a critical factor in the survival of such a pathogen. It has been calculated that measles can only persist in densely populated human settlements of at least 300 000 to 400 000 people. Such large concentrations of people have existed for less than 2 000 years, suggesting that the measles virus has been a common and prevalent pathogen among humans for less than 100 generations, although it probably occurred sporadically for a long time before that. Two additional factors that affect the need for a high density of susceptible hosts are: individuals readily become immune to measles, and the measles virus is not readily transmitted from person to person, being very short-lived in the external environment.

● Conversely, a relatively *low* density of susceptible hosts is required to maintain sexually transmitted infections in human populations. Can you suggest why?

■ There are three reasons. First, the mode of transmission, sexual contact, is affected very little by population density (humans manage to mate with one another whether they are living far apart or close together in dense aggregations). Second, transmission is very efficient, because the pathogen does not need to survive in the outside world at all. Third, immunity to most STDs is very weak (as mentioned earlier), so virtually everyone in the population who is not already infected is susceptible.

Macroparasites, such as flukes and tapeworms, tend to have very long latent and infectious periods; most species have a life expectancy of more than one year in the adult stage and produce eggs for most of their adult life. The nematode worm *Onchocerca volvulus*, which causes river blindness, lives for eight to ten years in humans. Because of their very long infectious periods, these macroparasites tend to be very persistent, and are prevalent even in very small and highly dispersed human populations.

5.7   Instability in host–pathogen relationships

Over long periods, in terms of tens or hundreds of years, the balance of relative advantage between a pathogen and its host changes; as a result, certain pathogenic diseases have had a greater impact on human populations at some times in history than at others. These fluctuations have many underlying causes, but two arise from the biology of the host species. Hosts have two distinct forms of defence against infectious disease, *resistance* and *immunity*, which must be considered on different timescales.

Immunity was defined earlier, and is a property of an *individual*. It develops during the life of that individual and is not passed on to its progeny. **Resistance** is a property of a *species*, or of a *population*; it evolves by natural selection and is passed on from generation to generation. Resistance is largely a consequence of genes that contribute to a fast and effective immune response to common pathogens. Over many generations, natural selection favours those individuals that are most resistant to the common pathogens in that environment; resistant individuals have greater reproductive success than more adversely affected members of the population, and so the genes that contribute to the resistance have a greater chance of being passed on. Over time, genes that confer some resistance to infection spread through the host population.

A source of instability in host–pathogen relationships arises from the fact that a pathogen sometimes invades a new host species, which has no evolutionary history of interaction with it and, hence, has not evolved resistance. As mentioned above, and in Chapter 2, several human pathogens are thought to be derived from animal parasites. There is compelling evidence that HIV is derived from a virus of monkeys, for example. As described earlier, these *zoonotic* diseases are especially virulent in their newly acquired human hosts, who have not had time to evolve effective resistance.

5.7.1   The coevolution of host resistance and pathogen virulence

The example of myxomatosis, described above, is one in which greater resistance has evolved in the host, rabbits. This effect, combined with the evolution of decreased virulence in the virus, typically leads to a relatively stable state in which pathogen and host coexist, with only a relatively small proportion of the host population being adversely affected by the pathogen. This situation is not truly stable, however, because at any time a mutation may occur in the pathogen population, producing a more virulent form.

● What effect do you think this might have, over time, on the relationship between the pathogen and the host?

■ The more virulent form of the virus will spread through the host population, killing the least resistant individuals. Since only the most resistant survive to pass on their genes ('survival of the fittest'), this favours the gradual evolution of greater resistance in the host population as a whole. Eventually a stable state of coexistence between host and pathogen is restored, until the next significant mutation occurs in either.

The instability of host–pathogen relationships is of profound importance for medical and social intervention to reduce the incidence of infectious diseases. The fact that pathogens are continually evolving means that the 'war' against them may never be won. An example is provided by TB, which we referred to earlier.

The bacterium *Mycobacterium tuberculosis* kills about 2 million people each year throughout the world and, in parts of some developing countries, infects about 95 per cent of the population. In the aftermath of World War II, TB was almost eliminated from most developed countries by improved nutrition and housing across the whole population, coupled with the use of drugs, vaccination and isolation of infected people. However, TB is now increasing in most countries of the world and the WHO estimate that, in the absence of any new therapeutic compounds to fight the disease, the bacterium will have newly infected another 1 billion people and caused 35 million deaths by 2020 (WHO, 2000a).

There are a number of reasons for this increase, including the spread of another pathogen, HIV. People with a very poor immune response (whether due to HIV infection or some other cause, such as chronic malnutrition) are more likely to develop infectious diseases, including TB.

A change in the TB bacterium itself has also contributed to its increased prevalence. Strains of the TB bacterium that are resistant to all drugs have evolved in recent years, known as **multi-drug resistant (MDR) strains**. The evolution of drug-resistant strains has occurred in many different types of pathogenic bacteria, and also in the malarial parasite (*Plasmodium*), a fact that has contributed to its increase in parts of the world where malaria had been eradicated in the 1960s. The existence of drug-resistant strains of bacteria and parasites provides the basis for prescribed antibiotics being dispensed with the instruction to 'finish the bottle', that is, to continue taking the antibiotic after the symptoms have been alleviated.

● Can you explain the rationale for this instruction, based on your knowledge of natural selection and the discussion (above) of the evolution of resistance?

■ Among the population of bacteria infecting a person, there will typically be much variation between individual bacteria in their degree of resistance to a given antibiotic. The first few doses of the drug will kill the least resistant bacteria, leading to a rapid alleviation of the symptoms, but more resistant bacteria will remain alive. These may eventually be killed by subsequent doses of antibiotic. People who do not finish a course of antibiotics risk a renewed bout of the disease, caused by a population increase among the more resistant bacteria that have not been killed at the beginning of the course of treatment. Such people are also carriers of those resistant bacteria, which can be passed on to others. Over time, with repeated but inadequate prescription of a common antibiotic, strains of bacteria can evolve which are completely resistant to it.

You can see how the constant re-balancing of the equilibrium between ourselves and our pathogens has occurred as new medical therapies such as antibiotics have been discovered and used in large amounts around the world. What will our next line of defence be when resistance to all our current drugs is reached? You will see in Chapter 6 how knowledge of the genomic DNA sequence of pathogens (such as *Mycobacterium tuberculosis*) might help us to develop new weapons in this battle.

5.7.2 Cyclic outbreaks of infection

Diseases to which hosts develop immunity, such as measles, typically show cyclic outbreaks (Figure 5.9) because, during each outbreak, a large proportion of the host population becomes immune. When the proportion of immunes relative to susceptibles in the population is high (as shown earlier, in Figure 5.7c), the prevalence of the pathogen inevitably declines. It does not usually die out, however, because new susceptibles are being added to the host population.

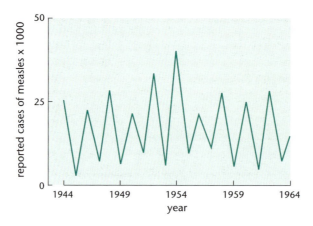

Figure 5.9 *Reported cases of measles in New York City from 1944 to 1964. (Source: Begon, M., Harper, J. L. and Townsend, C. R., 1990,* Ecology: Individuals, Populations and Communities, *Blackwell Scientific Publications, Oxford; after Yorke, J. A. and London, W.P., 1973, Recurrent outbreaks of measles, chickenpox and mumps: II Systematic differences in contact rates and stochastic effects,* American Journal of Epidemiology, **98**, *pp. 469–82)*

● There are two sources of new susceptibles: what are they?

■ New hosts are born who have not been exposed to the pathogen and so have not developed immunity. Immigration from other host populations brings in non-immune individuals from areas where the disease is not present.

The incidence of measles in New York shows a two-year cycle. This is much shorter than is typical for viral infections in natural populations, and is probably due to the high rates of immigration of people into this large population centre.

The best documented example of an infectious disease with a much longer cycle is *plague*, caused by the bacterium *Yersinia pestis* and transmitted to humans via rat fleas. Rats were originally infected by transfer of bacteria from other species of rodent, including some that were trapped for their fur. A disease resembling plague was first recorded in the Middle East in about 1100BC, and swept around the world as the 'Black Death' until about AD644, when it disappeared from Europe for about 700 years. The second pandemic (a term signifying worldwide spread affecting large numbers of people) began in the fourteenth century and 'burnt itself out' in around 1670, following the Great Plague of 1665, when at least 70 000 people died in London alone. Plague reappeared in Europe in the eighteenth century, reached Glasgow in 1900 and broke out in East Anglia in the years before World War I. It killed over 13 million people in India in the first quarter of the twentieth century, and remains a significant threat to life in some parts of the developing world today. Plague also illustrates the importance of cultural evolution as a factor in cyclic patterns of infectious disease.

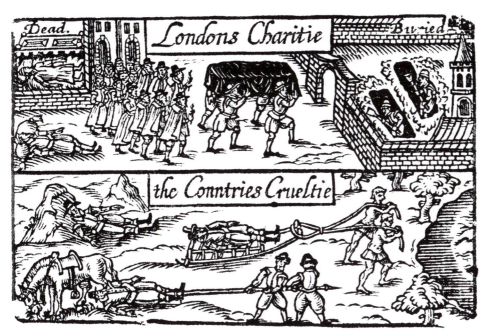

This engraving contrasts the burial of plague victims in London and the English countryside in the great plague epidemics of the seventeenth century. (Photo: Private Collection/Bridgeman Art Library)

5.7.3 Impact of cultural evolution on infection rates

Cultural changes taking place during the transition from hunter–gatherer societies to settled agricultural, and later urban, communities underlie the pandemic waves of plague in Europe.

● Can you suggest some cultural developments that contributed to outbreaks of plague?

■ Settled communities attracted rats to their food stores; rat fleas live well in the woollen clothing worn by early pastoralists; in later centuries the fashion for furs brought trappers in direct contact with the primary hosts of plague bacteria; international trade carried infected rats around the world.

Various aspects of the impact of cultural evolution on patterns of infection, and also the inherent instability of the relationship between humans and their pathogens, are well-illustrated by the history of infectious diseases introduced to North America from the Old World. The process began with the arrival of Christopher Columbus in October 1492 (the article by Meltzer, 1992, listed under Further sources tells the story). Following the arrival of Europeans, more Native Americans died of a variety of infections than were born, a situation that has not been reversed until very recently. Estimates for the Native American population in 1492 range from two to 18 million; by the end of the nineteenth century it had fallen to 530 000. (These figures refer to pure-bred Native Americans; there were, and still are, many people descended from interbreeding between Native Americans and Europeans.) The diseases that devastated the Native American population included smallpox, measles, influenza, bubonic plague, diphtheria, typhus, cholera, scarlet fever, chickenpox, yellow fever and whooping cough.

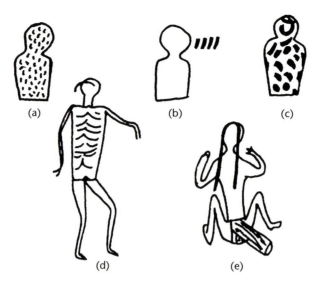

These Sioux Indian drawings were used to record the numbers who died primarily in epidemics of infectious diseases imported by European colonists and as a result of starvation through land loss. They represent (a) measles, (b) whooping cough, (c) smallpox, (d) starvation, and (e) cholera. (From American Indian Holocaust and Survival: A Population History since 1492 *by Russell Thornton. Copyright 1987 by the University of Oklahoma Press, Norman, Oklahoma and London, Figure 4.2, p.81)*

This example raises two questions. The more obvious one is: why did Native Americans have so little resistance to the pathogens that caused these diseases? The less obvious question is: why did the invading Europeans not contract infectious diseases from the Native Americans? The answers are thought to lie in the rather different cultural histories of the two human populations before they collided in 1492.

Another feature of the gradual abandonment of the hunter–gatherer form of subsistence, and the development of village life, was that several species of wild animals were domesticated, including pigs, cattle and chickens, from which humans contracted certain infectious diseases. Smallpox is believed to be derived from cowpox, measles from rinderpest (a disease of cattle) or canine distemper, and influenza from viruses that originated in pigs. Over hundreds of years, these diseases had sporadically devastating effects on settled agricultural and pastoral populations. The individuals who survived infection had a high level of resistance to the new diseases; as a result, settled populations of humans came to coexist with the pathogens derived originally from their domesticated animals.

The transition from hunter–gatherer to agricultural and pastoral societies did not happen everywhere at once. It occurred much earlier in the regions we know today as Africa and Europe than it did in Asia. Evidence from the nature of their language, from anatomical features, and from analysis of their genes, suggests that Native Americans originally came from Asia, crossing to America via a land-bridge across what is now the Bering Strait about 12 000 years ago. They settled in a land that had a very diverse range of large mammals, such as mammoths, giant sloths, lions, sabre-toothed tigers and bears. Some 10 800 years ago, 80 per cent of these large mammals became extinct.

There is much debate as to whether these extinctions were caused by humans, or were due to climatic change, or a combination of the two. Whatever the cause, Meltzer suggests that one outcome of these extinctions was a shortage of species suitable for domestication by the immigrant humans. Most of the surviving mammal species, such as the American bison, could not easily be domesticated and, in any case, were so abundant that they could easily be obtained by hunting. Native Americans, as a result, did not domesticate animals and so did not acquire infectious diseases from them or evolve resistance to their pathogens. Thus the European explorers brought America a wide range of infectious diseases of relatively recent origin, to which the Native Americans had never been exposed. Their lack of history of domestication of animals meant that they had few unusual pathogens of their own with which they could return the compliment.

5.7.4 Genetic bottlenecks

The history of interactions between European colonists and Native Americans illustrates some interesting points about the rate at which host–pathogen relationships evolve. When a new pathogen enters a host population, it tends to cause very high mortality, especially if the population is very dense and the infection is transmitted directly. The resultant rapid decline in the size of the host population creates what is called a **genetic bottleneck**. The small population that survives a very serious epidemic contains a very high proportion of individuals that have high resistance to the pathogen, because they are descended from genetically resistant parents. As a result, as the host population increases again, it has a much higher rate of resistance than before the epidemic. This is exactly the same as we described earlier for the evolution of drug-resistant strains of bacteria.

Total resistance, however, does not evolve. There is always variation in resistance among individuals in the host population, and genetic variation in virulence in the pathogen population, leading to the kind of unstable situation described above, in which minor outbreaks occur from time to time as mutations arise and more virulent varieties of pathogen emerge. The evolution of host–pathogen relationships tends, therefore, to be a slow process, with erratic shifts one way and then the other, punctuated by periods in which, through population crashes and genetic bottlenecks, evolutionary change may be very rapid in the short-term (Figure 5.10).

During the coevolution of a pathogen and its host, adaptation by one and counter-adaptation by the other lead quite rapidly (in evolutionary terms) to their coming to coexist in unstable equilibrium. During the course of evolution, a single host

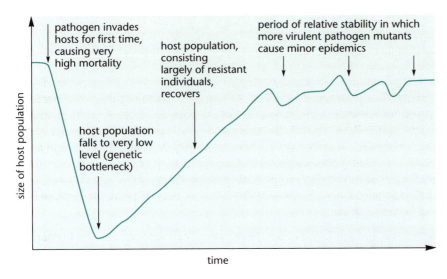

Figure 5.10 *Schematic diagram of the evolution of a host–pathogen relationship over time.*

species may undergo a series of events like that summarised in Figure 5.10, so that a host coexists with a large number of different pathogen species, with some of which it has an ancient association, with others a more recent one.

We turn next to examine the long-term evolutionary results of this interaction between host and species and a succession of diverse pathogenic parasites. It may surprise you to learn that sexual reproduction may have evolved as a consequence of our relationships with pathogens.

5.8   The evolution of sex

A current, unresolved problem in evolutionary biology is the evolution of sex. Relatively few pathogens reproduce sexually, that is, by fusion of gametes from a male and female (see Chapter 4), but do so by some form of asexual reproduction, such as just dividing into two (there are types of asexual reproduction, but they do not concern us here). Many macroparasites, such as the tapeworm, reproduce sexually at some times in their life history, asexually at others. What evolutionary pressures determine which form of reproduction occurs?

● Consider a female in a sexually reproducing species. Whenever she reproduces, she passes on 50 per cent of her genes to each of her progeny, the other 50 per cent being provided by their father, or fathers. If she were to abandon sex and produce young asexually, what effect would this have on her offspring's genotype?

■ Each of them would contain 100 per cent of her genes. Thus, an asexual female in a normally sexual population has a twofold advantage over other females: she passes her genes on to the next generation twice as effectively.

This leads to the general argument that, at the level of *individual* organisms, natural selection should favour asexual reproduction over sexual reproduction. This fundamental 'cost of sex' is often referred to as the cost of producing males. Much of the current debate amongst biologists about the evolution of sex is directed at identifying advantages that could offset this fundamental disadvantage of sexual reproduction.

5.8.1 Sexual reproduction and host–pathogen coevolution

Sexual reproduction differs from asexual reproduction in two important respects when viewed from an evolutionary perspective. First, as described in Chapter 4, the production of gametes (eggs and sperm) involves a form of nuclear division called *meiosis*, in which *half* the genes in the egg-producing or sperm-producing cell are passed on to each new gamete. Because the genes can be divided into a huge number of different 'halves', this generates great diversity in the genotype of each egg or sperm that a single individual can produce. Second, the fusion of two gametes, from genetically different parents, creates completely new combinations of genes. As a result of these two processes, sexual reproduction produces offspring that are much more genetically diverse than those produced by asexual reproduction. Asexually produced progeny are genetically almost identical to their single parent and to one another ('almost' because small errors can occur when the genes are copied before cell division).

In the coevolution of pathogens and hosts, pathogens have a distinct advantage, as noted earlier. They typically have a very short generation time and a very high reproductive rate; remember that a bacterium in the human gut can generate several dozen generations in a single day. Bacteria and viruses typically reproduce asexually and so show very little genetic variation between individuals of the same type. However, their genotype is subject to mutation, so there is some genetic variation on which natural selection can act. Certain viruses, such as HIV and influenza virus, have very high mutation rates and so generate many, slightly different 'strains'. As a result, pathogens can evolve, that is become better adapted to the defences of their host, *within the lifetime of their host*. This is the key to the disadvantage of asexual reproduction among host species.

● Can you suggest what it is?

■ If the host reproduces asexually, it produces offspring genetically identical to itself and for which there is, therefore, a population of pathogens that are already adapted to infect it.

No such population of 'ideal' hosts (from the pathogen's viewpoint) is available if the host reproduces genetically variable offspring by sexual reproduction. The hypothesis, then, is that sexual reproduction is an adaptation against pathogenic organisms. It ensures that at least some progeny are produced that are less susceptible to attack by those pathogens that have evolved during the lifetime of their parents.

Another important role for pathogenic parasites in the evolution of their hosts has been identified in the context of host sexual behaviour. W. D. Hamilton and Marlene Zuk published a highly influential paper in 1982 in which they suggested that exclusively male characteristics in certain species, such as bright coloration, elaborate visual displays, courtship songs, mating calls and odours, often act as 'revealing handicaps'. The argument is, first, that animals are subject to potentially debilitating parasites; second, that resistance to such parasites is heritable; and, third, that only those individual males that are resistant to parasites are able to express their sex-related characteristics fully. Consequently, females should evolve a mating preference for those males that have the best-developed sexual characteristics, because the offspring that result from such matings are likely to inherit greater resistance to parasites from their father.

In recent years, numerous studies of a diverse array of animal species have demonstrated that females do prefer those males with the most highly developed sexual characteristics. Examples include long tail plumes in birds, complex calls in frogs and bright coloration in fishes. A number of studies have confirmed the predicted relationship between such characteristics and parasite infestations but, to date, only a small number of studies have confirmed that females preferring males with well-developed sexual characteristics produce progeny that are relatively free of parasites.

5.8.2 What use are males?

This line of argument has recently been taken further than accounting for the evolution of sex, by addressing the question 'What value are males?'. In many animal species, males make no contribution to reproduction other than the provision of sperm. In such species, there is typically intense competition among males for access to females, with a relatively small proportion of males actually mating, either as a result of being successful in fights with other males or by being very attractive to females. To achieve matings, males have to undertake energetically very demanding activities, like fighting and prolonged courtship, and only a few are successful. Males can thus be regarded as a 'dispensable caste' whose genotypes are 'screened' for disadvantageous genes during energetic sex-related behaviour.

At first sight, these arguments are of little, if any, obvious direct relevance to humans, though the general question 'What value are males?' is not without interest in a human context! Human males do not develop the kind of extravagant sex-related characteristics that are seen, for example, in peacocks and birds of paradise. Furthermore, at least during the early stages of human evolution, men probably contributed more to reproduction than the donation of sperm to women, though modern people vary greatly in the extent to which fathers contribute materially or culturally to raising their children.

Men and women do, however, look different; they show a number of secondary sexual characteristics that distinguish the two sexes. As described in Chapter 2, these differences are based largely on differences in the skeleton, the distribution of adipose tissue (fat), and patterns of hair growth. To some extent, these differences reflect the different roles of men and women in reproduction; the wider hips of women are an adaptation for giving birth to babies with large heads, for example. However, it is widely argued that certain sex differences in humans have become 'exaggerated' during evolution because of their role in sexual attraction.

This process is called **sexual selection**, which is a form of natural selection that favours any characteristics that enhance an individual's ability, not to survive, but to obtain matings. For example, adult women differ from all other mammals in having prominent mammary glands (breasts) at times when they are not feeding babies. In many cultures, breasts are attractive to men; evolutionary theory suggests that they have evolved as a 'permanent fixture' outside feeding periods because they increase the female's chance of obtaining a mate and passing on her genes.

Yet more controversial is the suggestion that female sexual preferences may have favoured in men the accentuation of characteristics commonly identified by heterosexual women as being sexually attractive. The fact that these characteristics vary somewhat from one population to another does not undermine the theory. Thus, while humans are clearly not as flamboyant in their secondary sexual characteristics as peacocks, they may, by a similar process, have evolved sex differences for which the sole basis is sexual attraction.

5.9   Biodiversity and the place of micro-organisms

The inevitable focus on human infectious disease in this chapter may have further reinforced the widespread misconception that micro-organisms are *generally* harmful to other life-forms. Bacteria in particular among the micro-organisms have had a bad 'image', which is at odds with their essential role in maintaining the rich diversity of life on Earth. Here we step back from the emphasis on disease and consider the diversity of organisms and their lifestyles and life histories. What is the relative importance of humans and micro-organisms in the wider scheme of things?

The word **biodiversity** has become part of the lexicon of environmentalism and 'green' politics in recent years, but what does it actually mean? In general terms, it refers to the fact that a given type of habitat — such as a tract of tropical forest, a seashore or a hedgerow — supports a large number of animal and plant species that vary greatly in terms of their way of life and their interactions with each other. As described at the beginning of this chapter, species interact with one another in many different ways. For example, plants are fed on by herbivores and in turn herbivores fall prey to predators. Such interactions are often depicted as a 'food chain' with plants, described as **primary producers**, at the bottom and predators, called **consumers**, at the top (see Figure 5.11). This analogy, however, is a poor

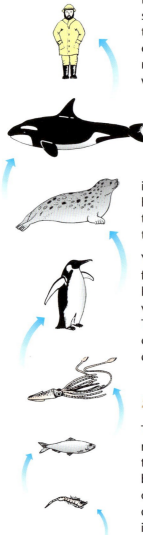

Figure 5.11 *An example of a food chain, in the oceans around Antarctica, involving plankton, krill, fish, squid, penguin, leopard seal, killer whale and human.*

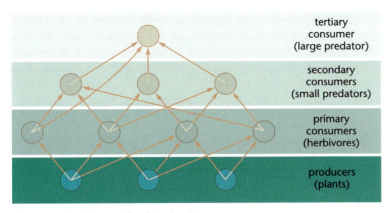

Figure 5.12 *A generalised food web.*

one; such is the number of species and the complexity of interactions among them that the phrase 'food web' is now more commonly used (see Figure 5.12).

The organisms in a **food web** can be arranged in a vertical series of categories, according to how they obtain nutrients; these categories are called *trophic* levels. At the lowest trophic level are the producers; these are plants and phytoplankton, which use energy from the Sun to convert simple chemicals into sugars, amino acids and other complex substances and, in the process, produce vast amounts of oxygen. Phytoplankton are plant-like single-celled organisms that drift in the sea and are the basis of most marine food chains, like the one shown in Figure 5.11. These primary producers are eaten by small, primary consumers, which are in turn eaten by larger secondary consumers, and so on. They are also major producers of oxygen, so they contribute to the atmosphere that other organisms require to sustain life.

When the number of species, and the total number of individuals at each trophic level is calculated, what is revealed is a broad-based *pyramid of numbers* (Figure 5.13a), in which there are many more species and individuals at lower levels than there are at the higher levels. More importantly, when account is taken of the body mass (or **biomass**) of all the organisms at each level, what emerges is a *pyramid of biomass*, which shows that the total biomass of small organisms at the lower trophic levels greatly exceeds that of the larger organisms further up the food web (Figure 5.13b).

Humans occupy a position at the top of the global food web and we share this position with other large-bodied animals, but we and they are relatively insignificant in terms of total biomass. It is easy to lose sight of the enormous and vital importance of bacteria and other microscopic organisms simply because each individual is so small.

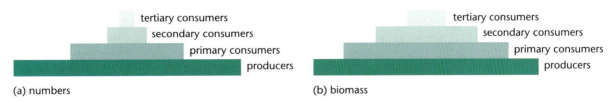

Figure 5.13 *(a) A typical pyramid of numbers. (b) A typical pyramid of biomass.*

The shape of the pyramid of biomass arises largely because the transfer of energy from one trophic level to the next is very inefficient. As a rough estimate, only about 10 per cent of the energy potentially available at any one level actually finds its way up to the next, the rest being dissipated in various ways, including heat. This is shown graphically in Figure 5.14.

These simple ways of depicting biodiversity and the interaction between species make an important point. Communities of organisms are based ultimately on microscopic organisms, such as bacteria and plankton, which are so numerous that, despite their microscopic size, they make up much the largest proportion of the total mass of life on Earth. The main business of bacteria is feeding off dead plants and animals, not in causing disease in humans and our crops and livestock. Only a small minority of species and a tiny fraction of the bacterial biomass are symbiotic on or in larger animals and only a few of them are pathogenic.

In the next chapter in this book, we turn our attention to the mechanisms that have evolved in humans (and, indeed, in all animal species) to defend themselves from these pathogens.

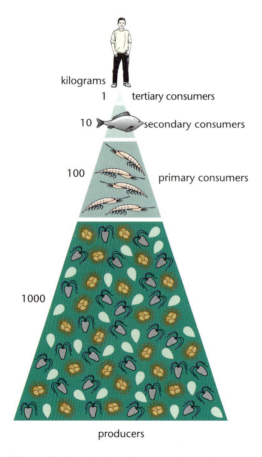

Figure 5.14   *A schematic view of a marine food web that supports humans. Such is the inefficiency of transfer of nutrients and energy from one trophic level to the next that, to produce one kilogram of a human, it requires 1 000 kilograms of plankton.*

OBJECTIVES FOR CHAPTER 5

When you have studied this chapter, you should be able to:

5.1 Define and use, or recognise definitions and applications of, each of the terms printed in **bold** in the text.

5.2 Give examples of the diversity of the pathogens that cause communicable diseases in humans, and illustrate methods of classifying them in terms of their size, site of infection, mode of action and mode of transmission.

5.3 Explain what is meant by coevolution and give examples of different kinds of host–pathogen relationships that have evolved by coevolution, emphasising the interaction of latency, virulence transmission routes and host density.

5.4 Give a general account of the evolutionary consequences of the fact that pathogenic organisms have much faster generation times than their hosts, and explain the role of factors that lead to instability in host–pathogen relationships, using examples of specific diseases.

5.5 Illustrate the importance of micro-organisms in maintaining the biodiversity of the global ecosystem.

QUESTIONS FOR CHAPTER 5

1 (*Objectives 5.1 and 5.2*)

Give brief definitions of the following terms: microparasite, vector, virulence.

2 (*Objective 5.2*)

Look at Box 5.2 and for each of transmission routes 1–4, identify a pathogen *in addition* to those named in Box 5.2 that is transferred to new hosts by that route.

3 (*Objective 5.3*)

Define the term coevolution and give an example of it in the context of host–pathogen relationships.

4 (*Objective 5.4*)

Identify three adaptations of host species, such as humans, that are defences against pathogens, explaining in each case the significance of that defence.

5 (*Objective 5.4*)

Briefly describe four factors that may cause host–pathogen relationships to become unstable over time.

6 (*Objective 5.5*)

Summarise the principal reasons why micro-organisms can be said to 'support' all life on Earth.

CHAPTER 6

Surviving infectious disease

Study notes for OU students

Before commencing this chapter, it would be helpful to refresh your memory of the structure and functions of cell membranes, and the nature of 'lock-and-key' interactions at the cell surface or between enzymes and molecules in biochemical reactions — look again at Figures 3.5 to 3.11. During your study of Section 6.9.1, you will be asked to revise the article by Marc Strassburg, entitled 'The global eradication of smallpox', which was set reading for *World Health and Disease* (Open University Press, second edition 1993; third edition 2001), Chapter 3, and can be found in *Health and Disease: A Reader* (Open University Press, second edition 1995; third edition 2001).

6.1   The threat of infectious disease

The fact that numerous species of pathogenic organisms coexist with the human population in an unstable equilibrium in which neither becomes extinct, is a matter of no interest to an individual suffering from an infectious disease. At the personal level, the important questions are 'Will I survive? And if I do, will I suffer permanent harm?' As Chapter 5 described, over 17 million people die from communicable diseases worldwide every year (WHO, 2000b, Annex Table 3); there are almost 4 billion cases of diseases caused by parasitic animals and protoctist (single-celled) parasites, and 6–7 times this number of episodes of bacterial and viral infections resulting in illness, disability and death — particularly among children under five. As the twentieth century progressed, infectious and parasitic diseases became a relatively inconspicuous cause of mortality in high-income countries, but they still produce significant bouts of illness for most people throughout their lives, and newly emerging infectious diseases (most notably, AIDS) have brought the threat from infection closer.

In this chapter, we will look inside the human body at the highly varied defence mechanisms which have evolved in response to the threat of infection and at the counter-measures evolved by different types of pathogen. You will get some idea of why certain pathogens are mildly inconvenient while others kill, and why it is that certain individuals seem more susceptible to infectious disease than others. We will also briefly review some of the ways in which medical science is attempting to tilt the balance in favour of human survival.

6.1.1   Immunology and 'military metaphors'

The branch of biomedical science known as **immunology** studies the cells and molecules that interact in the bodies of animals to protect them from infection. This network of cells and molecules is collectively called the **immune system**. When it works successfully to eradicate pathogens in the body *before* they cause symptoms of disease, we say that the host has **immunity** to that type of pathogen. 'Host' is a general term meaning an organism that has pathogens living on or inside it, which will already be familiar to you from Chapters 2 and 5.

First, a word of caution about the language of threat and counter-attack which permeates every discussion of the biological responses to infectious disease. Elsewhere in this series, we discussed the usefulness and the pitfalls of biological *metaphors*[1].

[1] See the discussion of biological metaphors in *Studying Health and Disease* (Open University Press, 2nd edn 1994; colour-enhanced 2nd edn 2001), Chapter 9.

A prime example is the use of military terms as metaphors for the biological processes that occur when pathogenic organisms enter the body. Pathogens are often described as 'invaders' or 'foreign cells' which sneak through the body's defences like undercover agents; ranged against them is an 'arsenal' of biological weapons, which search out and attack the invader with deadly accuracy, like a 'smart bomb' homing in on its target. These are exciting images and close enough to some important features of the actual biological processes to justify their limited use.

However, overuse of military images has one serious drawback. It reinforces the wholly mistaken view that pathogens and the defensive mechanisms in the human body are literally engaged in warfare, with each side trying to outwit the other. In this make-believe world, as one side develops a new strategy, so the other counters it with an opposing move. Cells are portrayed as though they are knowledgeable entities capable of intentional actions. For example, the human immunodeficiency virus (HIV) is frequently represented as an adversary of frightening cleverness, which has 'disarmed' our biological defences and rendered them powerless to protect us.

● What biological error can you identify in this use of military metaphors? You will need to think back to earlier chapters and the processes that underlie evolutionary change.

■ HIV has not been cleverly designed to evade biological defences that it somehow 'knew' the details of in advance. It is the product of random mutations which occurred over time in the genetic material of 'ancestor' viruses. Mutation generated a range of slightly different viruses and HIV is simply the present-day survivor of a competition between earlier versions, which were 'selected against' because they were less successful at reproducing new virus particles and transmitting them from one host to the next. In evolutionary terms, the strains of HIV we see today are the versions *best adapted* to survive and reproduce under *present* conditions.

Later in this chapter (Section 6.6.3), we will look more closely at the specific interaction between HIV and human biology,[2] but we begin by taking a more general view of pathogenic organisms and the defences of their human hosts against infection. The first level of defence does not involve the immune system at all.

6.2 Physical and chemical barriers to infection

The most effective way to survive an infection is not to let pathogens get into the body in the first place. Intact skin forms an impenetrable barrier to most pathogenic organisms and the acidity of sweat also inhibits the growth of many kinds of bacteria on the body surface. But we have to breathe, drink and eat, so it is inevitable that infection will enter in contaminated air, water and food, as well as through breaks in the skin. Humans reproduce sexually, which creates more opportunities for infection to be transmitted. Figure 6.1 (overleaf) illustrates the range of passive physical and chemical barriers to infection; most are in the respiratory and reproductive tracts and gut, as you might expect.

An example of a chemical barrier is an enzyme called *lysozyme*, which splits the chemical bonds that hold together the molecular components of bacterial cell walls. (Look back at Chapter 3, Figure 3.11b and imagine that the enzyme pictured

---

[2] HIV/AIDS is the subject of an interdisciplinary case study in a later book in this series, *Experiencing and Explaining Disease* (Open University Press, 2nd edn 1996; colour-enhanced 2nd edn 2001), Chapter 4.

Figure 6.1 *Physical and chemical barriers to infection in the human body.*

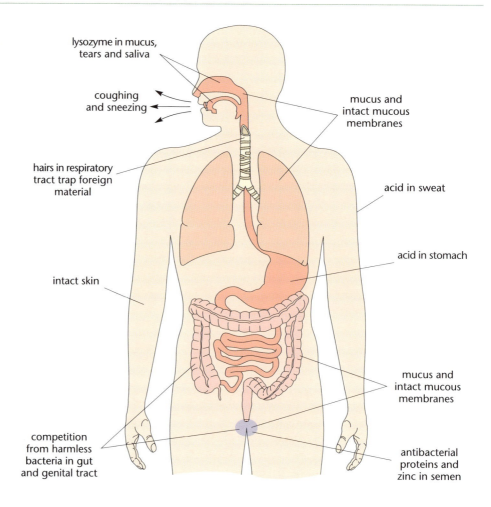

lysozyme in mucus, tears and saliva

coughing and sneezing

mucus and intact mucous membranes

hairs in respiratory tract trap foreign material

acid in sweat

acid in stomach

intact skin

mucus and intact mucous membranes

competition from harmless bacteria in gut and genital tract

antibacterial proteins and zinc in semen

is lysozyme.) Bacteria have a 'wall' of sugar-rich molecules outside their cell membrane, which gives some protection from chemical attack and dehydration in the often inhospitable conditions inside the body (as mentioned in Section 5.3.3). These sugars are unique to bacteria, so the presence of lysozyme in blood, sweat and tears (and nasal secretions and breast milk) has no effect on human tissues, but it digests holes in the cell wall of many bacteria.

However, some types of bacteria have evolved yet another protective layer, a capsule of protein outside the sugar-rich cell wall, which lysozyme cannot penetrate. This example illustrates the point made earlier about the evolution of defensive mechanisms which in their turn are rendered ineffective by later evolutionary developments. Note, in passing, that viruses also have a tough outer envelope of proteins which is resistant to digestion.

6.3   Why is the immune system so complicated?

As you will see shortly, once pathogens breach the physical and chemical barriers and get into body tissues and fluids, they meet a range of cells and molecules that interact in a defensive network of bewildering complexity, collectively known as the immune system. In this short chapter we can do no more than sketch in some of the major features of the immune system and its response to infection, but before embarking on this task, it is worth reflecting for a moment on why such a complex system of defences has evolved.

6.3.1 A multiplicity of targets

The world is populated by millions of different organisms competing for habitats in which they can survive and reproduce. The bodies of animals contain numerous suitable niches for smaller organisms to colonise; the larger and more complex the body of the host, so the more varied are the habitats it contains and the greater the number of species of smaller organisms it can support. Humans are composed of huge numbers of specialised cells of many different kinds with a stable temperature and constant food supply, so the opportunities for colonisation by bacteria, viruses, fungi, protoctists and larger parasites are endless, as a glance back at Figure 5.1, will confirm. Some of these organisms are harmless, some are even beneficial (for example, certain bacteria in our guts are essential partners in the process of digestion, as Chapter 7 will describe), but many cause damage and disease.

Pathogens come in many shapes and sizes; their bodies are composed of a wide range of chemical substances, some of which are exactly the same as molecules found in the body of their host, but others (like the sugars in bacterial cell walls) are unique to that type of organism. Moreover, they have very different 'lifestyles'; for example, some reproduce *inside* the cells of their host (these *intracellular* pathogens are particularly difficult for the host to detect), whereas others live in the gut or the bloodstream; some reproduce very rapidly, whereas others are slow-growing or even lie dormant for many years before becoming active. And, most important of all, different pathogens have evolved quite different mechanisms to protect themselves from the host's defensive responses.

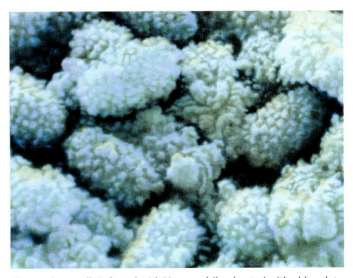

Human lung cells infected with Haemophilus *bacteria (the blue dots; the colour has been added artificially to reveal the extent of the infection); this bacterium causes a respiratory illness with some similarities to viral influenza. (The electronmicrograph was taken at a magnification of 6 200.) (Photo: NIBSC/Science Photo Library)*

The biological inevitability of extensive infection by such a varied array of organisms has given a 'selective advantage' to animals which have evolved an equally extensive network of biological protection. The success of the human species can be attributed partly to the effectiveness of our immune system in detecting and destroying or inactivating all these different pathogens. In this book we are concerned primarily with the health of the human species, so the account in this chapter focuses on the human immune system. But in describing the mechanisms by which we are protected from infection, you should bear in mind that the immune systems of other mammals, birds and adult amphibians are similar to those of humans. If humans have any advantage, it is in the size of the 'repertoire' of pathogens to which our immune system can respond.

● Compared to other mammals, humans are long-lived and produce few offspring, who mature very slowly (Chapters 2 and 5). How might these features of our life history have contributed to the evolution of an exceptionally sensitive immune system?

■ In the course of our long lives, humans encounter a huge range of pathogens which, in the absence of a sensitive defence system, could damage our reproductive success. Juveniles must survive the long period before reproduction takes place, if they are to pass on their genes to the next generation. Natural selection will have favoured the survival of individuals with the most efficient immune systems and, over many generations, the genes responsible for encoding these adaptations will spread through the species as more of the 'best adapted' offspring survive.

● In what ways has human *cultural* evolution been facilitated by a complex immune system capable of responding to a huge range of pathogens? (Think back to Chapter 2.)

■ This ability has contributed to the successful colonisation by a single species, *Homo sapiens*, of nearly every terrestrial habitat, from snowfields to deserts and tropical rainforests. It has also enabled humans to eat an enormous variety of animals and plants, which carry micro-organisms and macroparasites into our bodies, and survive because the immune system (and the digestive system, the subject of Chapter 7) usually provide adequate defence. Most humans now live in settled communities in close contact with other humans and with many species of domestic animals — eating, sleeping, expelling waste and depositing rubbish in close proximity; an effective immune system is essential in a situation that so encourages the transmission of pathogens between people and between ourselves and other species.

Other developments in human culture such as mass migration of labour during times of economic disaster, famine or war, cheap air travel and package holidays to every part of the globe, and international trade in foodstuffs including livestock, have brought increasing numbers of people into contact with pathogens that were formerly restricted to a few locations. HIV is the prime example, but the spread of malaria carried by mosquitoes in the clothes and luggage of air travellers is another.

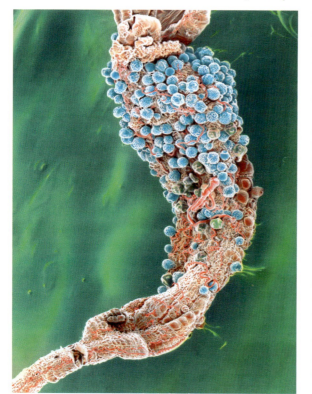

Moreover, the very fast generation time of most micro-organisms means that their genetic makeup (genotype) can change quite rapidly as mutations or 'mistakes' occur when DNA is copied during cell division. As Chapter 5 described, high rates of reproduction and mutation give pathogenic organisms an advantage in that they can evolve a succession of new varieties, a few of which will be better adapted than their predecessors at surviving inside the human body. Thus, the human immune system not only has to cope with all the existing pathogens, but also with any that may evolve in the near future.

*Electronmicrograph of the gut of a mosquito covered in malarial parasites (*Plasmodium*; the colour has been added artificially); a single infected mosquito hidden in an aeroplane can re-import malaria into areas where it had been eradicated, including Western Europe. (The electronmicrograph was taken at a magification of 300.) (Photo: London School of Hygiene and Tropical Medicine/ Science Photo Library)*

6.3.2 The need for self-tolerance

There is another vitally important reason why the human immune system (like that of other mammals and many vertebrates — animals with backbones) has evolved such complexity. In the jargon of immunology, the immune system must be able to tell the difference between 'self' and 'non-self'. Like the pathogens that penetrate its outer barriers, the human body is composed of many different kinds of cells, and many of the molecules of which these cells are composed are common to humans and pathogenic species. Despite their structural similarities, the immune system has to distinguish accurately between the body's own cells and a harmful bacterium, virus or parasite, and differentiate between an essential protein such as an enzyme or hormone and the harmful proteins (toxins) that certain bacteria secrete. More difficult still, it must detect any of its *own* body cells that are infected with viruses or other intracellular pathogens, yet leave untouched all neighbouring uninfected cells.

When the immune system is in good health, it can maintain **self-tolerance** while mounting a vigorous destructive attack on pathogenic cells and their harmful secreted molecules. Self-tolerance is the highly selective *unresponsiveness* of the immune system to the cells and molecules that make up the natural body of the host. Later in this chapter (Section 6.5.5) we will briefly describe how self-tolerance is achieved. For now, it is enough to note that self-tolerance is a property of all forms of active defence against pathogens throughout the animal kingdom.

We turn next to the most ancient defence mechanisms evolved millions of years ago in animals without backbones (invertebrates). This may seem an odd place to start a discussion of the human immune system, but we still use all these mechanisms too!

6.4 Innate immunity

Even the most simple *invertebrates* (such as worms, jellyfish, sponges, insects and shellfish) can actively defend themselves from infection, using mechanisms that have striking similarities to those found in *vertebrates* (such as fish, amphibians, reptiles, birds and mammals — including humans and other primates). These shared defence mechanisms have been given a collective name, **innate immunity**.

'Innate' means inborn or evident in all members of a particular species without the need for any prior learning experience. The term was chosen by the biologists who first began unravelling the mechanisms of the immune system because the similarities in the defences of animals as diverse as mice and earthworms were so striking that they seemed to have been 'programmed' into the earliest evolution of life on Earth. Indeed, when the DNA of very diverse animals is closely examined, similarities are found in the nucleotide sequences of some of the genes involved in generating these innate immune responses. The suggestion is that these gene sequences appeared quite early in evolutionary history, and conferred such an advantage on their possessors that they were preserved as new species evolved from their common ancestors.

The basic mechanisms that contribute to innate immunity can be broadly divided into those based on defensive cells and those based on defensive proteins, and we will look briefly at each of these in turn. Then we will 'sum up' by describing what happens if these mechanisms are all triggered at the same time in the same place, producing a chain-reaction known as an *inflammatory response*.

6.4.1 Defensive cells

In humans, all the defensive cells of the immune system are collectively called the **white cells** (or *leukocytes*).[3] White cells are often misleadingly referred to as white 'blood' cells because they are most easily detected in the bloodstream, but in reality they occur throughout the body. Innate immunity rests on three general types of white cell — the phagocytes, the cytotoxic cells, and the inflammatory cells. (Note that within each of these broad categories, there are several different named cell types, the details of which are beyond the scope of this book; if you are interested in learning more about immunology, then consult the list of further sources at the end of the book.)

Phagocytes

Phagocytosis roughly means 'eating cells'. In Chapter 3, you learned about the process called *endocytosis* in which cells take in large molecules or particles of food by enclosing a portion of the outside world in a bag of cell membrane (a vesicle) and drawing the bag and its contents into the interior of the cell. (You may wish to look back at Figure 3.9a.) All animals have **phagocytes**, cells that use endocytosis to draw pathogenic organisms into their interior, where they are rapidly destroyed. The vesicle containing the pathogen fuses with small membrane-bound packets called *lysosomes* (Figure 3.5 showed several within a liver cell). Lysosomes contain digestive enzymes and chemicals — some of which are akin to domestic bleach! — which break up the molecules of the pathogen. Some of the breakdown products are simply used as nutrients by the phagocyte and the rest are dumped outside the cell by the reverse process of exocytosis (Figure 3.9b). Figure 6.2 shows phagocytes at work.

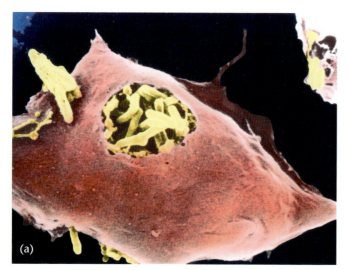 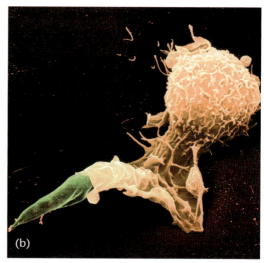

Figure 6.2   *(a) The phagocyte's surface membrane has been disrupted to reveal the bacteria (*Mycobacterium tuberculosis*) it has engulfed (photographed at a magnification of 2 700). (Photo: Juergen Bergen, Max Planck Institute/ Science Photo Library); (b) The surface membrane of this phagocyte has the characteristically 'frilly' appearance seen when it is actively engulfing a large object — in this case, a* Leishmania mexicana *parasite (green, bottom left) (photographed at a magnification of about 2 000). (The colours in both photographs have been artificially added.) (Photo: Professor S. H. E. Kaufmann and Dr J. R. Golecki/Science Photo Library)*

[3] You may need some help with pronouncing the names of cell types and processes given in this section: *leukoctyes* ('loo-koh-sights'); *phagocytes* ('fag-oh-sights') and *phagocytosis* ('fag-oh-sigh-tosis'), but note *phagocytic* ('fag-oh-sit-ic'); *cytotoxic* ('sight-oh-tox-ik') and *cytotoxicity* ('sight-oh-tox-iss-itee').

Phagocytosis is a major contributor to defence against infection throughout the animal kingdom and is possibly the most ancient of the active defence mechanisms to evolve. Some phagocytes are highly mobile and 'rove' around the body, squeezing between other cells to penetrate every tissue; others remain stationary in parts of the body where infection is likely to occur.

Cytotoxic cells

Cytotoxic cells are another general category of defensive cells; their method of attacking pathogens is not well represented by their name (which means 'cell poisoning'). In fact they do not kill pathogenic cells with poisons, but by a simple mechanical device. They manufacture cylindrical tubes of protein that penetrate the outer membrane of the pathogen's cells, even if the outer membrane is protected by a wall of sugars or a protein envelope (as it is in some bacteria).

The fluids inside a cell generally contain a more concentrated mixture of dissolved molecules than the fluid outside. This concentration gradient between the inside and the outside of the cell is maintained by the intact cell membrane, which acts as a highly selective barrier to the passage of molecules in both directions.

●   What do you predict would happen to a cell that has been punctured many times by cylindrical tubes pushed through its cell membrane?

■   The cell would be unable to prevent the collapse of the concentration gradient as dilute fluids from outside the cell rush in through the punctures. (If you are unsure about why, then look back at Figure 3.8). In the absence of an intact barrier, the concentration on both sides of a permeable membrane equalises as the molecules 'spread out' evenly through the available space.

A cell that has been punctured in many places becomes so leaky that it swells and bursts under the pressure of in-rushing fluid. Cytotoxic cells can be found in all animals. Several different types exist in humans, including the memorably named *natural killer cells* (or NK cells for short); they are all members of the white cell population. They are particularly active against any of the body's own cells that have been invaded by intracellular pathogens (all viruses, some bacteria and certain protoctists live and reproduce *inside* the host's cells). This ability to attack cells that appear to be 'altered self' is also demonstrated in the curious phenomenon of **graft rejection**.

If tissue is transplanted from the body of one person to that of another, as in a skin graft or kidney transplant, the graft is attacked and destroyed primarily by cytotoxic cells, even when the donor is closely related to the recipient. This ability is surprising since tissue transplantation is not a natural event, so why should a 'defence' against it have evolved? The likely explanation is that it is a side-effect of the ability to distinguish between self and non-self with such exquisite accuracy that even the cells of another member of one's own species are recognised as 'foreign'. You will see later (Chapter 9) how various genetic and cellular methods are being used to overcome this problem in human organ transplantation, raising a number of ethical dilemmas.

Graft rejection can be demonstrated in many kinds of invertebrates, including sponges, which may give a clue to an earlier evolutionary function. If two sponges are bound tightly together by a clamp, cytotoxic cells in each animal migrate into the area of close proximity and attack the cells of the other sponge, until a zone of dead cells is produced between them. This mechanism forces sponges to 'keep their distance' and may serve to prevent overcrowding of habitats. It is a sobering thought (if true) that the problems faced by medical science in persuading a human body to accept a transplant from another person may partly be a consequence of mechanisms that first evolved in invertebrates like the sponge.

Inflammatory cells

Another group of cells involved in innate immunity trigger local *inflammation* around an infection site. There are several kinds of inflammatory cells, but the best known are the **mast cells**, which are abundant in the airways and around the eyes. When activated, inflammatory cells release a 'cocktail' of intensely irritant chemicals, including *histamine,* which cause the walls of nearby blood vessels to swell and become very leaky, so that fluid and white cells flood out. The inflamed area feels puffy and hot and looks red because of the high blood flow.

- ● Explain why this uncomfortable inflammation is 'adaptive' in the evolutionary sense, i.e. gives some survival advantage to organisms that possess it?

- ■ The inflammatory response causes the area of an infection to be flooded with phagocytic and cytotoxic white cells and a whole range of defensive proteins. Despite the temporary discomfort, this response can eradicate an infection before the pathogens have time to multiply sufficiently to cause damage and disease.

Unfortunately, the inflammatory response is easily triggered in some people by harmless plant and animal material such as pollens and cat fur, as any allergy sufferer can testify. In such cases, the person makes a special kind of antibody that binds to the **allergen** (a general term for whatever substance the person is allergic to) and this in turn binds to and activates the *mast cells.* You will learn more about antibodies shortly. In Chapter 10 we consider the possibility that chemical pollutants in modern industrial environments contribute to the incidence of allergies. But for the moment, we focus on the effectiveness of the inflammatory response against pathogens.

6.4.2 Defensive proteins

Another major contribution to innate immunity comes from the many different proteins that directly or indirectly damage or inhibit pathogens. You met one of them earlier in the chapter (Section 6.2) — lysozyme, the enzyme that attacks unique sugar molecules in bacterial cell walls. Another protein that combats viruses is called *interferon,* so named because it 'interferes' with the process of making new virus particles inside infected host cells. We will briefly look at two more categories of defensive proteins which play an important role in innate immunity.

Antisomes: precursors of antibodies?

All invertebrates have phagocytic and cytotoxic cells as part of their defences against infection, but proteins that damage pathogens are not found in the earliest animals to evolve (sponges, corals, jellyfish and flatworms). In more complex invertebrates like the octopus, sea-urchins, insects and shellfish, proteins can be detected that bind onto pathogens but do not bind to the animal's own cells. These *antisomes* do no direct harm to the pathogen, but they are believed to be the evolutionary precursors of the *antibodies* found in all vertebrate species.

Antibodies are discussed in Section 6.6.1, but their general function is to 'label' suitable targets for destruction by other mechanisms in the immune system. For example, phagocytic cells are able to engulf bacteria much more rapidly if the pathogens have antibodies bound to their surface. In invertebrates, the antisomes seem to have the same effect. Note that the binding protein does not *directly* damage the pathogen; it simply makes the pathogen more likely to be destroyed by other mechanisms.

Complement

Another important example is a 'protein cascade' known as complement. Before we describe its action, it is worth dwelling for a moment on the general principle because **cascade reactions** are common in biological systems and you will meet another later in this chapter. In a cascade reaction, a series of molecules or cells exists in an *inactive* form; they remain inactive until a specific 'trigger' activates the first member of the series, which in turn activates the second member of the series, and so on, until the last member is activated. The final component of the series brings about a major change in the system. Generally, a 'scaling up' takes place as the sequence progresses, so that whereas only a few molecules or cells of the first member of the series were activated, they are able to activate many more molecules or cells of component two, and so on.

● What advantages can you see in cascade reactions?

■ First, the reaction can very rapidly generate a high concentration of the final component, because all the elements were pre-formed in the system just waiting to be activated. Second, the large number of steps in the sequence gives several opportunities for 'negative feedback' (Chapter 3) to influence whether the cascade proceeds beyond that step. When the outcome of a completed cascade is a major change in the system, there is an advantage in having built-in failsafe mechanisms that could switch it off at an early stage.

The complement cascade reaction is a good example of why such failsafes are advantageous. The term 'complement' refers to over 20 different inactive proteins found in certain body fluids including blood. Once activated, the proteins in the cascade build up on the surface of pathogens until the final component is activated. The final component is a cylindrical molecule rather like the protein tube produced by cytotoxic cells (described in Section 6.4.1) and with just the same function; it punctures the pathogen's cell membrane (Figure 6.3). It is vitally important that the cascade is *only* triggered by non-self cells, to avoid damaging the body's own cells, but if it *was* set off inappropriately at least there are several steps at which it might be stopped. There are two main mechanisms for triggering the complement cascade: it can be set off by unique configurations of sugar molecules found only in the walls of bacteria; also, when antibodies bind to the surface of non-self cells, they can trigger the cascade at that location.

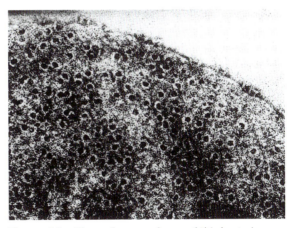

Figure 6.3 *The surface membrane of this bacterium (Escherichia coli, a causative agent of intestinal infections, including potentially fatal diarrhoeal disease) has been punctured many times by complement proteins activated by unique sugar molecules found in the surface layers of many bacteria. (The photograph was taken with an electron microscope at a magnification of 400 000.) (Photo: Courtesy of Professor Robert Dourmashkin, St Bartholomew's and The Royal London School of Medicine and Dentistry, London)*

6.4.3 Limits to the innate response

The white cells and defensive proteins described above do not occur in isolation; if pathogens get into the body, all these mechanisms are triggered at once. Most of the mechanisms of innate immunity are more effective against bacteria and protoctists than against viruses and larger parasites, which is one reason why viral infections are difficult to treat and parasitic infestations are generally long-lasting and may cause chronic illness and disability. The large parasites escape complete destruction primarily because they *are* large: it is a tall order for the immune system to destroy a worm or fluke composed of millions of cells. Viruses are simple protein boxes containing little more than a strand of genetic material (DNA or RNA), and are far less vulnerable to the puncturing techniques that damage true cells.

●   Can you think of a reason why phagocytosis may not be an adequate defence against virus infection?

■   If a phagocyte engulfs a virus it may simply aid the progress of infection, since the virus can only replicate inside a host cell.

6.4.4 Non-specific recognition of pathogens

Throughout the foregoing discussion of innate immunity, there has been a question lurking in the background, which you may now be able to answer.

●   How does a phagocyte, or a cytotoxic cell, or a protein that binds only to pathogens, accurately recognise 'legitimate' targets and attack them without harming the body's own cells? (The discussion of cell membranes in Chapter 3 may help you suggest an answer — look back at Figure 3.10.)

■   Interactions can be restricted to very specific 'partners' if a lock-and-key fit is required between the partners before a reaction occurs. Phagocytes and cytotoxic cells 'recognise' pathogens because pathogens have molecules in their structure that exactly fit the shape of receptors on the surface of the white cell (as in Figure 3.10c). These molecules must be unique to pathogens and not found in the host's cells and body fluids. Similarly, a protein that binds selectively to or damages only pathogens, does so because it can only bind to molecular shapes unique to pathogens, which are not present 'naturally' in the host.

The molecules found only in the structure of pathogens, but not in the structure of animals, are complex sugars, or sugars joined to proteins (glycoproteins) or fats (glycolipids). There are relatively few different kinds of these 'pathogen-sugars' and they are commonly found in the structures of a wide variety of different pathogens, so the ability to recognise a *few* unique sugars enables the innate immune system to recognise a *lot* of different pathogens. Recognition is *non-specific* in the sense that the animal cannot distinguish between one kind of pathogen and another, since all it is able to 'recognise' are the unusual sugars that are common to both.

Non-specific recognition of pathogens is a *defining characteristic* of innate immunity. Invertebrate animals are only able to recognise pathogens in this non-specific way, but it seems to give adequate protection from the relatively limited range of pathogenic organisms that infect invertebrates. Remember that 'adequate protection' simply means that, even though some individuals in the host species may die from the infection, many survive.

6.4.5 The evolution of innate immunity

During the long evolution of animal species in close interaction with pathogens — particularly the bacteria, which were the first to evolve — animals that were able to recognise pathogens and attack them were at a *selective advantage*; that is, they were more likely to survive and reproduce than animals that could *not* defend themselves as effectively from infection. This statement is an expression of how evolution by natural selection operates at the level of 'whole organisms' in the hierarchy of biological organisation.[4] Another way of saying the same thing, but at the *molecular* level, is 'animals whose cells carry receptor molecules, which exactly fit the shapes of complex sugars found only in the structures of pathogens, are at a selective advantage'.

● Can you rewrite the last sentence to describe how selection would operate at the *genetic* level?

■ Animals whose DNA includes genes that encode the instructions for making receptor molecules, which exactly fit the shapes of complex sugars found only in the structures of pathogens, are at a selective advantage.

The unique sugars commonly found in the structures of pathogens have probably been extremely stable components of these organisms over millions of years of evolution. We can infer this from the fact that the relatively small number of different receptors required to fit (and hence recognise) all of these unique molecules can be found on the surface of defensive cells in animals throughout the animal kingdom. The widespread existence of these receptors and the genes that code for them are evidence for the coevolution of pathogens and their hosts over a very long time-scale; so long that, even as new animal species evolved, they preserved the genes involved in recognising pathogen structures.

However, a feature of evolution that you should recall from Chapter 5 is increasing diversity. As time passes, so more species evolve and though some become extinct, new species are continuously forming. By 500 million years ago, all the major kinds of animals alive in the world today were already present. The evolution of vertebrates created extremely varied habitats in which new strains of pathogen could evolve. The strategies that had evolved to protect invertebrates from infection were not adequate to defend vertebrates from this rapidly increasing and diversifying array of pathogenic organisms. Reinforcements were required!

6.5 Adaptive immunity

6.5.1 The evolution of adaptive immunity

Much of the current understanding of the cells and molecules involved in defensive reactions to infection in the human immune system has been worked out by extrapolating from research done on rats and mice.[5] It may seem rather implausible at first glance that these animals have much in common with us, but think again! Like us they are highly successful *mammals* (warm-blooded, hairy animals that give

---

[4] The hierarchy of biological organisation is illustrated and discussed in *Studying Health and Disease* (Open University Press, 2nd edn 1994; colour-enhanced 2nd edn 2001), Chapter 9, particularly Box 9.1 and Figure 9.1.

[5] The practical and ethical issues raised by the use of animals as substitutes or 'models' for humans in biomedical research is discussed in *Studying Health and Disease* (Open University Press, 2nd edn 1994; colour-enhanced 2nd edn 2001), Chapter 9.

birth to immature offspring, which are fed initially on their mother's milk); brown rats and house mice live in communal groups in close contact with humans in virtually every habitat on Earth, and they eat an enormous variety of foods. Inevitably, they too have evolved a complex immune system to cope with the wide range of pathogens they encounter in their daily lives. They have the added practical advantage of breeding prolifically in laboratories as well as in their natural habitats.

You will recall that *Homo sapiens* was a late-comer on the evolutionary scene, arriving less than 2 million years ago, but worms had already been here for around 750 million years and reptiles preceded us by at least 500 million years. The innate mechanisms they evolved to cope with infection can be found in the human body today. This is not to imply direct lineage between ancient species and modern humans; it may simply be that similar solutions to the same problem have evolved independently in several different parts of the animal kingdom, in much the same way that birds, insects and bats independently evolved wings as a means of flight. But looking at other organisms gives an insight into the selection pressure exerted by the evolution of an increasingly varied array of pathogenic organisms. As time passed and yet more species of pathogen evolved, so the complexity of the immune systems in their host species increased because only the 'fittest' survived to reproduce and pass on their genes.

Innate immunity only recognises the *major* molecular differences between host and pathogen, such as unique sugars and proteins shared by many different types of bacteria and viruses, but never found as part of the host's cells. A more difficult problem for a complex animal's immune system is to recognise and attack a pathogen that is *itself* an animal (such as a tapeworm), rather than a bacterium or a virus, and which is therefore constructed from molecules that are mostly the *same* as those of the host's own body. Moreover, as more and more different kinds of microscopic pathogens evolved, many of them took to colonising the *inside* of the host's own cells, making them much more difficult to detect. Exquisite precision is necessary in these circumstances to distinguish between the cells and molecules of which the pathogen is constructed and those of the host.

6.5.2 Specific recognition of pathogens

The *additional* pathogen-recognition mechanisms evolved only by vertebrates, which enable them to achieve this 'fine focus', are known collectively as **adaptive immunity**, for reasons that will emerge later. They reinforce and extend the capabilities of the innate mechanisms already described, which remain the foundation of our own defence against pathogens.

Animals with adaptive immunity are capable of detecting extremely small variations in the surface contours of molecules; they can recognise any molecular shapes that are even very slightly different from quite similar molecules normally found in the host. These tiny unique 'non-self' molecular shapes are clusters of a few amino acids (the building blocks from which proteins are made; Chapter 3) and are collectively known as **epitopes**. Note that adaptive immunity is based on recognising unique fragments of *proteins*, in contrast to innate immunity which recognises unusual *sugars*.

Any large molecule or cell that contains epitopes in its structure is called an **antigen**. The toxins produced by certain bacteria typically contain several different epitopes, each constructed from tiny sections of the large protein molecule as it coils in space (see Figure 6.4a). Virus particles and whole cells, such as bacteria or protoctists, and the cells of larger parasites, may have hundreds of different epitopes in their structure (Figure 6.4b).

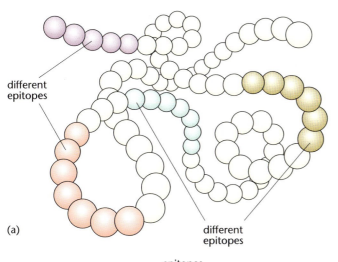

different epitopes

different epitopes

(a)

Figure 6.4 *An antigen is a large molecule or cell with one or more unique areas (epitopes) in its structure, which are recognised as 'non-self' by the host's adaptive immune system. (a) In this sketch, a large molecule contains four different epitopes, each of which is recognised as non-self because cells in the host's immune system have antigen receptors that exactly fit these epitopes. The rest of the molecule does not trigger an immune response because the host's own body contains these same molecular configurations; they appear to be 'self'. (b) A single-celled pathogen has many copies of several different epitopes in its structure.*

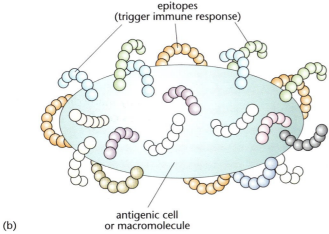

epitopes
(trigger immune response)

antigenic cell
or macromolecule

(b)

Each organism has a characteristic array of epitopes, which together make up a sort of 'call-sign' for that pathogen. Thus, the epitopes on the influenza virus are different from those on the measles virus; those on the bacteria that cause tuberculosis are different from those on the bacteria that cause pneumonia, and so on.

The adaptive immune system can recognise these epitopes because the defensive cells on which it relies carry **antigen receptors** with binding sites that exactly 'fit' the shapes of pathogen epitopes. The principle of lock-and-key interactions between antigen receptors on the host cells and unique molecular shapes on the pathogen's surface is the same as in innate immunity, but the adaptive immune system has to generate *millions* of different antigen receptors in order to recognise the millions of tiny molecular differences between itself and all the pathogens the host might encounter in its lifetime.

The massive 'repertoire' of different antigen receptors involved in adaptive immunity is in sharp contrast to the relatively small range of receptors found on the cells involved in innate immunity. Innate immunity only operates at the 'broad brushstroke' level of distinguishing self from non-self, without being able to recognise more subtle distinctions between (for example) two strains of bacteria. But the adaptive immune system is capable of such exquisite recognition of tiny molecular differences between cells that it can, in effect, 'tell one pathogen from another' because each pathogen has a unique set of epitopes and can be recognised quite *specifically* by the host's immune system. The adaptive immune system in humans is the most sensitive in the animal kingdom. It has been estimated that each of us can detect at least *100 million* different epitopes that occur in the structures of cells other than our own.

So great is the capacity for non-self 'pattern recognition' that individuals can also distinguish between the molecules on the surface of their own cells and those of their closest family members. This capacity is demonstrated by the rejection of transplants, even between first-degree relatives, unless the graft-recipient's immune system is suppressed by drugs. The only exception is when the graft-donor and recipient are identical twins; since their genes are identical, all the molecules on the surface of their cells are also identical and the graft appears to be 'self' to the recipient.

6.5.3 Millions of antigen receptors

The extraordinary capacity for recognising vast numbers of different non-self molecular shapes (epitopes) ensures that vertebrates have a high probability of detecting any pathogen they may encounter during their relatively long lives. Although humans can generate the largest repertoire of differently shaped antigen receptors, and so can recognise the greatest range of different epitopes, other mammals and birds are not far behind. The range of recognition gets steadily more restricted in the earliest vertebrates to evolve, such as reptiles and sharks and, as described earlier, in invertebrates recognition is restricted to a few large and unusual sugar molecules commonly found in many bacteria and viruses.

However, the need to recognise at least 100 million different epitopes poses the human genotype with a packaging problem. If you think back to the lock-and-key analogy of shape recognition, then we need 100 million different 'keys' to fit these 100 million different 'locks'. As each unique epitope fits into the binding site of just *one* unique receptor shape, this means in practice that there must be at least 100 million differently shaped antigen receptors on the surface of cells in the human immune system, each of which exactly fits an epitope that might occur somewhere in nature — past, present or future.

● What does this imply about the number of genes required to encode these antigen receptors?

■ 100 million different antigen receptor shapes ought to mean 100 million different genes, each one encoding the structure of one receptor.

Human DNA only contains about 40 thousand genes altogether, with much else to do besides detecting pathogens. How can so few genes contain the codes for so many different receptors? The solution to this problem takes us back for another look at DNA.

6.5.4 Shuffling genes to create receptor diversity

In Chapters 3 and 4 we described the way in which the instructions for making a unique protein are contained in the sequence of nucleotides of a single unique gene. At this point we have to confess that the notion that 'one gene makes one protein' is an oversimplification. The study of the adaptive immune system brought about a minor revolution when it was recognised that certain large and complex proteins involved in the immune response to pathogens were actually assembled from several smaller proteins, each coded for by different genes. This discovery proved to be the key to the puzzle of how the human adaptive immune system could make 100 million different receptor proteins with apparently far too few genes for the task.

Imagine that you had just a few hundred different genes to play with, but you needed 100 million different proteins. If each of those proteins was assembled from sections encoded by about six different genes, then how many unique combinations of six genes could you get from a pool of several hundred? Hundreds of thousands of different proteins could be generated by 'shuffling' the combinations of a few hundred genes. Then imagine that when the sections of protein were assembled, they could be spliced together in a variety of ways. This process introduces yet more diversity, more than enough to produce over 100 million different receptor proteins, each one capable of binding to just one epitope shape.

The genes that code for the receptors involved in pathogen-recognition are 'shuffled' early in embryonic development in members of the white cell population called **lymphocytes** ('lim-foh-sights'). The lymphocytes are the principal cells on which *adaptive* immunity rests.

Humans contain versatile bone marrow **stem cells**, so-called because they give rise by cell division to all the lymphocytes and to the many other kinds of white cell that take part in immune responses (such as phagocytes and cytotoxic cells), and also to red blood cells and platelets, which are part of the blood-clotting mechanism. (We will discuss these stem cells further in Chapter 9, when we consider their potential uses in medical treatments for a wide range of degenerative diseases.)

In their DNA, these stem cells have several hundred genes that contain the coded instructions to make several hundred different sections of possible antigen receptors that could bind to different epitopes. As the stem cells divide and mature to give rise to new lymphocytes, all but five or six of these several hundred receptor-genes are lost from the DNA that is passed on to each of the 'daughter' cells. The losses are random and as a result each daughter lymphocyte inherits a *unique* set of five or six genes, just enough to code for a single uniquely shaped antigen receptor. The surviving genes are 'spliced' together by special enzymes that join the broken pieces of DNA (see Figure 6.5).

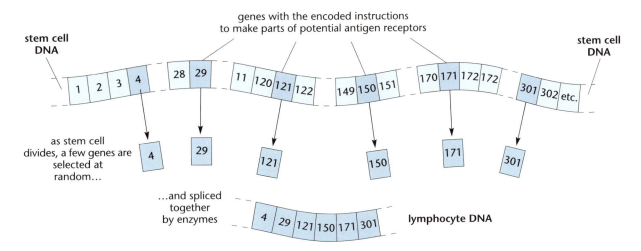

Figure 6.5   *Each lymphocyte inherits a unique combination of a few receptor-genes from the pool of several hundred receptor-genes in the stem cell's DNA. It then has the coded instructions to make one receptor shape and hence to bind to one specific epitope. (The dashed lines indicate where long sections of DNA have been omitted from the drawing to save space.)*

The joins are somewhat haphazard, which introduces yet more variation into the nucleotide sequence that each lymphocyte inherits. By shuffling a few hundred genes and 'dealing them out' to the lymphocytes in random combinations, at least 100 million different antigen receptors can be generated, enough to fit every epitope likely to be encountered in a lifetime. But the random nature of the shuffle creates another problem: it is inevitable that it will also generate receptor shapes that 'fit' parts of the molecules from which the host's own body is made. Unless these 'self-receptors' are eliminated, the adaptive immune system will turn on the host.

6.5.5   The induction of self-tolerance

Early in embryonic life, when millions of different antigen receptor shapes are being randomly generated as new lymphocytes form, these receptors inevitably collide with complementary shapes on cells and macromolecules in the embryo. In the protected world of the embryo, unless one of the few infections that cross the placenta strikes (e.g. rubella), all the molecular shapes that these receptors encounter are part of the embryo and thus part of 'self'. Each time a receptor binds to part of a self-molecule in the embryo, the lymphocyte that carries that receptor undergoes profound changes in its ability to respond to that epitope. The mechanisms underlying this 'self-learning' process are complex and beyond the scope of this chapter, but the overall effect is that by the time of birth, all the lymphocytes in the body have become *unresponsive* to the body's own cells and molecules.

● Explain why the cells involved in *innate* immunity do not need this process of 'learned unresponsiveness' to self.

■ None of the receptors on phagocytes or other cells in the innate immune system 'fit' self-molecules; they only bind to the relatively small number of unique pathogen sugars.

By contrast, learned unresponsiveness is essential if the adaptive immune system is to remain self-tolerant for the lifetime of the host. The breakdown of self-tolerance is a serious business. Several important **autoimmune diseases**, including rheumatoid arthritis, multiple sclerosis and juvenile-onset diabetes, involve self-destruction of body tissues by the host's own immune system, because the mechanisms that maintain self-tolerance have failed.

In the normal course of events, lymphocytes are responsive only to cells or molecules that have, in their structure, 'non-self' epitopes that are recognised by antigen receptors. Once a lymphocyte has bound to its matching epitope, a series of reactions is set off in the immune system which culminate in the destruction of the pathogen or the toxic molecule of which that epitope was a part. As you will see later, the adaptive response crucially also involves the full range of *innate* defences which are recruited to join the attack.

6.5.6   Scaling up the adaptive immune response

It may have been puzzling you why the additional protective mechanisms evolved by vertebrates are called 'adaptive'. The term is a little unfortunate because it has one meaning in evolutionary biology, which is already familiar to you, but another in immunology which has yet to be explained. Adaptive in its evolutionary sense describes a characteristic that increases the likelihood that an organism will survive long enough to reproduce, and this is clearly true of all aspects of the immune response to infection. Having an immune system is certainly 'adaptive' in that sense of the term. But immunologists use it to describe an adaptation which takes place in response to infection *during the lifetime* of an organism. In other words, the term is being used to describe a *developmental* rather than an evolutionary feature. So how does the adaptive immune system *adapt*?

Think back to the previous discussion about shuffling genes and remember that each lymphocyte carries on its surface many copies of the *same* antigen receptor, which can bind to just *one* shape of epitope. Although each individual lymphocyte can only recognise a single epitope shape, *between them* the entire population of lymphocytes has receptors for at least 100 million different epitopes. A useful new term can be introduced here: identical lymphocytes carrying the *same* antigen receptors — and hence capable of binding to the same epitope — are said to be members of the same **lymphocyte clone**. It follows that there must be at least 100 million different lymphocyte clones in the human immune system — each capable of recognising a *different* epitope.

This leads to another 'space' problem. Imagine a pathogen such as a bacterium, which has (say) 10 different epitope shapes in its structure, each recognised by the members of a different lymphocyte clone which carry the matching antigen receptors. Ten lymphocytes would not be enough to mount an effective immune response against a pathogen that was actively reproducing (some bacteria can double their numbers every 20 minutes!) — in reality many millions of lymphocytes are required. But the human body is not large enough to accommodate 100 million different clones of lymphocytes, *each* consisting of millions of cells. Moreover, if it *did*, this would be a very wasteful use of precious resources, because only those lymphocytes that recognise the pathogens which the host actually encounters during its lifetime would ever be called upon for protection. All the rest would be a waste of space and energy. A much more economical solution has evolved, which is known as **clonal selection**. Figure 6.6 (overleaf) shows the sequence of events.

First, the few lymphocytes that had the correct antigen receptors to bind to unique epitopes on the pathogen (clonal selection) are triggered by the encounter to multiply by numerous cell divisions (**clonal expansion**). We should note at this point that clonal expansion *also* requires several chemical signals from other types of white cell, to which we will return shortly. Every daughter cell derived from this replication process is identical to the parent, so all the new lymphocytes in the expanded clone have the *same* antigen receptors, which bind to the *same* unique epitope shape, and hence bind to the pathogen that triggered the original cell.

When a particular pathogen is encountered for the first time, it takes a few days before a large enough clone of defensive lymphocytes has been generated to mount an effective attack; this is called the **primary immune response**. During the delay, the pathogen could multiply sufficiently to cause illness in the host. Once all the pathogens have been destroyed, the defensive lymphocytes engaged in the original attack die within a few days, so they are unable to contribute to an immune response if the same pathogen re-enters the body. (This 'programmed cell death' is an example of a phenomenon to which we will return in Chapter 8.)

However, as the original clone is expanding, thousands of the new lymphocytes *differentiate* (change) into a more specialised cell type known as **memory cells**, which survive for months or even years after the pathogen has been eliminated. If that same pathogen gets into the body again, the memory cells can multiply far more quickly than was possible the first time around. The enhanced

secondary immune response may be fast enough to prevent symptoms from occurring, and it generates even more memory cells so that a third infection has even less chance of taking hold. This ability to adapt and improve the defensive response as a consequence of an encounter with a specific pathogen underlies the term *adaptive* immunity.

● When children are immunised against common infectious diseases such as whooping cough and diphtheria, they are usually given three injections of the vaccine at intervals of several months. What do you think the vaccine might contain? Why do three, spaced injections give better protection than one?

■ Vaccines contain samples of the unique epitopes found in the structure of the pathogens you wish to protect the child against. The first injection triggers off a primary immune response, in which the few lymphocytes capable of recognising those epitopes multiply into large clones and long-lived memory cells are formed. The second and third injections trigger the production of even more memory cells, so that if the live pathogens ever get into the body they will be eliminated before they can cause illness. (We discuss vaccines in more detail at the end of this chapter.)

Adaptive immunity is a very specific form of defence. Pathogens that get into the body once are likely to get in again, so it is advantageous to be 'primed and ready' for them. But the adaptation that follows an infection or a vaccination with a specific pathogen (such as measles) does not change the number of lymphocytes capable of recognising most *other* pathogens. So, for example, immunity to measles does not improve the immune response to the polio virus, or the bacteria that cause TB, or the malarial parasite, or anything else you might think of. However, there are a few closely related pathogens that have some epitopes in common, so immunising against one of these pathogens gives some protection against the other. The most famous example is illustrated by the work of the English country doctor Edward Jenner who, at the end of the eighteenth century, protected people from smallpox by scratching their skin and introducing matter from cowpox pustules; the viruses that cause the two diseases are closely related.

6.6   Collaboration between innate and adaptive immunity

The principal way in which the adaptive immune system protects us from infection is by directing the mechanisms already described for innate immunity to much greater effect. To see how they do this, we must look at lymphocytes more closely.

Lymphocytes come in two main 'families': the *T cells* and the *B cells* ('T' and 'B' refers to 'thymus' and 'bone marrow' respectively, the sites in the body where these cells mature). Each of these families of lymphocyte has a very diverse range of functions, which are the subject of weighty textbooks; we have space here for only the most basic details. What they have in common is that each T cell or B cell has antigen receptors on its surface that can bind to a single epitope shape, and they all undergo clonal selection, clonal expansion and memory cell formation after the original contact with their matching epitope (as in Figure 6.6) and other activating signals. They all interact with the innate immune system in various ways.

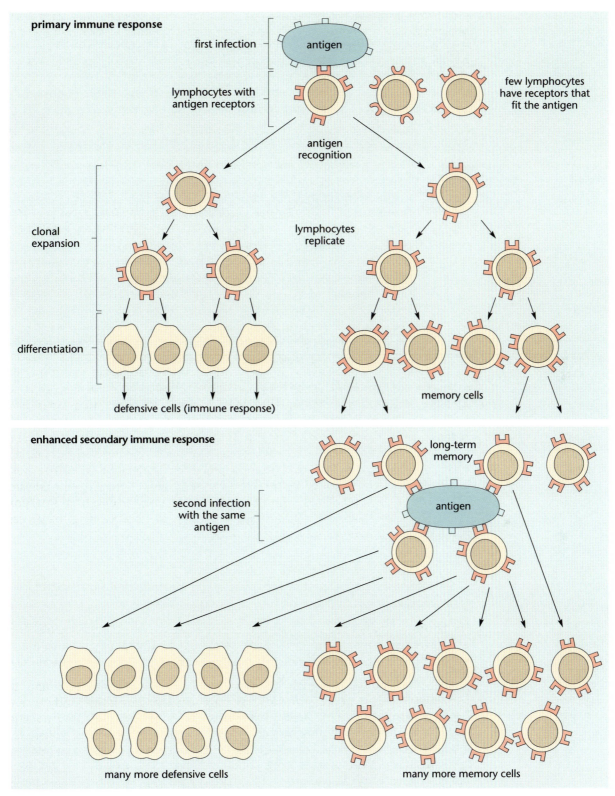

Figure 6.6   *Clonal selection is a defining characteristic of adaptive immunity. It enables the immune response to a pathogen to be highly specific and rapidly 'scaled up' as the original lymphocyte replicates to give a greatly expanded clone of active defensive cells. The formation of memory cells during the primary immune response enables any subsequent encounters with the same pathogen to trigger an even faster secondary immune response.*

6.6.1 B cells and antibodies

B cells are a type of lymphocyte which, when activated by contact with the correct epitope and certain chemical signals, synthesise and secrete complex proteins known as **antibodies**. Each B cell produces only one type of antibody, which has in its structure two identical binding sites that fit a single epitope shape (Figure 6.7). Each activated B cell synthesises millions of identical antibody molecules, all of which bind to the same epitope and hence to the same pathogen, leaving the 'stem' of the antibody molecules exposed on the pathogen's surface.

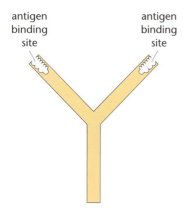

antigen binding site   antigen binding site

Figure 6.7 *Schematic diagram of an antibody molecule; the two identical binding sites at the tips of the 'arms' have a three-dimensional structure that exactly fits the shape of a specific epitope.*

The importance of antibodies in an immune response to an active infection is that they 'label' pathogens for destruction by the mechanisms of innate immunity. Antibodies themselves are harmless, but a pathogen that has antibodies bound to its surface is rapidly detected by phagocytes and cytotoxic cells, which might otherwise fail to recognise it. Remember, the cells of innate immunity can only detect a relatively few unusual sugars in pathogen structures, but they all have receptors that bind onto the exposed 'stem' of antibody molecules which stick out like flags when the antibodies are bound to epitopes. The antibodies act as 'bridges' between the antigen and the defensive white cells, enabling them to get a better 'grip' on their target. Antibody molecules bound to a pathogen are also potent triggers of the complement cascade, with results already illustrated in Figure 6.3.

The fact that the interaction between an antibody molecule and its matching epitope is highly specific has enabled them to be used in diagnostic tests. The presence of antibodies in a person's body that can bind to the epitopes of a certain pathogen demonstrates that the person is, or has recently been, infected with that pathogen. This is the basis of the HIV test, which detects antibodies in the person's bloodstream that bind selectively to samples of HIV particles in a laboratory test. The virus particles themselves are not detected directly, but their presence is inferred from the presence of specific 'anti-HIV' antibodies in the blood.

Antibodies have become an important research tool because of their ability to 'pick out' their matching epitope and bind to it in laboratory tests, even when the epitope is in a complex mixture of other molecules. This is precisely what happens in life, where antibodies bind only to their matching epitope even though faced with a massive array of other molecular shapes on all the cells and molecules of the body. At the end of this chapter, we will look briefly at ways in which this specificity may be harnessed by medical science.

6.6.2 T cells

The other family of lymphocytes on which adaptive immunity depends are the **T cells**. There are two basic types. **Cytotoxic T cells** function in much the same way as the cytotoxic cells described earlier under innate immunity, but with much more precision in their selection of targets. They have evolved in response to pressure from pathogens that replicate inside the host's own cells, where only the most subtle recognition systems can detect them. But as you will see shortly, they cannot do this without collaboration from the innate immune system.

● Which types of pathogens are the cytotoxic T cells best adapted to attack?

■ All viruses, intracellular parasites such as *Plasmodium* (which causes malaria), and some of the smallest bacteria which replicate inside the host's cells (e.g. those causing TB and leprosy).

Helper T cells secrete over 20 different signalling molecules (cytokines) with the general property of enhancing the effectiveness of all the other contributors to an immune response (Figure 6.8) — the phagocytic, cytotoxic and inflammatory cells of the innate immune response *and* the B cells and T cells of the adaptive immune response. They are thus the principal 'conductor' of the immune orchestra. They also secrete *interferon*, a defence molecule we mentioned earlier, which 'interferes' with the construction of new virus particles within host cells; and they synthesise some of the components of the *complement* cascade.

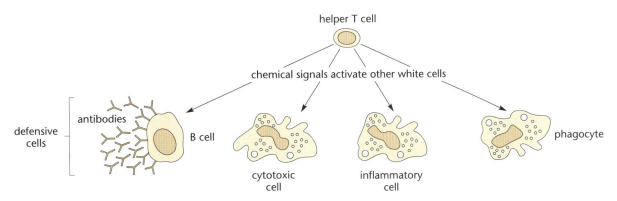

Figure 6.8 *Both the innate and adaptive mechanisms of the immune response are regulated by the activity of helper T cells. Although many other regulatory mechanisms exist, the immune system cannot function effectively without the helper T cells.*

It would be misleading to suggest that the helper T cells are the only regulatory influence on the immune system (for example, the helper T cells themselves require a whole range of chemical signals from certain phagocytes, which are in evolutionary terms a much 'older' type of cell), but they are pivotal in tilting the balance of survival in the host's favour.

6.6.3 Policing the body

So now you have a general picture of innate and adaptive immunity and can view the adaptive mechanisms as a later evolutionary development that can 'piggy-back' on the older innate responses to infection, giving them more direction and impact. But there is a vitally important aspect of the immune response in which the adaptive mechanisms are *reliant* on the innate mechanisms; this has to do with maximising the chances of a pathogen that gets into the body 'meeting' the few lymphocytes that can recognise it.

Before the primary immune response to a certain pathogen is triggered by the first encounter with a specific pathogen, there are only a few thousand mature lymphocytes in the body with the correctly shaped receptors capable of binding to it. If you consider that there are normally around 2.5 million lymphocytes in total in each ml of blood, and the average adult human has a blood volume of 5 litres, then the total number of mature and immature lymphocytes in the bloodstream alone is roughly 12.5 billion. But there are about 900 billion in the lymphatic system (Figure 6.9 overleaf) and roving through the tissues!

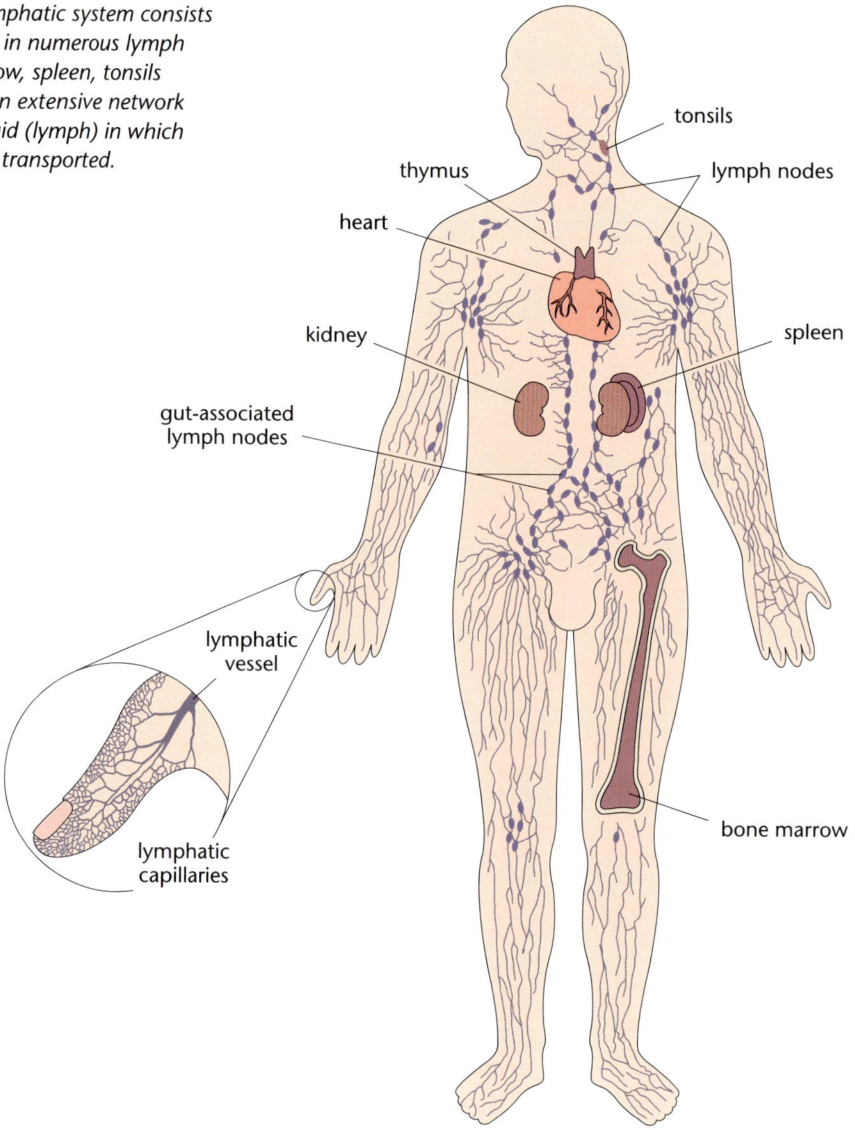

Figure 6.9 *The human lymphatic system consists of solid masses of white cells in numerous lymph nodes and in the bone marrow, spleen, tonsils and thymus, connected by an extensive network of capillaries containing a fluid (lymph) in which white cells and nutrients are transported.*

Against this background, you can see that the chance of a random encounter between a certain pathogen and one of the few lymphocytes that can recognise it is not high.

Lymphocytes (both T cells and B cells) spend less than 10 per cent of their lives circulating around the body in the bloodstream or lymphatic vessels. The rest of the time they stay in the various *lymph nodes* (solid masses of white cells, bounded by a membranous wall) which can be found throughout the body, but are particularly noticeable in the neck, armpits and groin (they can be felt as 'swollen glands' during certain infections), or in major lymphoid organs such as the spleen, thymus and bone marrow, or in the sheets of membrane that join together loops of gut in the abdomen (Figure 6.9).

All these sites of static lymphocytes have a blood supply and a lymphatic supply, so any pathogens that get into either of these circulatory systems will be swept along and eventually reach a lymph gland or organ. There the pathogen may 'bump into' a lymphocyte that has the correct receptors on its surface to fit its unique epitopes, which all sounds rather 'hit and miss'. The human body is a vast assembly of suitable habitats for a huge variety of different organisms, some of which are lethal if allowed to reproduce. It would not be an adequate strategy simply to wait for a chance encounter with the immune system. A better method of policing the body that evolved quite early in evolutionary history, is based on the highly mobile *phagocytes.*

Phagocytic cells can move freely around the body, either in the bloodstream or by squeezing between the cells of which all our tissues are made. Apart from the cornea (lens of the eye) there is nowhere they cannot reach; they can even get into the brain. Phagocytes come in different kinds, each of which has a particular 'territory', but all take the same action whenever they encounter a pathogen. First they engulf it (look back at Figure 6.2), then they break down its structure into small sections and transport those sections back to the cell's own surface, where they expose bits of pathogen (with its various epitopes) on their *own* cell membrane. Finally, they head for the nearest lymph node or lymphoid organ, to 'present' the pathogen epitopes they have acquired to the helper T cells.

This essential step in the immune response is known as **antigen presentation**. Without it, the precise mechanisms of the adaptive immune response fail to operate. For example, B cells cannot produce antibodies without chemical signals from helper T cells, but the T cells are not triggered to produce these signals until they have been presented with the correct epitopes by phagocytes. Similarly the cytotoxic T cells also require epitopes to be 'presented' to them before they are correctly activated and can destroy host cells infected with internal pathogens.

Moreover, in the act of presenting epitopes to the T cells, the phagocytes also give information about where the original infection can be found. We mentioned earlier that each type of phagocyte has a particular territory, so the T cell has only to identify which type of phagocyte has arrived to know something about its 'usual address'. This mechanism assists in directing the adaptive immune response to the correct location, and is another example of collaboration between the evolutionarily 'ancient and modern' branches of the immune system.

6.7 Pathogens fight back

The versatility of the human immune system, combining both innate and adaptive mechanisms, has exerted selection pressure on the array of human pathogens. Those that have evolved strategies to counteract the host's immune response are at a selective advantage and increase in the population, generation by generation. As we described in Chapter 5, humans and their pathogens have *coevolved.* A vast number of different mechanisms have been evolved by successful species of larger parasites, protoctists and bacterial or viral strains, which increase their chance of survival. We have space here to review only a few of these so-called pathogen *escape mechanisms*, but their variety testifies to the random nature of the mutations that generated such diverse solutions to the same problem: how to survive in the hostile environment of the host's body.

● Can you think how an invading pathogen might evade detection?

■ You might have thought of several ways, including 'covering over' an epitope so the host's antigen receptors cannot bind to it, or changing the actual shapes of the epitopes frequently, so the pathogen stays 'one step ahead' of the immune response.

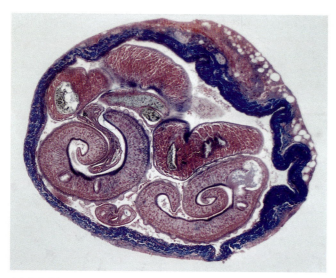

Adult Schistosoma mansoni *flukes blocking a blood vessel leading from the liver (maximum diameter of the larger male worms in the section is about 1 mm); one reason for the success of these parasites, which infect over 200 million people worldwide, is that they disguise themselves from the host's immune system by concealing their own epitopes under a layer of molecules 'borrowed' from the host. (Photo: Courtesy of Professor John Lewis, Royal Holloway College)*

Some pathogens conceal their unique epitopes from the immune system under a coating of other molecules that resemble those of their host. *Ascaris lumbricoides*, the most common roundworm infesting the gut, has a coating of molecules that closely resemble human collagen, a component of human cartilage and the deeper layers of the skin. More effective still are those pathogens that 'borrow' molecules from their host to coat themselves with. The surface layer of the bacterium *Staphylococcus aureus*, which causes abscesses, secretes an enzyme that coagulates clotting components in human blood, which then adhere to the bacteria. Various species of *Schistosoma* flukes, which cause the tropical disease schistosomiasis, coat themselves with a whole range of their host's proteins and sugars.

An entirely different strategy is to change the shapes of the unique epitopes on the pathogen's surface very frequently, a process known as **antigenic drift**. This is one of the escape mechanisms displayed both by HIV and the influenza virus.

- How would it help a pathogen to evade destruction by the immune system if it changed the shapes of its epitopes?

■ The first time the host's lymphocytes encountered that pathogen, they would mount a relatively slow and ineffective *primary* immune response, which usually gives the pathogen enough time to replicate successfully and move on to a new host. If the same pathogen is encountered again, the *secondary* immune response may be strong enough to eradicate the pathogen. But if it has changed the shape of its epitopes between the first and second encounter, the immune system responds to it slowly, as though meeting it for the first time.

In HIV, the genes that encode the surface epitopes are highly unstable and prone to mutate. HIV changes its epitopes so fast that, even within the same person, an increasing number of new strains of the virus are generated the longer the infection persists. The waves of influenza that sweep across a country from time to time are the result of a new variant of the influenza virus that no one has encountered before. Antigenic drift is an illustration of the fact, emphasised in Chapter 5, that pathogens can evolve faster than their hosts because of their much shorter generation time.

- How does the 'escape' mechanism of antigenic drift create difficulties for vaccination programmes to prevent outbreaks of influenza?

■ The vaccine can only contain samples of epitopes from influenza strains that already exist. It cannot protect people from new variants that arise by mutation. (If a vaccine against HIV is ever to be developed, it will have to overcome the same problem.)

The most common pathogen escape mechanisms might be summed up as 'resisting arrest'. Many kinds of pathogens synthesise and secrete chemicals that deter phagocytes or cytotoxic cells from approaching or getting a grip on them. Others secrete enzymes and 'blocking' proteins that break down or inhibit the important molecular defences in the immune response, such as complement, lysozyme and antibodies. Viruses, protoctists and bacteria that reproduce inside the host's cells are more difficult for the immune system to detect or attack without causing substantial damage to neighbouring healthy tissue. These varied escape mechanisms illustrate the delicate balance that has been struck between 'host kills pathogen' and 'pathogen kills host'.

6.8   Variations in immune responsiveness

Before leaving the inner world of infection and response, we return to the territory of Chapters 4 and 5 and the information contained there about variation in the susceptibility of populations and individuals to disease.

6.8.1 Genetic variation and immunity

Each of us has a unique genotype and just as this affects our ability to withstand or sustain lung damage from tobacco smoke, or to produce the enzymes necessary for adequate digestion and nutritional health, so too it affects our resistance to infection. The frequency with which a population encounters a certain pathogen over many generations results in the selection of genotypes that confer some *resistance* to that pathogen (Section 5.7.1). Similarly, where a pathogen is rare, there is only a very weak selection pressure to favour the increase in the population of genes that confer some protection against this pathogen. Thus, the arrival of colonists in the Americas resulted in devastating infection among the indigenous populations from pathogens to which the settlers were relatively immune.

Even within a single population, there is enormous variation between individuals, as you might expect. At one end of the spectrum can be found rare individuals with genetic defects in their immune system that are so severe they can only survive in highly protected environments. At the other end of the spectrum, the differences between one person's susceptibility to infection and another's are so subtle that they can only be inferred by extrapolation from studies of laboratory rats and mice. In rodents, it is clear that the immune responsiveness of each animal has a 'personal profile' in which certain pathogens are attacked more effectively than others. Thus, each individual may be a 'good responder' to certain pathogens, but have less effective responses to certain others, and may not be able to respond at all to a very few. The pathogens that provoke high or low responses vary from one individual animal to the next. It seems likely that the same is true for humans.

6.8.2 Variation across the lifespan

Immune responsiveness varies not only between individuals, but within the same person at different times in their lives.

● When would you expect a person to be most vulnerable to infection in their lifetime and why?

■ In early life, when every pathogen is being encountered for the first time, so that all responses are of the slower *primary* type.

Babies and infants are also more vulnerable to infection because certain features of the immune system take up to two years to mature. But they are born with pre-formed antibodies already circulating in their bloodstream, which came across the placenta from their mother's circulation. Her immune system makes antibodies to any pathogen she has encountered in the previous few months, which she 'donates' to the baby while still in the uterus and, after birth, in her breast milk (which, by the way, is pathogen-free). The antibodies in breast milk survive digestion in the baby's gut and give some protection against those pathogens most likely still to be in the local environment. (We discuss the role of breast milk in infant nutrition in Chapter 7.)

At the other end of the lifespan, the effectiveness of the immune system to respond to encounters with new pathogens gradually declines in old age. Elderly people usually retain their immunity to any infection they have previously encountered and successfully eliminated, but may succumb to new infections, particularly those affecting the respiratory system. This vulnerability may partly be due to a lifetime of breathing pollutants (particularly tobacco smoke) and partly due to 'shallow' breathing which leaves parts of the lungs inadequately inflated and creates suitable habitats for bacteria to multiply. Other aspects of changed biology in old age are discussed in Chapter 8 of this book.

6.8.3 Stress and the immune response

A possible cause of variation in susceptibility to infection that has created much speculation is *stress*. This 'catch-all' term has so many different meanings that it is extremely difficult to be certain whether or not the normal stresses encountered in everyday life have any *significant* effect on immune responsiveness.

It is commonly believed that at times of emotional stress, people are more likely to get minor coughs and colds, but this effect has been very hard to demonstrate conclusively in well-designed experiments on human subjects living 'normally' stressful lives. Too many other variables get in the way. However, several studies of university students show that they have higher concentrations of common bacteria and viruses in throat swabs during exam periods than at other times of the year; certain parameters generally taken as indicating the level of immune responsiveness (e.g. antibody levels in the blood) are also depressed (see, for example, Maes *et al.*, 1998; Marshall *et al.*, 1998). One interpretation of these findings is that exam stress made the immune system less efficient and allowed more pathogens than usual to grow in the students' throats.

●   Can you think of an alternative explanation?

■   The students may have been *behaving* differently during the exam period than at other times of the year, with the result that they were more exposed to infection; for example, they may have smoked more cigarettes than usual, creating a sore throat where bacteria could get in.

Even though the experimental data linking everyday levels of stress to suppression of the immune system are not conclusive, the mechanisms by which stress could *in theory* increase vulnerability to infection are at least understood. A defining characteristic of the response to stress is the secretion of hormones (corticosteroids) from the adrenal glands, which increase the mobilisation of stored fats and sugars and their conversion into usable energy. This is an adaptive response to stress (adaptive is used here in its evolutionary sense), and is part of what is generally known as the 'fight or flight' reaction. However, it seems to have an unfortunate side-effect in that these same adrenal hormones reduce the effectiveness of the immune response.

● Think back to Chapter 5 and suggest an evolutionary explanation for such an apparently risky consequence of the physiological reaction to stress.

■ There appears to be a *trade-off* going on: the resources required for defence against an immediate short-term threat (such as the arrival of a predator) are being diverted from another, less immediate use — readiness to repel an infection that might not in fact materialise.

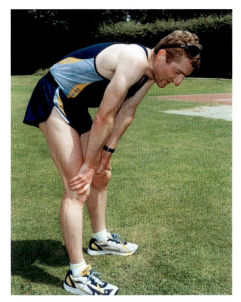

Although there is no consensus about whether short-term inhibition of the immune response actually results in greater susceptibility to infection, *chronic* stress lasting weeks or months has many adverse effects on health, including elevated risk of heart disease, hypertension, gastric and duodenal ulcers, stroke, anxiety and depression. Seen against this list of consequences, increased vulnerability to infection may be among the least problematic outcomes.

Heavy exertion can result in suppressing the immune system for between 3 hours and 3 days, particularly if the exercise is unfamiliar, or is prolonged as in the case of athletes in intensive training. (Photo: Mike Levers)

Evidence concerning the effects of intense or excessive *exercise* on the immune system is more convincing. Several studies have shown increases in the rates of infection among elite athletes in training for major competitions, especially for endurance events like the marathon; similar results have been recorded in unfit individuals who begin strenuous training for an unfamiliar sport (see, for example, Brines *et al.*, 1996; Mackinnon, 2000; Nieman, 2000). But moderate *regular* exercise may boost the immune system.

6.9   Harnessing the immune response

Finally, we offer a glimpse into the many ways in which medical science is attempting to harness the immune response in the prevention and treatment of disease — not all of which are caused by pathogens.

6.9.1 Conventional vaccines

Earlier in the chapter we mentioned **vaccination**, using fragments of pathogens (sub-unit vaccines) or whole killed pathogens (e.g. heat treated or freeze-fractured and dried). These are the easiest vaccines to produce, as long as you can grow sufficient quantities of the pathogen in otherwise sterile conditions, i.e. uncontaminated by other pathogens, yeasts, toxins, etc. More difficult technically are the *attenuated* vaccines, containing live pathogens from a less virulent strain than the usual disease-causing organism; generally, these attenuated strains have been produced in the laboratory by inducing the original pathogen to mutate and then selecting those with low virulence.

Conventional vaccination programmes have achieved some remarkable successes, most notably in 'The global eradication of smallpox', the title of an article by

Marc Strassburg.[6] The smallpox story illustrates the extent to which the biology of the pathogen can profoundly affect the ability of medical science to act against it.

● What features of the smallpox virus made it particularly vulnerable to eradication by a vaccination programme?

■ It can only reproduce in humans; there are no reservoirs of infection in other species. It has a short incubation time and it does not produce 'carrier' states in which people who seem well are actually infectious (which is the case with many other infections, e.g. typhoid, HIV), and it spreads from person to person fairly slowly. It was also possible to produce a stable 'freeze-dried' vaccine containing smallpox virus epitopes.

Vaccination against polio — another viral infection — has also been remarkably successful: down from 350 000 cases worldwide in 1988 to under 1 500 in 1999. The polio vaccine is very stable and has the additional merit of surviving digestion in the gut, so it can be given by mouth. Other pathogens have proved harder to counter by vaccination because they have none of the advantageous features described above. An additional problem arises where it is difficult to obtain adequate or stable samples of the pathogen's epitopes to use as the basis of the vaccine. This is the case with leprosy and malaria where the pathogens have proved extremely difficult to grow in bulk.

However, there are disadvantages with conventional vaccines. Sub-unit vaccines and those based on intact killed pathogens tend to elicit relatively short-term immunity, so they need 'boosters' at frequent intervals. And although they trigger the production of specific antibodies in the immunised person, they are generally rather weak at triggering immune responses from cytotoxic cells. This means that they give less effective protection against pathogens that hide inside the host's own cells.

● 'Live' attenuated vaccines, by contrast, generate long-lasting cytotoxic immunity, but they have one serious drawback. Can you suggest what it is?

■ There is always the danger that one of the attenuated pathogens could mutate again and recover its original virulence.

The difficulty in producing attenuated strains of HIV has held up the search for a vaccine to protect the world's population against AIDS.

6.9.2 Genetically engineered vaccines

Genetic engineering is providing a new approach to this problem. The gene coding for an epitope that is unique to a certain pathogen can be removed from the pathogen's DNA and inserted into the DNA of harmless, fast-growing bacteria, which then manufacture the epitope in bulk as though it was one of their own proteins. It should even be possible to generate all the mutations of a gene that encodes a pathogen epitope, and induce bacteria to synthesise all these different epitope variants, which can then be delivered in a vaccine.

[6] Reproduced in *Health and Disease: A Reader* (Open University Press, 2nd edn 1995; 3rd edn 2001); this article was set reading for *World Health and Disease* (Open University Press, 2nd edn 1993; 3rd edn 2001), Chapter 3.

● What pathogen escape mechanism will a vaccine produced in this way overcome?

■ The genes encoding the epitopes of some pathogens (e.g. HIV and the influenza virus) undergo *antigenic drift*, i.e. they mutate frequently, changing the epitope's structure slightly each time. If a genetically engineered vaccine already contains all the possible mutant forms of the epitope, then even if new variants arise in pathogens in the future, the immune system of vaccinated individuals will already have been primed to respond.

The feasibility of producing genetically engineered vaccines has greatly increased in recent years, as complete DNA sequences for the genomes of many pathogens have been worked out, including those of many pathogenic viruses and bacteria. In addition, at the time of writing (late 2000), geneticists were close to completing the genomes of the parasites that cause malaria (*Plasmodium*) and sleeping sickness (*Trypanosomes*). A team from the French Pasteur Institute and Britain's Sanger Centre have identified the 4 000 genes of the TB bacillus (*Mycobacterium tuberculosis*), a breakthrough that will provide a wealth of new vaccine and drug targets to be tested against the increasingly drug-resistant TB strains which have emerged around the world. As well as providing a source of potential vaccines, the knowledge of the many genes within pathogenic organisms might enable drug companies to design targeted pharmaceutical agents.

6.9.3 DNA vaccines

One of the most recent developments in vaccine design is called *DNA vaccines* (reviewed in Weiner and Kennedy, 1999). Instead of splicing the DNA coding for a pathogen epitope into a harmless bacterium (which, as described above, then makes the protein that goes into the vaccine), medical scientists have discovered that delivering the DNA *itself* directly into the person to be immunised will do the job just as well — in fact more efficiently. The DNA can be injected into the skin or propelled through it by a high-pressure 'gene gun'. Once the gene encoding the pathogen epitope gets into a host cell, its nucleotide sequence is translated into new proteins which resemble the epitope. The body responds by producing antibodies *and* cytotoxic T cells directed against the epitope. These responses may be sufficient to protect the recipient from infection with that pathogen, although in early trials the effect is relatively short-lived.

However, this approach is promising because large quantities of DNA vaccines could be readily produced, containing the codes for thousands of different epitopes at once. A further advantage is that DNA is a relatively stable molecule, so it can be stored and distributed easily. In 2000, trials were underway into DNA vaccines against TB, HIV, malaria, influenza and herpes virus.

6.9.4 Vaccines against cancers?

Perhaps the most exciting and unexpected applications of knowledge about the immune system relates to the major degenerative diseases, in particular to cancers. It used to be thought that the immune system was on general 'surveillance' for abnormal cells arising by mutation during an individual's life, which might become malignant. It turns out that the immune system has only a limited role in cancer control in humans, except for those cancers which are themselves triggered by pathogens that the immune system can detect. Cancer cells are not 'foreign' material, but self-cells that behave in an abnormal manner (we return to this subject in Chapter 8), and are ignored by the immune system which is self-tolerant. However, it might be induced to attack cancers by a variety of manipulations.

In theory, it might be possible to generate anti-cancer antibodies from B cells which have been given additional genes in the laboratory. Or *hybrid* antibodies can be made — with human 'stems' to the antibody molecules (see Figure 6.6), linked to antigen-binding sites taken from mouse antibodies that recognise epitopes on human cancer cells.

●   If mice can be induced to produce antibodies directed against human cancer cells, why can't mouse antibodies be used as therapeutic agents in people? What is the reason for developing mouse–human hybrid antibodies?

■   Mouse antibodies would be identified as 'non-self' and destroyed by the human immune system if they were used as a vaccine; the hybrid antibodies have human protein 'stems' so they are much less likely to trigger an immune response.

If antibodies can be made that bind only to cancer cells, they might also be used as carriers of toxic molecules or radioactive isotopes, which could then be targeted onto the cancer very precisely (a so called 'magic bullet' therapy). It might also be possible to harness the many chemicals involved in inflammatory reactions and direct those more effectively against cancers. If genes can be identified which are cancer-cell specific, the use of DNA vaccines which generate both antibody and cytotoxic T cell responses against malignant tumours might prove powerful tools.

In Chapter 9, we explore further the manipulation of human biology for therapeutic ends and ask what ethical dilemmas are raised by 'tinkering with nature'? But this book has other aims before we turn towards the future. The story of human evolution and its impact on human health and illness is more than the interaction between humans and their pathogens. In the next chapter, we move on to a completely different, but equally vital aspect of human biology: how people deal with food and the products of digestion and absorption.

OBJECTIVES FOR CHAPTER 6

When you have studied this chapter, you should be able to:

6.1 Define and use, or recognise definitions and applications of, each of the terms printed in **bold** in the text.

6.2 Describe the basic mechanisms involved in the innate and adaptive responses of the human immune system to an infection, and comment on the evolutionary pressures that may have shaped this system.

6.3 Illustrate the general features of the primary and secondary immune responses to pathogens and give examples of states of deficiency or inappropriate activity of the immune system.

6.4 Give examples of ways in which variation in the biology of either the human host or the pathogen can affect the outcome of an infection, illustrating the unstable equilibrium between survival and destruction.

6.5 Outline how a knowledge of pathogen genomes or pathogen epitopes could be exploited to harness the immune response for therapeutic purposes.

QUESTIONS FOR CHAPTER 6

1   (*Objective 6.2*)

The human immune system is capable of recognising at least 100 million different epitopes, which may occur in the structures of pathogens or the molecules they secrete. What other features of human biology and culture have contributed to the evolution of this enormous repertoire, or have been facilitated by it?

2   (*Objectives 6.2 and 6.3*)

The common cold is caused by rhinoviruses, of which there are several hundred different kinds. Children suffer repeated colds, often several in one year, but adults get fewer and fewer colds and they have generally become a rarity in old age. Explain this phenomenon in terms of the immune response to infection.

3   (*Objectives 6.3 and 6.4*)

In what ways does the human immunodeficiency virus (HIV) 'escape' destruction by the immune system?

4   (*Objective 6.5*)

How might a knowledge of the genome of HIV help in the search for an effective vaccine?

CHAPTER 7

Digestion and dietary change

Study notes for OU students

This chapter is about the biological mechanisms that convert food into biochemically usable nutrients. It relates to changes in the human diet during the last 10 000 years, including the impact of agriculture and pastoralism (Chapter 2). Chapter 3 gave essential background on how molecules pass across cell membranes (Section 3.3.4), and the importance of negative feedback in regulating homeostasis (Section 3.8.2, particularly Figure 3.18). Chapter 4 discussed phenotype, genotype and the inheritance of dominant and recessive alleles. The discussion of blood glucose regulation builds on earlier material in *Studying Health and Disease* (Open University Press, second edition 1994; colour-enhanced second edition 2001), Chapter 9. The present chapter also relates to *World Health and Disease* (Open University Press, third edition 2001), Chapter 11, which discusses the contribution of diet to growth and maturation, its role in certain diseases, and the genetic modification of crop species.

7.1 Food — a biological challenge

All living organisms need food; most plants can synthesise nutrients from water and other minerals when they are exposed to light, but animals eat only other organisms, either while they are still alive (e.g. the animal tissues eaten by certain parasites, and plants eaten by grazing and browsing animals) or when they are dead. Eating and digesting other organisms presents three major kinds of biological problems.

First, all organisms consist of large, chemically complex molecules, which are at least as complex, and often chemically very similar, to those of the eater. So digestion requires breaking down food without harming oneself.

Second, food is often available only infrequently and in large chunks — more so, of course, for lions or polar bears, which eat perhaps twice a week, than for humans who generally eat several times a day. However, *metabolic activity* (all the biochemical activities necessary for breathing, moving, thinking, etc.) goes on continuously: we use a bit less biochemical energy while asleep in a warm bed, and more during strenuous exercise, but most of the processes that keep us alive go on all the time. So the mammalian body faces a dilemma: its food supplies arrive intermittently, but usage of the nutrients is more or less continuous.

Third, intimate contact between the eater's tissues and those of potentially harmful organisms in our food is almost unavoidable. Consuming living or freshly dead micro-organisms can be very risky. Fresh or inadequately cooked meat, and animal products such as milk and eggs, may harbour many symbiotic bacteria; in many parts of the world meat may be infested with macroparasites or with prions (see Chapters 2 and 5). Cooking kills most living organisms (and freezing kills some of them), but all fresh or cold food is 'contaminated' with micro-organisms that fall on it from the air. Most of these are harmless, and some foods, such as cheese, yoghurt and beer, are made by culturing micro-organisms, which give them a distinctive taste and texture. Even if micro-organisms are excluded or killed, our food contains 'foreign' proteins, which in some individuals can stimulate the immune system to make an allergic response.

● What food (other than very hot food) is normally completely free of micro-organisms? (We mentioned it in Chapter 6.)

■ Breast milk, as long as it passes directly from the mother to the infant.

However, milk is an excellent culture medium for micro-organisms and most animal milk is contaminated by the time it reaches the human consumer — one reason why an essential part of the process of digestion even for babies is inactivation of potentially harmful organisms.

This chapter explains how human digestion and metabolism deal with these three problems.

7.2 Digesting food

Most food consists mainly of large, chemically complex molecules that, for reasons outlined below, must be *digested* (broken down) into much smaller molecules before they can be *absorbed* into the body and utilised. **Digestion** and **absorption** are separate processes and it is important to consider them individually.

From the point of view of digestion, the constituents of food can be classified as *fats* or *lipids* (including oils), *carbohydrates* (starches, sugars) and *proteins* (e.g. lean meat, fish, egg white). Most natural foods are mixtures of these major constituents, plus smaller quantities of *vitamins*, *minerals* (sodium, iron, calcium, etc.) and various non-nutritive components that are discussed later.

7.2.1 Enzymes

The principal agents of digestion in all organisms (micro-organisms, fungi and some green plants as well as all animals) are *enzymes*, protein molecules that facilitate the making or breaking of chemical bonds between other molecules (a look back at Figure 3.11 will remind you of how they *catalyse* — speed up — chemical reactions). Most enzymes are effective only for one particular, or a few very similar, kinds of chemical reactions, and particular molecules can usually only be joined or severed by one unique enzyme. The first step in enzyme activity is specific binding of the enzyme to certain parts of the molecule (or molecules) involved in the reaction. Once in use, a typical enzyme remains active often only for a few minutes, or at most a few hours.

Most of the hundreds of different kinds of molecules that animals take in as food are so large and chemically robust that several different **digestive enzymes** operating in succession are necessary to break them down into fragments small enough to be absorbed. The names of most enzymes end in *-ase*. For example, the many enzymes that attack different parts of protein molecules are collectively known as *proteases*. The enzyme *lactase* binds to and splits one particular bond in the sugar lactose, breaking it into two almost equal-sized, but chemically slightly different sugars called glucose and galactose. Later in this chapter, you will learn the significance of this reaction for human nutrition.

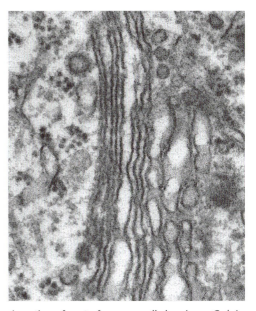

All enzymes are synthesised inside cells in the same way as other protein molecules. As soon as they are formed, the enzymes (often in a non-active form) pass to a structure called the *Golgi body*, where they are enclosed in an envelope of membrane. Thus parcelled up, they move to the edge of the cell and are *secreted* (expelled into the surrounding medium) when required.

● Why do you think digestive enzymes are thus parcelled up before being secreted into the fluid outside the cell?

■ The material to be digested is chemically very similar to the cells that produce the digestive enzymes. If the enzymes were not contained in this way, they would digest the cell itself.

A collection of cells whose main function is secretion is called a **gland**; sometimes individual secretory cells 'embedded' in other tissues carry out this function, and sometimes they are densely packed together into a secretory organ bounded by its own membrane. You will encounter both types of gland as we take a journey down the human digestive system.

A section of part of a nerve cell showing a Golgi body, magnified 15 000 times by an electron microscope. Golgi bodies are 'stacks' of internal membranes in which secretions such as digestive enzymes are modified, stored or wrapped in membrane before being expelled from the cell. (Photo: Heather Davies/The Open University)

7.2.2 The digestive system

The gut of all mammals is a series of chambers and tubes lined by cells with contrasting properties. As it passes along the gut, the food comes into contact with many different enzymes and different chemical environments. Our next task is to describe the structures and functions of the human gut from end to end. Figure 7.1 shows the main features of the **human digestive system** and the organs associated with it. The 'tube' from mouth to anus is generally referred to as the **gut**.

In humans, digestion starts in the *mouth*; chewing breaks up the food and an enzyme secreted from the salivary glands attacks certain bonds in starches. A complex muscular action called swallowing compresses the food into small balls and propels it through muscular, non-secretory portions of the gut called the *pharynx* and *oesophagus*, and down to the stomach. Swallowing is greatly facilitated by the secretion of **mucus**, a watery lubricant, which — in the mouth comes from the salivary glands (as you will see as we progress down the gut, *all* of it is lubricated by mucus secreted by specialised cells in the gut wall). Figure 7.1 shows that the pharynx is also the route through which air moves from the nose and mouth to the trachea (windpipe) on its way to the lungs.

● Look at Figure 7.1; what happens when we 'choke' on food?

■ A piece of food goes 'the wrong way', entering the top of the trachea where it immediately provokes powerful, unsuppressable contractions of the breathing muscles (coughing) which propel the food back into the gut.

A gulp of water stimulates swallowing, which helps to convey the misdirected piece of food down to the stomach. Choking is most likely to happen when we try to eat in strange postures, such as while lying down, and in infants, in whom coordination of swallowing and breathing is imperfectly developed.

Digestion in the stomach

The *stomach* is a highly distensible bag, expanding in adults from an empty volume of only about 0.05 litres to as much as 1.5 litres after a large meal. Special cells in the lining secrete water, hydrochloric acid and enzymes, particularly proteases that are adapted to work efficiently in an acid

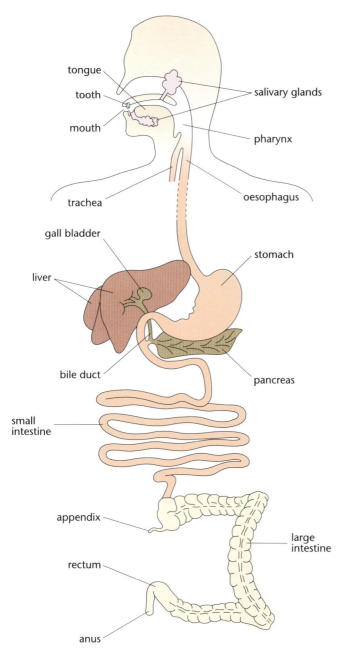

Figure 7.1 *The anatomy of the human digestive system and other organs with a role in digestion.*

environment. On a normal diet, the stomach lining of an adult secretes about 2 litres of fluid per day into the stomach. The digestive action of these secretions is assisted by rhythmic, sometimes powerful, contractions of the muscles of the stomach wall, which break up the food and mix it with the acid and enzymes. The hydrochloric acid makes the mammalian stomach one of the most acidic environments known in any biological system. Some components of food are broken down directly by the acid. Stomach acid dissolves pieces of bone, tooth or eggshell, in the same way as vinegar or bleach dissolves chalk. And, of course, all but a very few kinds of micro-organisms die instantly in a strongly acid environment.

● What happens to the remains of the micro-organisms killed by the stomach acids?

■ Micro-organisms are chemically very similar to plant and animal tissues, so the dead cells are digested in exactly the same way as 'proper' food.

The cells lining the stomach wall are protected from the acid and their own digestive enzymes by secretions of thick *mucus*. Most nutrients cannot cross this protective layer but a few, notably alcohol and certain fats, diffuse through it and the cellular lining of the stomach, whence they pass into the blood.

● What are the implications of this property for the action of alcoholic drinks?

■ Alcohol enters the blood, and hence reaches the brain, within a few minutes of being swallowed, much faster than most other components of meals.

Under some abnormal circumstances, the mucus layer is breached and the enzymes and hydrochloric acid erode the stomach wall, causing a painful disorder called a gastric ulcer. You will see later how ulceration is enhanced by the presence of certain bacteria, which are capable of colonising this mucus.

Passage through the stomach takes 2 to 6 hours depending upon the quantity of food and its chemical composition. Food consisting mainly of carbohydrate passes through more rapidly than that rich in protein, while fatty meals remain in the stomach for the longest time. The contents of the stomach leave in 'pulses' as the pyloric valve (which separates the stomach from the small intestine) opens and closes. At this stage, the homogeneous mixture of food and enzymes has the consistency of a fairly thick soup.

Digestion in the small intestine

The next structure in the digestive tract is the *small intestine*, which is a coiled, muscular tube approximately 6.4 metres long (21 feet!) and 2.5 centimetres in diameter, lined with many different kinds of cells. It is divided into three anatomically distinct segments: the *duodenum* (about 20 centimetres long), *jejunum* (2.5 metres) and *ileum* (3.7 metres).[1]

Secretions from the liver and the pancreas enter the duodenum through a shared duct a few centimetres from the pyloric valve. The liver secretes a yellow fluid called **bile** (about half a litre a day in adults) which is stored and concentrated in the gall bladder, a small sac under the liver, until eating stimulates its discharge. The active

---

[1] You may need help with pronouncing the names of these segments: *duodenum* ('dew-oh-deen-um'); *jejunum* ('jeh-joon-um'); *ileum* ('ill-ee-um').

ingredients of bile are not enzymes but complex salts that emulsify fats (emulsification breaks up fats so that they can mix with water, just as adding washing-up liquid does to fatty deposits on crockery); this process makes the molecules of fat accessible to enzymes that operate best in a watery, rather than a fatty, environment.

The *pancreas* is a much smaller gland than the liver (the pancreas of cattle and pigs used to be sold by butchers as 'sweetbreads'). It secretes about 1.5 litres of **pancreatic fluid** per day, containing a mixture of several different enzymes that digest fats, proteins and carbohydrates. Bile and pancreatic fluid also contain salts that neutralise the acid from the stomach, so the contents of the duodenum are only slightly more acid than the blood. The secretory cells in the lining of the small intestine itself also secrete over 1.5 litres of fluid daily, containing various enzymes that digest carbohydrates and proteins. All these enzymes can only function in a near-neutral (non-acidic) environment. Together they break up digestible carbohydrates into small sugars (mostly glucose and galactose), fats are broken down into fatty acids, and proteins into short chains of a few amino acids or into single molecules of the 20 different amino acids from which they are composed.

The scale of the operation is enormous: many common proteins in meat and grains contain thousands of amino acids, and the bonds that join them all together are severed during digestion. Mammalian digestion is very efficient; the combination of stomach acidity, enzyme activity and muscular churning at 37 °C breaks down food very fast and thoroughly. Consider how long meat, cabbage, etc. take to rot on a compost heap, compared to how long it takes a similar meal to go through you, or — even more impressive — through a cow or a sheep. Even at 100 °C, an Irish stew takes many hours to be reduced to a smooth soup!

● What do you think happens to the enzymes that were produced by the cells lining the stomach, when they reach the small intestine along with the food they have been digesting?

■ Stomach enzymes are adapted to work in a strongly acid environment, so they would be ineffective in the much less acidic contents of the small intestine. They are broken down by proteases of the small intestine in exactly the same way as the proteins in food, and thus their molecular constituents are 'recycled'.

As in the stomach, the secretions of mucus lubricate the food and protect the lining of the small intestine from being digested by its own enzymes. Rhythmic muscular contractions of the intestine wall, called **peristalsis** (pronounced 'perry-stall-sis'), aid digestion and absorption by stirring the gut contents and propelling them along at speeds of between 0.5–2.0 cm per second. The time spent by gut contents in the small intestine is very variable and difficult to measure. This region is the main site of absorption of nutrients from the gut contents and sometimes little of the original food remains.

7.2.3 Gut parasites and pathogens

● Why are endoparasites such as tapeworms and roundworms (see Chapters 2 and 5) more likely to settle in the small intestine than in the stomach?

■ The stomach is too acid for most parasites to live in. The small intestine is much less acidic and so is a more congenial environment.

The gut contents in the small intestine are also more thoroughly digested, making the nutrients in it more easily absorbed by the parasite as well as by the person. Parasites such as tapeworms (*Taenia*) and *Toxocara* (nematode parasites of dogs and cats, which can also affect people, Chapters 2 and 5) enter the body through the mouth, as eggs or dormant cysts, encased in a tough, impermeable shell that can resist hours of exposure to stomach acid and enzymes. After hatching in the small intestine, tapeworms attach themselves firmly to the gut lining, thereby resisting expulsion by peristaltic movements, and grow into soft, flattened 'tape'-shaped animals, which gain maximum contact with the nutritious gut contents. A few bacteria, among them *Vibrio cholerae* (which causes cholera), have also evolved the ability to form cysts that protect them from digestion by their host.

In the 1990s, medical researchers identified another bacterium that has evolved ways of surviving even in the harshest environment in our digestive system — the stomach. This spiral-shaped bacterium, *Helicobacter pylori* (or *H. pylori* for short) can live in the thick layer of mucus which lines the stomach wall, feeding on local nutrients. It is now known to be a major cause of *gastric ulcers*. (An *ulcer* is a localised inflammation which becomes so severe and persistent that a wound opens in the tissue at its centre; *gastric* ulcers occur in the stomach and *duodenal* ulcers in the duodenum — together, they are sometimes referred to as *peptic* ulcers.) Colonies of *H. pylori* survive by generating chemicals to neutralise the acid surrounding the infection site.

H. pylori is also protected from the body's natural defences by the mucus lining the stomach; the immune system is triggered by the presence of bacteria to send phagocytes and cytotoxic cells to the stomach wall, but they cannot reach the bacteria harboured by the mucus layer. The immune response is continuously activated by bacteria which it cannot eradicate and local inflammation occurs, damaging the stomach wall and eventually causing a gastric ulcer. *H. pylori* can also grow in the duodenum (the first short segment of the small intestine) and nearly everyone with a duodenal ulcer is found to be infected. Once the link between *H. pylori* and ulcers in the gut had been made, an antibiotic therapy was developed which eradicates the infection and enables the ulcerated gut wall to heal.

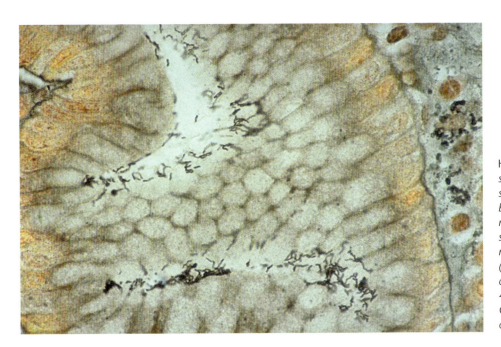

Helicobacter pylori *stained with a silver-stain appear as tiny black strands in the mucus lining the human stomach, in this microscope slide. (Photograph was taken at a magnification of 400.) (Photo: Joel K. Greenson MD, University of Michigan Hospitals)*

7.3 Absorption of nutrients

As well as completing the digestion of food, the small intestine is also the main site for absorption of the digested nutrients into the blood. On a regime of small, regular meals, most absorption takes place in the duodenum and jejunum, but the ileum is also absorptive, and acts as 'spare capacity' for absorption, becoming functional following very large meals. The whole of the small intestine is pleated and lined with tiny finger-like projections called *villi* (pronounced 'vill-eye', singular: villus, shown in Figure 7.2), whose surface is further frilled out to form microvilli, which maximise the surface area in contact with the intestinal contents.

The inner layer of cells forming a villus contains a mosaic of secretory and absorptive cells. The secretory cells are of two types. One kind secretes mucus that acts as a protective barrier against the digestive enzymes in the intestine, and the other secretes the digestive enzymes. At the base of the villi there is a layer of smooth muscle whose contractions churn the intestinal contents and move them down its length. The outermost layer of the small intestine (not shown in Figure 7.2) contains secretory cells, which lubricate its external surface, enabling the loops of gut to glide easily against each other and against other organs packed into the abdomen.

In the central region of the villus there are vessels of the blood system and the lymphatic system (these systems were depicted earlier, in Figures 3.21 and 6.8). In the gut, the lymph transports fats absorbed across the gut wall and eventually delivers them to the bloodstream. The lymphatic system also removes excess fluids, bacteria and the cell debris that results from the body's immune responses to

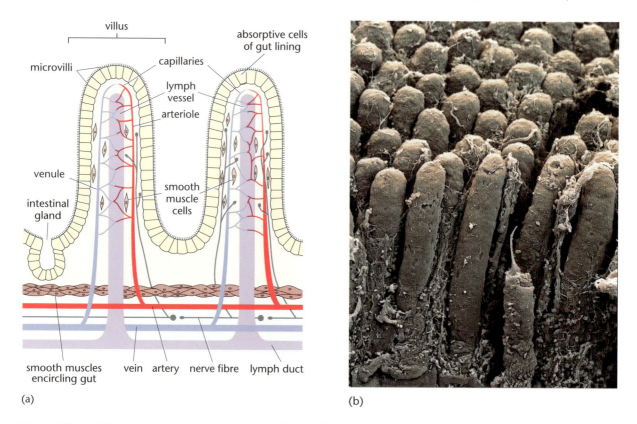

(a)

(b)

Figure 7.2   *(a) The general structure of the lining of the small intestine. (b) Scanning electron micrograph of villi in the human small intestine magnified about 100 times. Each villus projects about 1 mm into the gut cavity. (Photo: CNRI/Science Photo Library)*

infection. The small intestine is also richly perfused with blood, which then flows through the liver (where some of the newly absorbed nutrients undergo important chemical modifications), before passing through the heart and on to the lungs, limbs and peripheral tissues. After a heavy meal, a large proportion of the total blood volume in the body may be around the intestine and in the liver.

7.3.1 Passive diffusion and active transport

Cell membranes are made of fatty, rather than watery, materials (depicted earlier, in Figure 3.7), so the breakdown products of fats enter the gut lining quite well by passive diffusion, although they are mostly larger molecules than glucose and amino acids. Most other fat-soluble nutrients, such as vitamins A, D, K and E, are also absorbed passively through the cells lining the small intestine, as are the major ingredients of bile, which are taken up from the bloodstream by the liver and 'recycled' to produce more bile.

Some larger particles are actively engulfed by endocytosis (see Figure 3.9a); membranes of cells lining the small intestine form a vesicle around the particle into which digestive enzymes are secreted and the nutrients thus released are absorbed by the cell. Many other kinds of molecules do not enter cells by passive diffusion and can pass only through specific channels in the cell membrane. For some nutrients, including glucose and all the common amino acids, transport is not only restricted to particular sites on the cell membrane but is also 'active' in the sense that metabolic energy is necessary to convey each molecule from the gut contents into the tissues. Absorption of the minerals calcium and iron also involves specific transporter mechanisms. However, the gut of newborn infants is very much more permeable than that of adults and admits quite large molecules fairly indiscriminately.

The sites of active transport into the cells lining the gut are identified by specific protein molecules called receptors, which are embedded in the cell membrane and 'match' the chemical structure of their target molecules (as described in Chapter 3, see Figure 3.10). When the receptor has bound to the appropriate molecule in the gut contents, it transports it through the cell membrane and releases it into the cell. You should picture the lining of the small intestine as a mosaic of many different channels, each specific to a particular kind of molecule, that act as a sort of molecular 'escort service'. Nutrients are picked up from the gut contents and conveyed, molecule by molecule, into the blood.

As we noted earlier, the gut lining, liver and pancreas secrete large quantities of *water* into the gut, where it facilitates the digestion and movement of the food. Water is much too precious to be expelled with the undigested remains of meals, so most of it is reabsorbed. There is no active transport system, or indeed any specific channels, for water uptake, so you may wonder how it gets back into the body from the watery slurry of digested food in the gut.

● Salts (particularly sodium, potassium and chloride) are absorbed actively from the digested food and transported across the gut wall where they enter the blood and lymph. How does this process facilitate the reabsorption of water from the gut contents?

■ Active transport of salts produces a concentration gradient, with more on the inside of the gut wall than in the gut contents; water follows passively to equalise the concentration of salt solutions between the lining of the intestine and the gut contents (this process was depicted in Figure 3.8).

7.3.2 Disorders of digestion and absorption

As you have seen, digestion and absorption are both very complicated processes involving many different kinds of molecules, some of which (e.g. enzymes and receptor molecules) are unique proteins, each coded for by a different gene. If the gene is absent or (more commonly) significantly modified, either no protein is produced, or it is present but malformed, so it cannot do its job properly. You will not be surprised to learn that *disorders of digestion*, arising from the inability to synthesise certain digestive enzymes, or *disorders of absorption*, due to the absence or abnormality of a receptor protein, are among the commonest kinds of genetic diseases in humans.

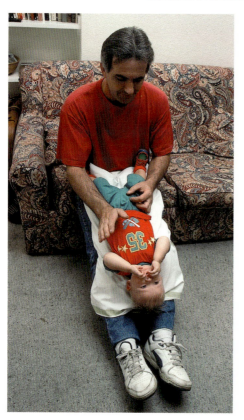

Children with cystic fibrosis need daily physiotherapy to help clear the mucus that builds up in their lungs; they also experience recurrent digestive disorders. (Photo: Courtesy of Camilla Jessel/Cystic Fibrosis Association)

The inherited disorder, cystic fibrosis, is an example of a disease that arises from a deficiency in a transport protein. As you saw in Chapter 4, the incidence of the disease in families and careful analysis of the DNA of affected people indicate that cystic fibrosis is due to the inheritance of two defective alleles of a single gene. The *CFTR* gene codes for a protein which is involved in salt transport across the surface membrane of cells lining the small intestine. The protein directly regulates the channel through which chloride (a constituent of common salt) passes across cell membranes. The most troublesome symptoms of the disease involve the accumulation of thick mucus in the respiratory system (facilitating the growth of pathogenic bacteria), but excessive mucus in the digestive system can cause recurrent diarrhoea, abdominal pain and even obstruction — all of which can be attributed to defects in chloride absorption.

Vitamins and minerals are essential to healthy nutrition, but the mechanisms by which they are absorbed are complicated and still incompletely understood. It is clear, however, that molecules produced higher up in the gut can be essential to the uptake of iron, and possibly other minerals, in the small intestine. If such factors are lacking, absorption may be so inefficient that, even if the diet contains more than enough of the essential mineral, almost none of it is taken up by the gut lining and into the blood. An example of the complexity of the steps involved in absorption of minerals is given by *pernicious anaemia*. The root cause is now known to be the lack of factors that enable the absorption of *vitamins*. These, in turn, facilitate the transport of *iron* from the diet, which is essential for the synthesis of *haemoglobin* (the oxygen-carrying pigment) and hence for the production of new *red blood cells.*

Absorption inevitably involves intimate contact between the intestinal lining and the gut contents. Although food always contains large amounts of 'non-self' proteins and other large molecules, they do not normally stimulate the immune system (Chapter 6) because by this stage, the food has been digested into molecular fragments too small to elicit an immune response. However, a certain amount of undigested material in the gut contents is normal, and indeed may be essential to maintaining strong peristaltic activity, which keeps the contents moving along the gut. If certain digestive enzymes are deficient or absent, or if the food contains much indigestible material, large proteins and carbohydrates may reach the ileum, and elicit an immune response in the gut wall. Such mechanisms may underlie 'intolerance' of certain foods in some individuals, who experience discomfort, flatulence and diarrhoea, for example if they eat processed wheat products.

Food intolerances are not to be confused with food *allergies*, which can be life threatening, and result from the inappropriate production of antibodies directed against certain proteins in foods (e.g. peanuts). In allergic individuals these antibodies trigger a *systemic* (whole body) inflammatory response, which results in constriction of the airways and a massive drop in blood pressure due to dilation of blood vessels. (The features of a *local* inflammatory response were discussed in Section 6.4.4.)

The delicate lining of the small intestine erodes rapidly, and so is continuously renewed. In adults, the entire lining is replaced with newly formed cells about every five days, with the loss into the gut of about 250 g of dead cells from the old lining. Because renewal of the lining of the small intestine is so dependent upon newly formed cells, any agents that impede cell division, such as starvation, high fever and certain anti-cancer drugs, quickly impair both the digestive and the absorptive functions of the small intestine.

7.4   The large intestine

The last section of the gut is the *large intestine*, so called because it is broad (about 6.5 centimetres wide), but relatively short (about 1.5 metres long). It includes the *colon* or bowel, which extends from the junction with the small intestine near a functionless protrusion called the appendix, followed by the *rectum* and the *anus*, through which the faeces are expelled (look back at Figure 7.1). Digestion and absorption are almost complete by the time the intestinal contents reach the large intestine, but there is still a variable quantity of undigested food remaining and material released from the gut, including secretions and debris such as dead cells from the lining of the small intestine. The brown colour of faeces is due mainly to a pigment in bile (formed from the breakdown of red blood cells) that is not reabsorbed or broken down and so is eliminated as waste.

7.4.1 Symbiotic bacteria

A distinctive feature of the colon is the presence of numerous symbiotic bacteria (Chapter 5). Surprising though this may seem, micro-organisms can often synthesise a wider range of enzymes than can larger, anatomically more complex organisms; this enables the normal gut bacteria to digest some components of the host's food, mostly carbohydrates, that human enzymes cannot break down. The bacteria take up the carbohydrates thus digested, metabolising them to gases (flatus) that distend the bowel and eventually emerge as farts. Adults on a mixed diet expel 1–3 litres per day of such gases.

The colonic bacteria are also an important component of faeces. Before being thus expelled, they help in the synthesis of several vitamins, including some B vitamins and vitamin K, which are absorbed passively through the lining of the colon. Cells in the lining of the large intestine may also take up and, with the help of phagocytic cells (see Chapter 6), digest whole bacteria.

● How would digesting these bacteria improve the nutrition of the host?

■ The bacteria are themselves nourished by the residues of the food that the human gut has not digested. Taking up such bacteria into the lining of the colon and digesting them is an excellent way of increasing the extraction of nutrients from otherwise indigestible food. (Such mechanisms may be particularly important for people on diets that are low in proteins and essential fats.)

You already know that almost all active micro-organisms are killed by the stomach acids and the digestive enzymes as they pass through the upper portions of the gut, so you may be wondering how the symbiotic bacteria survive to reach the large intestine. They form protected spores or cysts and only 'hatch' to proliferate when they reach the more benign environment of the large intestine.

At birth, babies have very few symbiotic or pathogenic bacteria, but they quickly acquire some from their mother. The process is quite efficient in newborns because their stomach is much less acid than that of adults, and they secrete only enzymes that are adapted to digest milk and are not very effective on bacteria. But in weaned children and adults, large or frequent doses of powerful antibiotics can destroy the symbiotic bacteria in the colon, causing abnormal faeces and, if doses are prolonged, vitamin deficiencies. The colon is only slowly re-colonised by 'new' bacteria taken in with food or water, because all but the best protected micro-organisms are killed and digested in the stomach and small intestine.

● What features of the infant gut make infants more susceptible to pathogenic bacteria that enter the body with water and food? Why are bottle-fed babies at greater risk than breast-fed babies?

■ The less acid stomach and the lack of 'generalist' enzymes that digest non-milk proteins make infants much more susceptible to intestinal infections. Breast milk is 'sterile' whereas infant feeding bottles are difficult to sterilise without using equipment or chemicals beyond the reach of most parents in low-income countries. Unpasteurised cows' or goats' milk may be heavily contaminated with bacteria, and formula milk may become contaminated when the milk powder is rehydrated with unsafe water.

7.4.2 The formation of faeces

The active absorption of salts from the gut contents into the tissues continues in the large intestine in much the same way as described earlier in the small intestine. Water in the gut contents diffuses across the gut lining into the tissues, thereby concentrating and drying out the gut contents, which are condensed to form faeces. The gut contents normally remain in the colon for about 18 to 24 hours, but the longer they remain, the drier the faeces become. Normal faeces contain about two parts water to one part dry solids. They move into the rectum, from where they are expelled by a complex series of movements called defaecation, which involve contraction of abdominal and thoracic (chest) muscles as well as those of the gut itself. Except in young children, these movements are normally under voluntary control.

● The gut responds to the presence of toxic materials and organisms by accelerating and strengthening peristalsis, speeding up the passage of the gut contents through the small and large intestines. How would the composition of the faeces be affected?

■ Shortening the time available for reabsorption of salts and water results in the production of the watery, unformed faeces that we know as diarrhoea.

Peristalsis sometimes become vigorous enough to override the voluntary control of defaecation. We are all familiar with the noticeable, sometimes painful, contractions of the gut muscles that precede diarrhoea, which sometimes happens uncontrollably.

● Why are brief bouts of diarrhoea an adaptive response to the presence of harmful materials or parasites in the gut?

■ The powerful contractions expel the potentially dangerous gut contents quickly, before their toxic components have time to be absorbed through the small intestine.

The presence of potentially toxic material in the gut often causes severe depression and distress, but as soon as it is expelled, the person feels better remarkably quickly, often within a few minutes, and recovers completely within hours. Mild diarrhoea is thus a natural, adaptive mechanism for preventing the absorption of toxic substances. In more severe forms of diarrhoea, notably that caused by the pathogenic bacterium *Vibrio cholerae*, the channels through which salts are reabsorbed in the lower intestine are also impaired.

● Why is diarrhoea potentially lethal, especially in babies and young children?

■ Salts and water are expelled as faeces instead of being reabsorbed. Secretion from the stomach, liver, pancreas and duodenum continues, so unless the salts and water are replaced, the body rapidly becomes severely dehydrated. Babies and young children have so few reserves of water and salts that they rapidly succumb to diarrhoeal diseases.

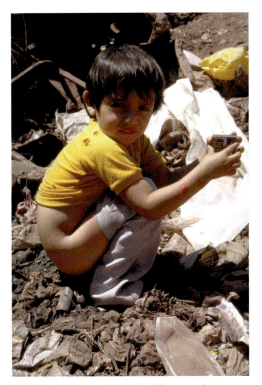

Diarrhoeal diseases kill 2.2 million people globally every year — 80 per cent of them are children under the age of five. (Photo: Courtesy of Carlos Gaggero/AMRO/WHO)

Earlier in this chapter (and in Chapter 4) we referred to the function of the *CFTR* gene as a regulator of chloride, and hence water, transport across membranes. When the gene is defective, it alters the transport of salts across the gut wall and *reduces* the loss of water from the gut contents. It should be clearer now why this gene may have persisted in the population; there may be a selective advantage to individuals who carry *one* defective copy of the gene, because it might prevent some of the effects of diarrhoeal-induced dehydration.

Over the last decade or so much attention has been paid to the role of dietary fibre in maintaining good gut function, with recommendations that fibre additives, such as bran, are included in the diet. Bran is a by-product of the process of milling grains like wheat. The bran residue, and many other plant fibres, consist of a carbohydrate called cellulose, which the human gut cannot digest. It retains water and adds bulk to the contents of the intestine, increasing the volume by 40–100 per cent, and it supports the growth of symbiotic bacteria in the bowel, many of which can digest cellulose. By increasing the volume of the gut contents, its presence gently stimulates peristalsis and so *decreases* the transit time of the intestinal contents, thereby slightly reducing the efficiency of digestion.

Absorbing fewer nutrients may not matter in well-nourished people, but consuming larger quantities of fibre can result in dietary deficiencies because fibre can absorb minerals such as calcium, iron, magnesium and phosphorus, making them unavailable for absorption into the blood supply. The advantage of faster transit is that food residues, some of which may be **carcinogenic** (cancer-causing or promoting), spend less time in the gut.

7.5   The brain and the gut

The gut is a major secretor of body fluids, a major user of proteins in the synthesis and secretion of enzymes, and an important interface between our bodies and the outside world. Not surprisingly, the activity of such an important structure is constantly monitored and controlled by the nervous system (depicted earlier, see Figure 3.22) and by numerous hormones (Section 3.9.3) — mostly in ways of which we are normally unaware. These elaborate and largely unconscious interactions between the brain and the gut mean that its secretions and muscular activity, and psychological factors affecting behaviour such as appetite and food preferences, are sensitive indicators of the well-being of the body as a whole. At least since the time of the ancient Greeks and probably much earlier, physicians have diagnosed illnesses by listening to and feeling the gut and studying its effusions.

7.5.1   Control of enzyme activity

The presence of food in the stomach triggers the release of various hormones that stimulate secretion of enzymes and bile, and activate peristalsis in muscles further down the gut. Thus many people find that eating breakfast stimulates defaecation about an hour later.

● Explain how the efficiency of digestion is increased by the secretion of enzymes being 'turned on and off' (stimulated and inhibited) by hormones.

■ Energy and materials are used for the synthesis and secretion of enzymes, and once free in the gut, each enzyme molecule does not remain active for very long. It is therefore more efficient to secrete enzymes only as and when required.

As mentioned above, small quantities of digestive enzymes are stored in the Golgi bodies of cells lining the gut for some time before being secreted. Digestion of a large meal always requires enzyme synthesis, which takes time — around 10 to 20 minutes. So 'early warning' signals to the gut, some generated just by seeing or smelling food, speed up digestion while also avoiding unnecessary wastage of the relatively large quantity of the body's energy and materials that are deployed in the synthesis of gut secretions.

● Why is precise coordination between secretions in different regions of the gut essential to efficient digestion?

■ Most enzymes work efficiently only in certain chemical environments and in the correct order.

For example, if the quantity of neutralising bile salts secreted does not match the acid produced in the stomach, the duodenal contents may be too acid (or not acid enough), thereby impairing the action of the many important enzymes secreted by the pancreas and small intestine. The pancreatic enzymes cannot digest fats properly until they are emulsified by the bile.

Control of gut activity by the nervous system and certain hormones is essential, particularly if, as is often the case with modern humans (and probably also our hunter–gatherer ancestors), each meal is different in composition from the last. Imperfect coordination between parts of the digestive system, if serious or prolonged, could lead to valuable reserves of protein, energy and water being squandered on synthesising secretions that are unable to digest food efficiently, as well as to pain and the various other unpleasant symptoms that we call indigestion.

7.5.2 Control of vomiting

Communications and interactions between the brain, and movements of the mouth and stomach (and to a lesser extent other parts of the gut) are numerous and complex, and frequently intrude into everyday life. The brain receives much information about the chemical composition, texture and quantity of food in the stomach as well as from the mouth and throat, although the exact mechanisms involved are far from clear. We have all experienced eating things that 'make you feel sick' almost at once (though rarely causing actual vomiting), and being aware that a snack is nutritious (or unsatisfying) within a few minutes of eating it.

● Why are such observations evidence for the existence of sensors that detect the presence of food in the stomach itself?

■ The sensations could not arise from absorption into the blood of significant quantities of nutrients from the food. Very little passes through the stomach wall and it takes hours rather than minutes for the food to pass into the absorptive regions of the small intestine.

Vomiting is a reversal of the muscular movements of the stomach and upper part of the duodenum, aided by powerful contractions of the breathing muscles of the chest. The primary function of vomiting is the expulsion of food that is sensed to be harmful before it reaches the absorptive region of the small intestine.

● What happens to potentially harmful gut contents that fail to stimulate vomiting?

■ They may be detected in the small intestine, where they may cause more vigorous peristalsis, perhaps leading to diarrhoea.

Many such substances elicit both mechanisms for expelling harmful materials from the gut. However, as described later, other toxins and pathogens evade detection, enabling them to enter the blood or establish themselves in the small intestine.

Many other factors, including excitement, pain, fear, motion sickness, noxious smells, some kinds of brain and spinal injuries and infections, and a variety of drugs, including many general anaesthetics and painkillers, often produce nausea (feeling sick) and vomiting, whether or not any food has been eaten. The physiological mechanisms are intricate and, in spite of intensive study, scientists know little about how they work, and why the connection between, for example, motion and nausea has evolved. Consequently, there are few really effective remedies for these unpleasant and inconvenient symptoms.

7.5.3 Regulation of appetite

Sensory feedback is very important in food selection and the regulation of appetite. Experience makes our responses quicker and more accurate; newly weaned children often have 'food fads' and have to be trained to eat 'what is good for them', establishing habits and preferences that last a lifetime. However, the mechanisms are not infallible: as the confectionery and 'junk' food industries know well, we are easily tempted to eat more of very appetising foods whether or not they are nutritious. Distortion of sensory perception of food leading to excessive (i.e. physiologically unreasonable) appetite is believed to be a major cause of overeating, and hence of obesity.

Some poisons, notably those in certain fungi, have no taste or smell and hence are undetectable. People, especially children, can often be persuaded to eat large quantities of foods that 'do not agree with them', sometimes with disastrous consequences. *Anorexia* (loss of appetite, not to be confused with anorexia *nervosa*, a mental disorder characterised by self-starvation) is a common symptom of a wide range of maladies from mild depression and anxiety to lethal fevers and chronic cancers.

●   In view of this account of digestion and its control by the nervous system, can you suggest why anorexia is such a common feature of feeling unwell?

■   Eating is an energetically expensive, often hazardous physiological process; digestion, absorption and the regulation of the concentrations of nutrients in the blood require large quantities of materials and energy, and there is always a risk of absorbing pathogenic organisms or toxic substances. Under almost all forms of stress, it is physiologically easier to live on reserves of energy and protein, at least for a few hours or days, than to embark upon the energetically expensive and risky activities of eating and digesting food and of absorbing the nutrients.

Babies and young children, and almost everyone else when feeling unwell, prefer bland-tasting food and small, nutritionally balanced meals. Alcoholic drinks, highly spiced dishes and large quantities of meat or sugary food may be appetising to healthy teenagers and adults but are much less attractive to, and suitable for, infants, invalids and elderly people. These dietary preferences arise from the intricate relationship between the brain and the gut.

7.6   Control of fuels absorbed into the blood

As we mentioned at the start of this chapter, one of the biological problems arising from eating irregularly is that *regulation* of the levels of nutrients absorbed into the blood is essential to efficient metabolism — the more so in animals such as humans, which eat large infrequent meals. Although digestion and absorption are relatively slow compared to the time taken to consume a meal, nutrients still enter the blood as abrupt 'pulses' rather than as a continuous trickle.

The major source of energy for movement and most biochemical activities is the precisely controlled breakdown of glucose and fats, in combination with oxygen obtained from the atmosphere as we breathe, to yield carbon dioxide, water and energy. This reaction is termed *oxidation*, so in biological language you would say that energy is obtained from the oxidation of glucose and fats.

7.6.1 Glucose regulation

On a normal diet of frequent meals rich in sugars and starch, much of the glucose that is oxidised to generate energy is absorbed directly from the gut. However, the liver can also *synthesise* (manufacture) glucose from amino acids absorbed from proteins in the diet, or — in periods of starvation — derived from the body's own tissues. The muscles, brain and other 'consumers' of the products of digestion work best with a steady supply of glucose and other nutrients. Both too much and too little glucose in the blood make one feel unwell and are harmful if prolonged. The most important reason for this is that the brain cannot use any other fuel; if glucose levels in the blood rise too high or fall too low, the outcome can be life-threatening. The normal functioning of the kidneys is also dependent on maintaining a constant optimum level of glucose in the blood.

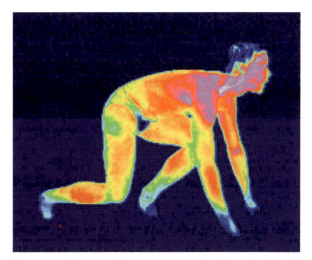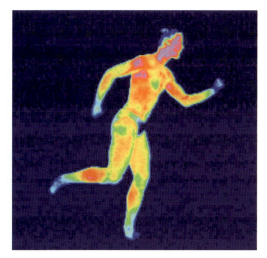

The energy for muscular movement and all the other metabolic processes in the body is obtained by breaking down glucose and fats in combination with oxygen taken in during respiration; the oxidation of fuels also generates heat, as these thermal images reveal — the hottest areas appear red and the coldest are blue. (Photos: Courtesy of Professor Francis J. Ring DSc)

As well as their roles in digestion, the liver and the pancreas make essential contributions to the **regulation of blood glucose levels**. (Other simple sugars, such as galactose, are also absorbed from the digestion, but the liver converts them at once into glucose, so in the following discussion we need only consider glucose.)

As noted earlier, digestion is coordinated and speeded up by *hormones* released by the early stages of eating, which stimulate the lower regions of the gut. Additionally, food intake triggers the release of **insulin** from secretory cells in the *pancreas.* Insulin is a vital hormone that stimulates adjustments in the metabolism of many tissues, including the liver, muscles and *adipose tissue* (the white or yellowish, greasy component of meat, popularly called 'fat'), which is specialised for storing energy as fatty molecules called *lipids*. Adjustments in metabolism in these tissues and organs counteract the sharp rise in glucose that results from a sudden flood of nutrients entering the blood through the small intestine shortly after a meal.

Mechanisms based on another pancreatic hormone **glucagon** ('glue-ka-gon'), counteract the decline in blood glucose to stop it falling far below its optimum level, which would otherwise occur after a period of several hours without consuming sources of glucose in food or sweet drinks.

The process as a whole is shown in Figure 7.3 (overleaf); the following discussion guides you around this flow diagram. Before we plunge into the details, you should note that the purpose of such precise regulation of blood glucose levels is to prevent damage to vulnerable organs such as the brain and kidneys from sharp fluctuations in blood glucose concentration. Glucose regulation is an example of *homeostasis* at work; (if you are unsure about this term, revise Section 3.8.2 and Figure 3.18 now).

The journey around Figure 7.3 starts where the orange see-saw tilts upwards. The passage of blood carrying even a slightly elevated concentration of glucose through the pancreas stimulates it to release more insulin into the blood. (Several other factors, including certain amino acids and some of the hormones produced by the gut, also stimulate insulin secretion, but we will not discuss these additional regulatory mechanisms.) Insulin has many different effects on several tissues, but the best known is the safe disposal and storage of excess glucose.

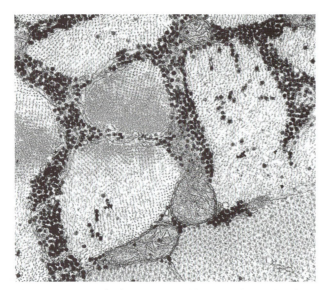

Electron micrograph of a fragment of human calf muscle taken soon after a meal rich in sugars and starch. Excess glucose in the blood has been converted into insoluble glycogen in the muscles (and liver), which forms tiny granules, here stained dense black. The contractile elements of the muscle are seen 'end-on', magnified 45 000 times life-size. (Courtesy of Dr M. J. Cullen, Muscular Dystrophy Research Group Laboratories, Newcastle General Hospital, Newcastle upon Tyne)

Insulin *stimulates* the muscles and the liver to take up the 'extra' glucose that cannot be used immediately for energy production. There the excess glucose is converted into harmless molecules such as *glycogen* ('glye-koh-jen') — a large, insoluble molecule formed from hundreds of glucose molecules linked together. Insulin also *inhibits* the release by the liver of glucose made from the breakdown of glycogen, and it greatly reduces the rate of breakdown of lipids stored in adipose tissue as alternative sources of energy.

● Why is curtailing the release of glucose from the liver, and of lipids from adipose tissue, important in regulating the concentration of glucose in the blood?

■ In the absence of fuels from these internal stores, all the other tissues (e.g. the muscles) have to get their energy from oxidising *dietary* glucose absorbed into the bloodstream from the gut, thereby helping to prevent its concentration in the blood from getting too high.

Insulin also stimulates the synthesis of fats made from excess glucose, which are then transferred for storage in the adipose tissue, and it enhances the rate at which fats from the diet are stored too.

● Explain how a person could become obese from persistently eating large quantities of sugar and starch, even if they only have a moderate intake of fatty foods?

■ Once absorbed into the blood, glucose derived from these energy-providing molecules is either oxidised (i.e. broken down as fuels for muscular movement, etc.) or converted into storage fats that accumulate in the adipose tissue, unless 'burned off' by exercise.

We turn now to the 'down' side of Figure 7.3. The muscles use large quantities of glucose (and fats) during exercise and shivering, and all of the biochemical reactions going on inside cells also require energy derived from glucose. In order to maintain supplies to important tissues such as the brain and the kidneys, the mechanisms that remove excess dietary glucose from the blood must be reversed as the concentration dips below the 'set point', i.e. the optimum safe level.

Insulin secretion is curtailed (it is almost impossible to stop any biochemical pathway completely and instantly), and the pancreas releases *glucagon*. It appears in the blood after about 24 hours of fasting, and stimulates the breakdown of glycogen in the liver and its release as glucose into the blood. Glucagon also promotes the breakdown and release of lipids from adipose tissue, and it stimulates some tissues (especially the muscles) to use more lipids as fuels, thereby preserving the limited supply of glucose in the blood for the brain and kidneys.

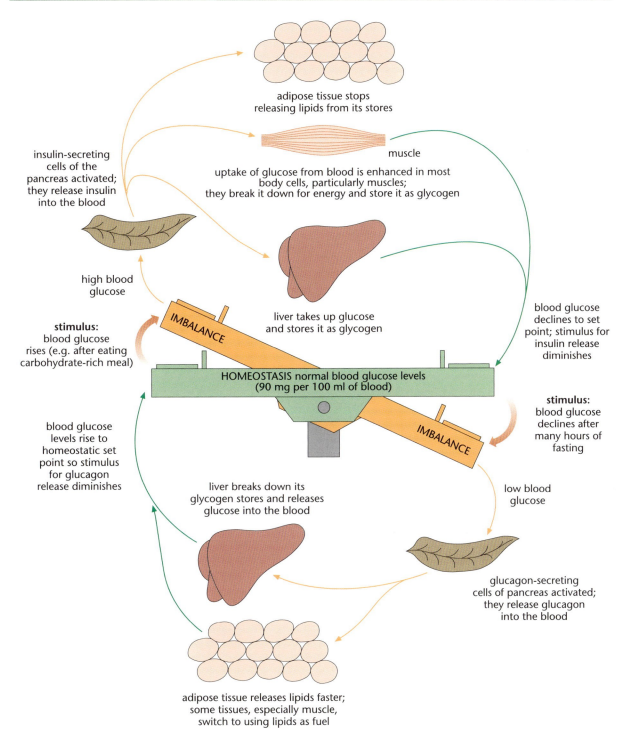

adipose tissue stops
releasing lipids from its stores

insulin-secreting
cells of the
pancreas activated;
they release insulin
into the blood

muscle

uptake of glucose from blood is enhanced in most
body cells, particularly muscles;
they break it down for energy and store it as glycogen

high blood
glucose

IMBALANCE

liver takes up glucose
and stores it as glycogen

blood glucose
declines to set
point; stimulus for
insulin release
diminishes

stimulus:
blood glucose
rises (e.g. after eating
carbohydrate-rich meal)

HOMEOSTASIS normal blood glucose levels
(90 mg per 100 ml of blood)

IMBALANCE

stimulus:
blood glucose
declines after
many hours of
fasting

blood glucose
levels rise to
homeostatic set
point so stimulus
for glucagon
release diminishes

liver breaks down its
glycogen stores and releases
glucose into the blood

low blood
glucose

glucagon-secreting
cells of pancreas activated;
they release glucagon
into the blood

adipose tissue releases lipids faster;
some tissues, especially muscle,
switch to using lipids as fuel

Figure 7.3 *See-saw diagram summarising the principal mechanisms in humans for homeostatic regulation of blood glucose. The orange arrows show what happens when blood glucose levels either rise too high (top left) or fall too low (bottom right); the green arrows show the mechanisms by which blood glucose is returned to the homeostatic 'set point', i.e. the optimum safe glucose level for efficient energy production. In reality, the 'see saw' is constantly oscillating up and down.*

● An important contribution to glucose regulation is not shown in Figure 7.3. What is it?

■ Information about the levels of glucose in the blood reaches the brain and contributes either to appetite and hence to replenishing the body's glucose supply by eating, or to the experience of satiation which causes most people to stop eating when the optimum glucose level has been restored.

Glucose regulation is an example of a *negative feedback* control system, in which changes away from the optimum 'set point' are *opposed* by mechanisms that restore the status quo. The classic example is the thermostat used to control domestic central heating. When the room temperature falls below the temperature setting on the thermostat, the boiler is switched on and when the set temperature is reached the boiler is switched off. The living situation is much more complicated than a simple thermostat!

As illustrated in Figure 7.3, there are *two* opposing negative feedback systems (secretion of insulin and secretion of glucagon) that combine to maintain the level of glucose in the blood within a range that safely supplies the body's immediate energy requirements.

7.6.2 Diabetes mellitus

Major deficiencies in the secretion of insulin, or in the tissues' ability to respond normally to the hormone, produce a disease called *diabetes mellitus* (commonly abbreviated to **diabetes**).

The form of diabetes that is due to defective insulin production usually manifests in childhood, and is known as *juvenile-onset diabetes*. It can be rectified, though not cured, by administering insulin by injection and taking small, frequent meals containing carefully controlled amounts of carbohydrate. However, insulin doses must be carefully regulated; too much insulin lowers the blood glucose too far, starving the brain of vital fuel and leading to fainting and coma. An excessive blood sugar level, sustained for long periods, caused by too little insulin (or a weak response to normal concentrations) is also harmful to the brain and to many other tissues, particularly the fine blood capillaries (e.g. in the eyes, kidneys, hands and feet). The initiating factor in this form of diabetes is not known, but is suspected to be a viral infection, which — in some individuals — triggers an autoimmune reaction; the person's own immune system attacks and destroys the cells in the pancreas that synthesise and secrete insulin.

Late-onset diabetes occurs in adults, usually after middle age; in most cases the person produces normal amounts of insulin, but the body cannot detect it because the insulin receptors in the muscles, liver, etc. have become 'resistant' to its signal. This form of diabetes can often be controlled by reducing dietary carbohydrates, and particularly by avoiding eating large quantities of glucose-containing foods in a short period of time.

In spite of the well-known defects in the storage and regulation of energy-releasing substances (glucose and fats), it is important to stress that they are stored in larger quantities, and their concentration in the blood is more efficiently regulated, than is the case for most other essential nutrients. An adult of average weight and body build has enough energy reserves to support at least six weeks of sedentary living on a total fast, as long as water is available. Protein is stored in the liver (and probably also in the muscles), but reserves are small, so symptoms of protein deficiency, such as shabby skin and hair, appear after only a few weeks on a very low protein diet.

Our brief account of the digestive system and the mechanisms of absorption, detoxification and energy balancing ends here. In the rest of this chapter, we take a wider view of the human diet and its effects on health via a case study which also illustrates the central theme of this book: the interaction of biological and cultural evolution.

7.7 Evolutionary adaptation to novel diets

As pointed out in Chapter 2, human habits and diet have changed greatly during the last 10 000 years with decline in large prey animals and the rise of agriculture and animal husbandry, from which we now obtain most of our food. Not merely the flavours but the dietary staples of our food have changed, and with them have come new toxins for the digestive system to cope with.

7.7.1 Dealing with toxins in food

Toxins are any substances that delay or disrupt any biological process in the cells or tissues of an organism. Just as too much glucose harms many tissues, too much of certain amino acids can also disrupt the functioning of the brain, kidneys and immune system. For example, a sudden excess of particular fatty acids or amino acids is probably the main cause of the headaches and general malaise that some people experience 4 to 12 hours after eating a lot of certain foods such as cheese, shellfish or chocolate. Symptoms disappear in a few hours as the liver takes up or detoxifies the culprit nutrients.

Many essential nutrients (e.g. iron, used in the synthesis of the red blood pigment haemoglobin, and many vitamins) are too toxic to be stored in large quantities. They must be supplied regularly in the diet in a readily absorbable way.

Many toxic substances only produce noticeable effects if present at high concentrations. The human diet, especially that of adults, includes a great many such potentially toxic compounds: indeed, we have come to like, at least in small quantities, the pungent flavours that they impart to our basic foods. Pure flour, rice or potato and unseasoned meat tastes bland and unappetising; most of the strong flavours we use in cookery come from plants, particularly seeds (e.g. coffee, pepper), leaves (e.g. tea, mint, sage and other herbs) and roots (e.g. ginger). Many fruits, by contrast, do not contain toxins and have evolved dispersal mechanisms that rely on their palatability to animals. Our hunter–gatherer ancestors must have been able to cope with a wide range of toxins in their varied and seasonal diets.

Simple flavours such as salt, sweet and sour (i.e. acidic) are due to small, simple molecules, but many others arise from chemically complex molecules that are either not digested at all or are only partially digested by the normal digestive enzymes, so they yield no nutrients. Some such large substances dissolve quite well in fats and hence pass through cell membranes and into the blood. Others, notably certain ingredients of tea and coffee, reach the small intestine almost unchanged, and inactivate enzymes by binding onto them.

● How would drinking a lot of tea or coffee affect a person's digestion and nutrition?

- Inactivation of enzymes would impair the efficiency of digestion and (since enzymes are proteins) would squander the body's protein reserves. However, this effect is only a significant cause of malnutrition if people drink very large quantities of tea or coffee, and eat very little.

Many non-nutritious molecules enter the blood, so reaching the brain (e.g. caffeine in tea and coffee) where, in small quantities, they may alter mood or the sensation of pain; in large doses they may produce serious mental and physical symptoms such as hallucinations and impaired control of movement. From a physiological point of view, such substances are toxins; the liver takes them up and converts them into harmless components (or wraps them up in protein molecules), which are then filtered out of the blood by the kidneys and excreted in the urine, or expelled in the faeces. Alcohol is an unusual toxin in that it both acts directly on the brain to impair movement and affect mood, and it is converted into glucose as a source of energy.

Inactivating and eliminating potential toxins uses both energy and proteins and the liver cannot cope with unlimited quantities or variety of such materials. Delicious though they are in small quantities mixed with bland-tasting foods such as meat or flour, one cannot live on a diet that consists only of sage, coffee, garlic, pepper, cinnamon, ginger, turmeric or similar ingredients.

As discussed in Chapter 2, cooking renders many potentially toxic foods more palatable and digestible. Indeed, the habit probably first developed as a means of dealing with plant foods rather than for cooking meat. Cooking enabled people to eat a wider range of plants, so their diet became more diverse, and hence more adaptable to changes in climate and season. The human diet changed even more rapidly during the last 10 000 years, with the rise of agriculture and animal husbandry.

It is very difficult to determine exactly when and why new foods were added to the human diet; plant fragments and even animal bones rot so quickly that few remains survive for us to study. Recently, anthropologists have tried to determine what ancient people ate by examining fine scratches and patterns of wear on teeth. Experts differ in their interpretation of these observations but everyone agrees that the human diet has changed in the recent past, and is still changing as new foods, and new ways of processing food, are discovered.

In view of the rapid, relatively recent changes in diet, we should not be surprised that certain natural and artificial flavours, preservatives and other non-nutritive ingredients of foods are indigestible for some people. More seriously, they pass unnoticed into the blood where they remain for some time because the person's liver cannot deal with them, and so they are only slowly excreted. Examples include certain artificial flavourings, preservatives and colouring agents that are apparently harmless to most people, but have been implicated in the causation of behavioural problems such as hyperactivity or depression in others.

7.7.2 Agriculture and dietary change

It is important to emphasise that *natural* substances in foods are often as indigestible and harmful as some synthetic food additives are believed to be. For example, some people (and many animals) dislike the taste of beetroot, which arises partly from the chemical that gives the plant its red colour. This substance is not digested and so passes unaltered into the blood, where it is usually harmless at low concentrations. Some people's liver can break it down and so they can eliminate it as colourless products, but that of others cannot, and so the red colour appears in their urine a few hours after eating beetroot. Such physiological differences do not matter for people's ordinary lives, but they illustrate the genetic diversity within the human population and help us to understand different people's food preferences and dietary needs.

In the transition to agriculture and pastoralism, we know that the teeth of *Homo sapiens* became smaller during its evolution and that dental caries, which were rare in hunter–gatherers, became much more common (Chapter 2). There may well have been changes to other parts of the digestive system as well, but such soft tissues are very rarely preserved in fossils, so we know nothing about them. In the absence of such information, we can deduce something about the adaptations that enabled people to live on the new diet from comparison of inherited adaptations of the gut and liver in different groups of modern people.

New crops and domestic animals were gradually introduced to different parts of the world, and they became established only where the climate proved suitable for them, so different groups of people did not all switch from hunting to farming at the same time. The modern human population is thus a rich mixture of diverse peoples who live in different climates, and have different cultures, diets, habits and genetically determined abilities to deal with foods. One of the most thoroughly studied examples of this diversity in diet, habits and physiological capacity is the ability of weaned children and adults to digest fresh milk — as the following case study illustrates.

7.8　Lactose intolerance: a case study

Milk is usually considered to be the most natural food. All female mammals suckle their young, sometimes for considerable periods, during which time the young grow rapidly. Milk consists of small globules of butterfat suspended in a solution containing **lactose** — the main sugar in milk — together with proteins and various minerals including calcium, chloride and sodium. In common with all other newborn mammals, human infants (with rare exceptions) are born with the ability to secrete

the enzyme *lactase* in the small intestine. This enzyme digests lactose, splitting it into two smaller molecules, galactose and glucose. Like other complex sugar molecules, lactose cannot pass through the gut lining, but the lining of the small intestine contains active transport sites that convey both galactose and glucose from the gut into the blood. So lactase converts the lactose in milk into a vital source of energy in young mammals.

Infants who are unable to produce lactase at all are very rare. Rearing them has only become possible in the last 30 years, with the development of synthetic substitutes for milk (e.g. manufactured from soya beans). The capacity to produce lactase declines after weaning, but some individuals lose it altogether, whereas others can still

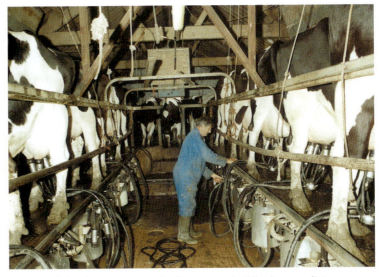

Cows' milk has become a standard component of the human diet, especially for infants and children in most parts of the industrialised world. But our ability to digest lactose as adults varies between individuals and between different populations. (Photo: Mike Levers)

digest lactose in whole milk throughout adult life. Various advertisers extol the virtues of 'getting enough bottle' for all age groups, but milk is not an adequate food for adults: for example, it is deficient in dietary iron and is an inadequate source of vitamin C. So there is a question to be answered about why some of us retain the ability to digest lactose at all. We explore the possible reasons at both the genetic, biochemical and evolutionary levels in this case study.

7.8.1 Lactose malabsorption and intolerance

The picture of milk as a 'natural' universal food suffered its first major blow in 1965 when Cuatrecasas, Lockwood and Caldwell published the unexpected findings of a study of teenagers and adults in Baltimore, Maryland, USA. They compared milk digestion in African Americans and in Whites and showed that the lactose was not efficiently digested by 73 per cent of the Black subjects and 16 per cent of the Whites. Further studies on different ethnic groups living in various parts of the world have revealed the existence of other populations with widely different proportions of people who can, or cannot, digest lactose after weaning.

People who cannot digest lactose are called *lactose malabsorbers* and the condition is known as **lactose malabsorption**. People who can digest lactose throughout their lives are called *lactose absorbers*.

● What do you think are the consequences of lactose malabsorption for the digestion of milk, and what effect might this have on the nutrients available to adults who are malabsorbers?

■ The fats and proteins in milk are digested and absorbed normally, but the lactose remains in the gut contents. The glucose energy supplied to the body that would normally be derived from milk is lost, but this is not a problem for lactose malabsorbers, since they are past weaning and can get plenty of glucose from other dietary sources.

However, gut contents that contain large quantities of lactose retain more water than is normal, thus diluting the digestive enzymes and disturbing normal digestion.

● What would happen to the lactose when it reaches the large intestine?

■ Like other residual carbohydrates, it would be digested by the symbiotic bacteria (most species of which can produce lactase).

● Could the resulting glucose (and galactose) pass through the gut lining and into the blood?

■ No. There are no glucose (or galactose) transporters in the lining of the large intestine.

The gut contents are not normally moved 'upstream' back to the small intestine, so instead of being absorbed into the person's blood, the products of lactose digestion mostly support the *proliferation* of the lactose-digesting bacteria. The abnormally large numbers of bacteria thus maintained produce much more carbon dioxide and other gases than is normal, leading to a condition called **lactose intolerance**. The symptoms include flatulence (wind), intestinal cramps and, in severe cases, diarrhoea, nausea and vomiting.

Lactose intolerance is usually mild in adults because many lactose malabsorbers have enough residual lactase activity to enable them to eat small quantities of whole milk (e.g. in a cup of tea, or as an ingredient of cake) without causing symptoms. But lactose malabsorbers who eat a lot of lactose-containing food over a short period may become ill.

● Would you expect lactose malabsorbing people to choose foods containing fresh milk?

■ No; there is efficient communication between the gut and the brain that makes people aware of and so avoid foods that, for one reason or another 'do not agree with them'. Under normal circumstances, it is possible to avoid such foods without fuss, and indeed many people do so without being aware of their physiological condition.

So, we have a paradox: there is apparently no *disadvantage* in being a lactose malabsorber, and no obvious *advantage* in being able to digest lactose as an adult — yet there is enormous variation in the proportion of both these phenotypes in populations around the world — as the next section describes.[2] The existence of major variation between populations strongly suggests that where the lactose absorbers *predominate* this phenotype has a selective advantage over the malabsorbers. Later in the case study we examine what that advantage might be.

7.8.2 Variation between populations and individuals

The proportions of lactose absorbers and lactose malabsorbers have been measured in a wide variety of human populations. Populations can vary between 0 per cent lactose absorbers, where no weaned children or adults produce sufficient lactase to digest lactose, and 100 per cent absorbers where everyone can do it. In a review of the distribution of lactose absorbers and malabsorbers from 197 populations, F. J. Simoons of the University of California concluded that:

> … high prevalences of lactose malabsorbers, from about 60–100 per cent of the persons studied, are typical of the overwhelming number of ethnic groups around the world … including all American Indians and Eskimos studied so far, some New World Mestizos, most sub-Saharan African peoples and their relatively unmixed overseas descendants, most Mediterranean and Near Eastern groups, most subjects whose origins are India, all peoples of Southeast and East Asia, as well as the two Pacific groups, New Guineans and Fijians, who have been studied. (Simoons, 1978, p. 964)

Conventionally, a population with 70 per cent or more lactose malabsorbers is described as *lactose malabsorbing*. Conversely, a minority of the world's peoples have high proportions of lactose absorbers (from 70 to 100 per cent). These *lactose absorbing* populations are primarily northern and western Europeans and their descendants in the Americas and Australia, but also certain peoples of the Mediterranean and Near East, three pastoral groups of Africa (Tussi, Hima and

---

[2] If you are unsure about the terms 'phenotype' and 'genotype', now would be a good time to revise them in Chapter 4; phenotype can be roughly translated as 'the way the person turned out'.

Fuiani), and several groups living in the western parts of the Indian subcontinent. Only a few present-day groups have intermediate prevalences of lactose malabsorbers (over 30 but under 70 per cent).

We can learn about the genetic aspects of lactose malabsorption by observing the frequency with which the children of normal absorbers and malabsorbers inherit their parents' characteristics. In Chapter 4, we described the typical pattern of inheritance of characteristics due to a single gene, which can occur in two alternative forms (alleles), one dominant and one recessive.

●   What would be the phenotype of a person who inherited both the dominant and the recessive allele of a gene, one from each parent?

■   The person's phenotype would be that produced by the dominant allele, which masks the effect of the recessive allele.

The observed frequency with which children inherit lactose malabsorption from their parents is typical of the inheritance of a characteristic due to the presence of two recessive alleles of a single gene.

●   About a quarter of the children born to parents who are *both* lactose absorbers turn out to be malabsorbers; what can you conclude about the genotypes of the parents?

■   The parents must be *heterozygous* (see Chapter 4) for the gene that controls lactase production after weaning; they each have one copy of the dominant allele and one copy of the recessive allele. A quarter of the offspring born to these heterozygous parents are homozygous for the recessive allele (they have two copies of the recessive allele, one copy inherited from each parent) and hence their phenotype is lactose malabsorbing.

●   Is lactose malabsorption likely to be due to a defect in the gene that codes for the lactase protein itself, or to a change in the mechanism that regulates the activity of this gene?

■   People in whom the gene that codes for lactase is defective would be unable to digest their *mother's* milk (or formula milk) and so would not normally survive infancy. The *normal* gene must exist in lactose malabsorbers and must have functioned effectively when they were babies, but it is 'switched off' after weaning so lactase is no longer produced, or only in very reduced amounts.

7.8.3 Selection pressures favouring lactose absorption

The hunter–gatherer peoples who lived before the rise of agriculture and pastoralism were all probably lactose malabsorbers. It is, of course, impossible to know for sure, but since all other weaned mammals are lactose malabsorbers, and there is no evidence that hunter–gatherers ever used animal milk in their diets, most were almost certainly lactose malabsorbers. Thus, lactose *absorbers* are the result of a relatively recent evolutionary change, which must have taken place *after* the first agricultural revolution when people began to domesticate milk-producing animals.

If the population was placed under some stress that gave the first adults with the ability to absorb lactose an advantage that led to greater reproductive success, then the genes involved would be favoured by natural selection and would thus gradually increase in frequency in the population. We will discuss what that selection pressure might be in a moment.

It is not known exactly when dairying cultures first emerged; a conservative estimate of the time since milk first became important in the diets of adults is 5 000 years or around 250 generations. If lactose absorbers managed, on average, to raise 1 per cent more children than lactose malabsorbers (which is not unreasonable), this period of time is sufficiently long for gene frequencies to have been altered substantially by natural selection.

What were the stresses that led to the genes involved in lactose absorption staying 'switched on' in particular populations? William Durham tried to answer this question in 1991 by choosing for detailed study 60 of the populations reviewed in Simoon's article (from which we quoted above), which between them represented the full range of ability to absorb lactose. Table 7.1 shows Durham's sample together with information about the normal diets those 60 populations had consumed for generations. The 60 populations in Table 7.1 are categorised by the presence or absence of dairying in their culture (rearing animals for their milk). The third column in Table 7.1 shows the percentages of lactose absorbers in each population category, and the fourth column shows the number of populations sampled in each category.

Table 7.1 The 60 populations chosen by Durham, categorised by their normal diet, showing the percentages of lactose absorbers in the populations in each category.

Category	Nature of subsistence	Lactose absorbers %	Number of populations sampled
I	hunter–gatherers traditionally lacking dairy animals	12.6	4
II	non-dairying agriculturalists	15.5	5
III	recently dairying agriculturalists	11.9	5
IV	milk-dependent pastoralists	91.3	5
V	dairying peoples of North Africa and the Mediterranean	31.8	16
VI	dairying peoples of northern Europe (above 40° N)	91.5	12
VII	populations of mixed dairying and non-dairying ancestry	56.2	13

Data derived from Durham, W. H., 1991, *Coevolution, Genes, Culture and Human Diversity*, Stanford University Press, Stanford, California, Table 5.1, p. 234.

● Look at the distributions of lactose absorbers among the seven populations I to VII in Table 7.1. Is there a relationship between the normal diet and the percentage of lactose absorbers?

■ Populations in categories I and II do not rear or use dairy animals and have low percentages of lactose absorbers, whereas the dairying cultures in categories IV and VI have high proportions of lactose absorbers. The 'mixed' populations in category VII have intermediate proportions of absorbers and malabsorbers.

● Do the data from the category III populations support or contradict the general pattern?

■ The finding that agriculturalists who have only recently turned to dairying have a low percentage of lactose absorbers is consistent with the relationship outlined above. The evolution of the ability to digest lactose, like all evolutionary changes, takes a relatively long time and it may not yet have happened in those populations that have recently adopted dairying.

● Milk has been a major food for the dairying peoples of North Africa and the Mediterranean (category V) for at least 5 000 years. Does the finding that they have relatively low proportions of lactose absorbers support or contradict the general pattern?

■ This finding appears to contradict the general pattern: it shows that the ability to digest lactose does not entirely depend upon that population using milk as a dietary constituent, even if the habit has been established for a very long time.

There is a cultural explanation for the apparently anomalous prevalence of lactose malabsorbers in North African and Mediterranean dairying populations, and it is to this aspect of the lactose digestion story that we now turn.

7.8.4 Cultural adaptations to avoid lactose intolerance

Dairying populations with a high proportion of lactose malabsorbers either do not collect milk from their domestic animals, or they routinely ferment it into cheese or yoghurt. Whole milk is generally regarded as 'baby food' and is not often drunk by adults or older children. The problem of lactose intolerance usually does not come to light until famine or mass migration force people to eat milk-containing food in abnormally large quantities.

Fermentation of milk into cheese is an ancient skill that probably began shortly after people domesticated large mammals. When milk is allowed to stand in a warm place, micro-organisms in the air colonise it, and their enzymes turn the lactose to lactic acid, which precipitates most of the protein and fats to form a thick, nutritious curd that is easily separated from the thin, watery whey. This ancient method of separating milk is still used to make pot cheese and cottage cheese.

Three processes may reduce the lactose content of cheese, making it edible to lactose malabsorbers: the micro-organisms convert the lactose into lactic acid; they secrete the enzyme lactase which splits lactose into glucose and galactose; lactose, like other sugars, is very soluble in water, so any remaining is removed in the whey.

Different conditions, especially temperature, favour the proliferation of different kinds of micro-organisms that confer different flavours and textures on the cheese. Thus, cheese production is a cultural practice that allows lactose malabsorbers in dairying populations to obtain most of the nutrients of milk without any of the symptoms of lactose intolerance. Important nutrients thus obtained from milk include calcium, which promotes the development of healthy bones and teeth, and fats, some of which have recently been shown to be essential for normal brain development and functioning.

7.8.5 Lactose absorption, latitude and vitamin D

As you have seen, some populations that have long practised dairy farming contain high proportions of lactose malabsorbers ,whereas others contain high proportions of lactose absorbers. This raises an interesting evolutionary question. A cultural solution (cheese-making) has long been available to allow dairying cultures to obtain adequate nutrition from dairy farming, and all of them do this. Yet in some (category V in Table 7.1) the ancient lactose malabsorbing phenotype has remained unchanged, whereas in others a new lactose absorbing phenotype emerged and increased until it became the norm in those cultures (categories IV and VI). This suggests that there must have been *additional* selection pressures that favoured the gradual increase in the proportion of lactose absorbers in dairying cultures IV and VI. You would not expect the proportion of lactose absorbers to rise so high (over 90 per cent), *unless* they derived an additional advantage from their ability. What could it be?

To answer this question, William Durham extended his earlier study to investigate the *locations* of the homelands of the 60 lactose absorbing and malabsorbing populations, which formed the basis for Table 7.1. He found an association between the proportion of lactose absorbers in a population and the *latitude* of their homelands; the majority of the populations with high proportions of lactose absorbers live in latitudes greater than 30 degrees North or South of the Equator. Exceptions to this relationship are milk-dependent peoples of East Africa and Saudi Arabia and the Inuit populations of Greenland. We will return to these anomalies later, after we consider Durham's evidence of a significant relationship between latitude and diet. But first we must describe the biology of *vitamin D*. The relevance of this vitamin to lactose absorption and latitude will soon become apparent.

Vitamin D

Vitamin D is very important to health and normal growth: it facilitates the transport of calcium through the lining of the small intestine into the blood, it controls the deposition of calcium in the bones during growth, and it maintains adult bone structure. The consequences of **vitamin D deficiency** are well known. With less calcium available, the skeleton fails to develop normally. The most obvious symptom is the bowing of the long load-bearing bones in the lower limbs, producing the condition called *rickets*. Children with vitamin D deficiency grow more slowly and may become smaller adults which, in women, has serious consequence because the pelvis may end up so small or misshapen that normal birth is severely impeded.

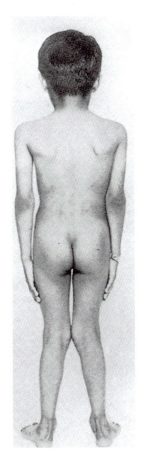

Vitamin D can be absorbed through the gut; dietary sources of vitamin D include fish and fish livers, mammal livers (e.g. pig, calf), shellfish and egg yolks. In the 1920s, Sir Edward Mellanby showed that vitamin D added to the diet could prevent the development of rickets, thereby providing a scientific basis for the folklore that cod liver oil (a rich source of vitamin D) is effective in preventing rickets.

Under the right conditions, the human body can also synthesise the vitamin for itself. A band of ultraviolet light called UV-B radiation promotes the synthesis of essential precursors of vitamin D in the human skin. The precursor molecules are transported in the blood from the skin to the liver and kidneys, where they are converted into the biologically active form of vitamin D. Under the control of

A child with rickets photographed in Scotland in the 1940s; without sufficient vitamin D, calcium is not properly absorbed from the gut so the growing bones cannot harden normally. The abnormally flexible bones bend under the child's weight, producing the characteristic bowed legs. (Photo: Professor G. C. Arneil)

hormones, vitamin D is released from the liver and kidneys into the circulation, where it has the same effects on calcium transport and bone structure as vitamin D acquired from the diet.

UV-B radiation and latitude

Until the invention of special kinds of electric lights in the twentieth century, the only source of UV-B was sunlight. The amount of UV-B (and other components of sunlight) to reach populations living at latitudes above 30 degrees North or below 30 degrees South of the Equator is up to 88 per cent *less* than the amount of UV-B experienced by people living in equatorial regions, depending on how far North or South they live (Figure 7.4). As a consequence, people living at *high* latitudes have a *lower* capacity to synthesise vitamin D in the skin than those living nearer the Equator. (Remember, the Equator has a latitude of 0 degrees, so latitude gets 'higher' the further you move away from the Equator to the North and to the South.)

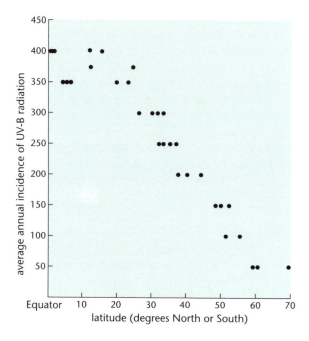

Figure 7.4   *The amount of UV-B radiation at the Earth's surface decreases as latitude increases, either North or South. (From Durham, W. H., 1991,* Coevolution, Genes, Culture and Human Diversity, *Stanford University Press, Stanford, California, Figure 5.8, p. 259)*

● What factors other than high latitude would inhibit the ability to synthesise vitamin D in the skin?

■ Dark pigments in the skin and wearing clothes both shade the skin from the UV-B light essential for forming the precursors of vitamin D.

If the skin is frequently exposed to plenty of sunlight, more than enough vitamin D is synthesised, even if the skin is partially shaded by dark pigments. Indeed, the pigment is essential to protect the skin cells from being damaged by too much radiation. Human ancestral peoples almost certainly had darkly pigmented skin. As explained in Chapter 2, humans evolved on the sunny grasslands of Eastern and Southern Africa, where protection from excess light and heat is essential and more than enough UV-B radiation reached the skin for vitamin D synthesis. Early people were probably as dark as their modern descendants now living in these regions.

However, if dark-skinned people migrate to a cloudy climate, and/or adopt the habit of wearing clothes that cover a large part of the body (as you would expect in colder climates), they risk suffering from vitamin D deficiency because they are not exposed to sufficient UV-B radiation.

● What adaptation do you predict is likely to have occurred in dark-skinned populations who migrated further and further away from the Equator?

■ There would be a selective advantage for those individuals with lower-than-average amounts of pigmentation in their skin, since this would facilitate their ability to synthesise vitamin D in latitudes with lower levels of UV-B radiation. The genes responsible for these lighter-skinned phenotypes could be expected to spread in the population over many generations, because the children of lighter-skinned parents had a survival advantage at these higher latitudes, particularly where the cold necessitated covering most of the skin with warm clothing.

As Figure 7.5 shows, this prediction is borne out by the relationship between latitude of origin and skin colour of the populations described in Table 7.1. The skin of indigenous populations is lighter in people native to higher latitudes (North or South). A comparison of Figures 7.4 and 7.5 shows that people's skin becomes paler with increasing latitude, which corresponds to the reduction in UV-B.

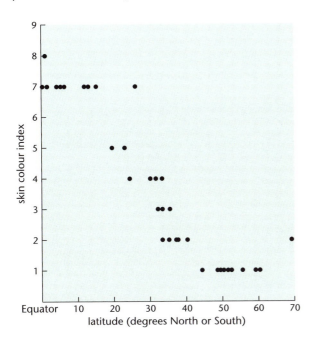

Figure 7.5 *The relationship between skin pigmentation and latitude of origin for the populations featured in Table 7.1. (The higher the skin colour index, the darker the skin.) (From Durham, W. H., 1991,* Coevolution, Genes, Culture and Human Diversity, *Stanford University Press, Figure 5.10, p. 262)*

Durham's hypothesis

We can now tie together all the strands of the lactose malabsorption story. William Durham (1991) suggested a causal link between the evolution of paler skin, the ability to absorb lactose after weaning and vitamin D deficiency. His theory (which is one of several possible interpretations of these observations) proposes that vitamin D deficiency in populations living in high latitudes gave a selective advantage to people who could absorb lactose from milk throughout their lives.

Durham argues that lactose malabsorption, which was the normal condition of our ancestors 10 000 years ago, became a 'problem' only after people adopted farming and animal husbandry as their major source of food. He believes that there was, from time to time, stress on populations caused by dietary deficiencies and by crowding and insanitary living conditions that fostered bacterial infection and parasitism. A cultural solution to this dietary stress in dairying communities was to make cheese and yoghurt, which lactose malabsorbers could digest. In this way, additional sources of calcium, fat and other nutrients in the milk became available, without the debilitating effects of lactose intolerance.

Despite this cultural adaptation, natural selection favoured the spread of the lactose absorption phenotype in those populations that migrated to higher latitudes. There was an *additional* stress on populations living in these cloudy colder climates where there was insufficient UV-B radiation to generate adequate vitamin D — even in pale skins.

As mentioned in Chapter 2, people began using animal skins as clothes when they colonised these Northern regions at the end of the last Ice Age, when the climate was even colder (and probably also cloudier) than it is now. When thus dressed, only a small fraction of the whole skin, perhaps only the hands and face, is exposed to sunlight, so vitamin D synthesis there must be as efficient as possible; most populations who wear heavy clothes never undress outside. It is important to point out that sunbathing is a modern habit. Pale-skinned people can produce several months' supply of vitamin D in an hour or two of sunbathing in bright sun, but at the potential cost of sustaining such severe skin damage that skin cancers are generated.

At the heart of Durham's hypothesis is the final biological paradox: why does the female mammal go to the 'trouble' and 'expense' of synthesising the lactose in breast milk from galactose and glucose, when it then has to be broken down again

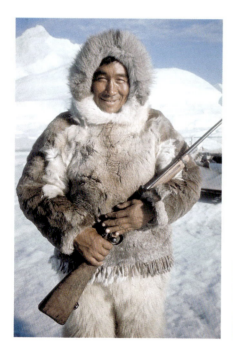 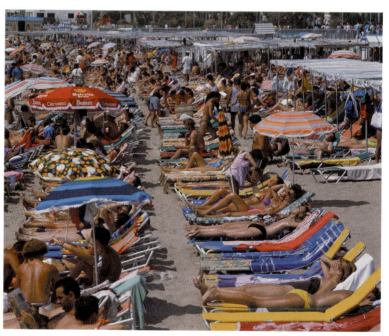

(left) Humans originally evolved in latitudes near the Equator and are not adapted to cold climates, where thick clothing is essential to survival; but so little skin is exposed that the ability to synthesise light-facilitated vitamin D in the skin is severely limited. (Photo: Camera Press) (right) Prolonged exposure to sunshine stimulates the formation of vitamin D and protective dark pigments in the skin. However, it also exposes light-skinned people to damaging levels of radiation; the fashion for suntans is believed to be a major cause of the recent increase in skin cancer among light-skinned populations. (Photo: Corbis Images)

by lactase into these constituents before it can be absorbed by the infant? The solution comes from the observation that suckling babies are *protected against vitamin D deficiency*. Lactose acts directly on the cells in the lining of the gut to facilitate the transport of calcium into the body and its incorporation into bones — in effect lactose in milk-fed infants is behaving like vitamin D. Recent research indicates that young children do not depend upon vitamin D for calcium transport while they are breast fed or given animal milk. Clearly, the ability to substitute lactose for vitamin D will confer the greatest advantage on infants in latitudes where the UV-B radiation is low and the coldness of the climate means that very little skin is exposed.

7.8.6 Exceptions to the lactose absorption hypothesis

Earlier in this story, two populations were identified as not conforming to the explanation for the selective advantage of lactose absorbers at high latitudes: the lactose malabsorbing Inuit populations of Greenland and the lactose absorbing dairying cultures of East Africa and Saudi Arabia.

The Inuit do not keep dairy animals and so have no sources of lactose after weaning. They are predominantly lactose malabsorbers who nevertheless live successfully at 69 degrees North with moderately dark skins, heavy clothing, and low and periodic levels of sunlight.

● Think back to the discussion of Inuit in Chapter 2. Can you suggest an explanation of how traditional Inuit societies avoided vitamin D deficiency?

■ They remained healthy because their native diet consisted almost exclusively of fish and meat, which are rich in vitamin D. Their natural diet compensated for the lack of UV-B, so there was no pressure for the evolution of lactose absorption persisting throughout life.

● In the last 40–50 years, most Inuit have abandoned their traditional diet and live almost entirely on food imported from southern Canada. How will this change of diet provide a 'natural experiment' testing Durham's hypothesis; (another way of putting this is to ask what *prediction* follows from Durham's hypothesis, that recent cultural changes in the diet of Inuits will put to the test)?

■ If the Inuit eat a diet containing less raw fish and meat, and hence less vitamin D, Durham's hypothesis predicts that over many generations the proportion of lactose absorbers in the population should *rise* in response to the selection pressure favouring this phenotype.

The existence of dairying communities in East Africa and Saudi Arabia who live at latitudes below 30 degrees (i.e. approaching the Equator), and have a long history of milk use, but who have high proportions of lactose absorbers in their populations, remains to be explained. These populations are inconsistent with Durham's hypothesis that all such cultures were originally lactose malabsorbing, and that lactose absorption spread only in *higher* latitudes as a result of natural selection. It might be argued that other conditions unique to the culture or environment of these Equatorial populations contributed to the selection of the lactose absorption phenotype. Alternatively, there may have been selection for some other (as yet unknown) consequence of inheriting the gene involved in lactose absorption.

The account given in this chapter of the association between lactose intolerance and vitamin D synthesis is still not universally accepted as the only possible interpretation of the facts (and doubtless new material will come to light in the future that might modify Durham's hypothesis), but it does illustrate some interactions between the physiology, geography and evolutionary history of our species. Collaborative research between anthropologists, biochemists and geneticists is helping to explain more of our habits and physiological capacities and limitations. The lactose story also shows that there is often more than one way of obtaining essential nutrients, so what is a healthy diet in one place could prove inadequate under other circumstances.

7.9   Food and the future

Humans are one of the most widespread large animals that have ever existed and our diet is correspondingly varied. People are still undergoing evolutionary change, and habits concerning diet are continuously changing as new foods and new ways of preparing existing foods are added to what we eat. Groups of people differ not only in their dietary preferences, but also in their genetic capacity to digest, absorb and metabolise certain foods. We end this chapter with a brief look at a development which has the potential to change human diets more radically than at any time since the switch from hunter–gathering lifestyles to agriculture and pastoralism.

7.9.1 Genetically modified foods

The use of *genetic engineering* to produce **genetically modified foods** (GM foods) is now widespread, despite generating a large amount of public and scientific interest and protest in high-income countries from the late 1990s. GM foods are produced from crop species in which one or more genes have been altered (mutated), or genes from an unrelated donor species have been 'spliced' into the recipient's DNA. Much of the public debate has focused on the impact that genetically modified crop plants could have upon the environment (such as the spread of artificial genes into wild species), and on the ethics of the food/biotechnology industry in creating crops resistant to its own herbicides or pesticides, or for creating monopolies on GM seed stocks.[3]

The nutritional aspects of GM foods have attracted much less public attention. GM soya, for example, is approved for use in 13 countries worldwide and by the year 2000 was being consumed by over 300 million people annually. In most cases, GM food plants have been engineered with the intention of altering one of the properties given in Box 7.1.

There are still relatively few GM foods on the market; although safety testing of many others is in the pipeline, it is too early to say (at the time of writing) what the outcomes will be. Perhaps the most that can be said is that some will turn out to be safe to eat and offer some nutritional advantage — at least to some of the world's populations — and some will turn out to be hazardous either to consumers or to the environment and its biodiversity. We cannot yet foresee the balance of advantages and disadvantages. However, we can dispel one persistent misconception.

● What happens to the components of a GM foodstuff (including the inserted DNA) which is eaten?

[3] These environmental and ethical issues are discussed in more detail in *World Health and Disease* (Open University Press, 3rd edn 2001), Chapter 11.

Box 7.1   Rationale for genetic modification of crop species

- Improving crop yields, e.g. by increasing the resistance of crops to agricultural chemicals, which can then be used at higher doses to control pests and weeds; or by improving drought tolerance or the ability to grow in poor or polluted soils.

- Prolonging the shelf-life of the crop, e.g. by increasing resistance to moulds.

- Improving the nutritional quality of the product, e.g. in 'golden rice', daffodil genes were added to the rice genome, resulting in vitamin-A enriched rice crops that may reduce the 100 million cases of blindness caused worldwide by vitamin A deficiency (mostly among children).

■ It is digested and broken down into its constituent components just like any other food, regardless of whether the GM component is in fresh produce eaten raw (e.g. GM tomatoes), or converted into a manufactured commodity (e.g. biscuits made with GM soya flour).

One concern about GM foods is that new enzymes, toxins or other potentially harmful molecules might be generated within a GM plant, which could cause food intolerance or allergies to develop within a proportion of the population. Of course, this problem could arise from any new food source, including plant material modified genetically by conventional selective breeding techniques, as is the case with wheat and many other common long-established foods.

In determining which GM products are suitable for human consumption, a rule of *substantial equivalence* is used; if a GM product is substantially equivalent in chemical composition to its natural antecedent, it is assumed to pose no new threat to our health. This criterion has been hotly debated between scientists. Opposing it are those who claim that not enough safety testing has been performed on these new foodstuffs — which might be eaten in large quantities — by comparison with the testing regimes for new pharmaceutical products — which are consumed in very small quantities.

Supporters of GM technology argue that it has several advantages: it may enable more efficient cultivation of crops with greater nutritional value, particularly in developing countries; some GM foods may require less cooking, so reducing the speed of deforestation for fuel; or they may require smaller areas of cultivated land, possibly helping to decrease pressures upon land usage. The use of GM technology has speeded-up the transfer of genes between plants, which farmers and plant breeders have been doing for many years. In the future, GM technology might be applied more widely to animals for both agricultural and medical use — an even more controversial subject to which we shall return in Chapter 9.

7.9.2 In conclusion

In summing up this complex subject, we return to the points we raised at the very beginning. Eating is one of the most expensive physiological processes in terms of the materials and energy required for digestion, the risk incurred of absorbing harmful organisms or substances, and the necessity to counteract abrupt changes in concentrations of nutrients in the blood. Food is not easy to deal with: the brain and its senses and the gut and associated organs such as the liver and pancreas work together to choose, digest and absorb nutrients from our diet and then to expel the waste products. Knowledge of the many different organs and biochemical processes involved in digestion and absorption may help you to appreciate why appetite, food preferences and eating habits can reveal so much about an individual's mental and physical health, and at the same time illuminate important interactions between the physiology, geography, genetics and evolutionary history of our species.

OBJECTIVES FOR CHAPTER 7

When you have studied this chapter, you should be able to:

7.1 Define and use, or recognise definitions and applications of, each of the terms printed in **bold** in the text.

7.2 Outline the gross structure and normal operation of the major components of the human digestive system, in relation to the digestion and absorption of proteins, fats, carbohydrates and non-nutritive components of food.

7.3 Give examples to illustrate the role of the nervous system and certain hormones in the control of eating and the passage of food through the gut under normal circumstances, and when food contains harmful components.

7.4 Demonstrate an understanding of the basic principles of homeostasis and negative feedback in a physiological system, and describe the roles of the major organs and hormones involved in regulating blood glucose levels.

7.5 Discuss the phenomenon of lactose absorption and malabsorption, cultural adaptations to overcome lactose intolerance, and the features of Durham's hypothesis about their possible relationship to latitude, vitamin D synthesis and the evolution of skin colour.

7.6 Summarise the main issues raised by the increasing availability of genetically modified crops and animals.

QUESTIONS FOR CHAPTER 7

1   (*Objective 7.2*)

Describe in a few sentences the roles of (a) the stomach, (b) the pancreas, (c) the liver, (d) the small intestine, and (e) symbiotic micro-organisms, in the digestion and absorption of food and/or the regulation of blood composition.

2   (*Objective 7.3*)

Describe some factors that contribute to appetite and food selection. Why are short-term anorexia, vomiting and diarrhoea considered to be adaptive mechanisms that protect the body?

3   (*Objective 7.4*)

List the factors that (a) increase, and (b) reduce blood glucose concentration.

4   (*Objective 7.5*)

Outline briefly the cultural and evolutionary changes involved in the origin and spread of (a) lactose absorption in adults, and (b) paler skin.

5   (*Objective 7.6*)

Using material in this chapter and *World Health and Disease* (Open University Press, 3rd edn 2001), Chapter 11, what are the potential benefits and risks from the widespread planting of 'golden rice'?

CHAPTER 8

On living longer

Study notes for OU students

This chapter briefly reviews the biological changes associated with ageing and contributes to the discussion of health and disease in older people in the UK, which occurs in two other books in this series: Chapter 9 in *World Health and Disease* (Open University Press, third edition 2001) presents data on patterns of disease and disability in later life (see Figures 9.2, 9.6, 9.7 and 9.11), and Chapter 10 reviews some explanations for them; *Birth to Old Age: Health in Transition* (Open University Press, second edition 1995; colour-enhanced second edition 2001), Chapters 9–11 discuss the sociological and cultural influences on the current health experience of the menopause and growing older in the contemporary UK.

8.1   Studying ageing

The wiser mind
Mourns less for what age takes away
Than what it leaves behind.
(William Wordsworth, 1770–1850, from
The Fountain, published 1800)

In Chapter 2 of this book you read that humans live longer than any other mammal. You also read that there are age-related changes in some physiological abilities, such as a decline in running speed and maximum grip strength. Scientists can measure the decline in function and describe the cellular changes that commonly occur as the body ages, but they have not yet identified a *core mechanism* of ageing. Biologists and doctors are still at the stage of cataloguing the physical and psychological changes without knowing if they are causes or consequences of age. Nevertheless, humankind still seeks the secret of eternal youth through an understanding of the mechanisms of biological ageing, in the hope that, once understood, it might be possible to prevent or at least delay these changes taking place. This chapter gives a brief review of ageing from a biological perspective, drawing on theoretical debates about the evolutionary significance of 'living longer' as well as laboratory research on the possible mechanisms that may underlie the ageing process.

8.1.1   Signs of ageing

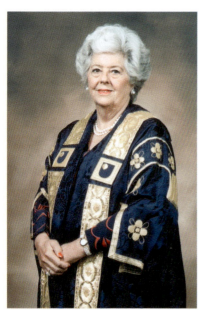

In some occupations or roles — for example Speaker of the House of Commons or Chancellor of the Open University — a person may need a 'mature' appearance in order to achieve promotion to a position of authority. (The Rt. Hon. Baroness Boothroyd of Sandwell is Chancellor of the Open University.) (Photo: Mike Levers)

A person's physical appearance changes during the course of their life. From maturity onwards these changes are often described as *ageing*, a word that has a negative connotation in some cultures and a positive one in others, where age is venerated.

● Can you give an example of an age-related change in physical appearance that is not necessarily socially disadvantageous, even in British society?

■ Changes in the distribution of body hair, hair colour and facial wrinkles can bring higher status (though more commonly to men than to women in present-day Britain); a man with grey hair is more likely to be described as 'distinguished looking' and a face with some wrinkles may be said to have 'character' or 'laughter lines'. A person may need a 'mature' appearance in order to achieve promotion or a position of authority.

People often refer to someone as 'not looking their age', the implication being that ageing is a sequence of milestones, each of which should be reached by a specific chronological age. The reality is different. Ageing does not start at any one time, nor does it proceed at a constant rate; rather, the gradual accumulation of cellular and tissue changes over time has external signs and effects that become increasingly evident with age. These changes can result from a number of biological phenomena, which we describe later in this chapter: there are changes in cells themselves and in proteins in the fluids between cells; 'degenerative' changes occur in whole organs; and the effects of diseases can contribute to the ageing process. But each of these manifestations of the ageing process does not affect everyone, nor do they occur in a specified order, even in people who do experience them at some stage in later life; there is considerable individual variation.

Ageing as a biological phenomenon could be defined as:

> a progressive, generalised impairment of function resulting from a loss of adaptive response to stress and in a growing risk of age-related disease. (Kirkwood, 1992, p. 35)

The correlation between the occurrence of these biological changes and chronological age varies between species. Similar changes occur in all mammals, but they occur at very different points in the lifespan when different species are compared, and do not correlate well with the closeness of death. Ageing is not, of course, a uniquely human phenomenon, but the physiological and behavioural manifestations of old age are very much *less* apparent in natural populations of other animals than they are among humans.

● Explain why this should be so (think back to the discussion of human growth and life history in Chapter 2).

■ Most animals die in the wild before they reach old age. Among those that do not, any slight decline in the ability to survive caused by ageing increases their risk of death through predation, starvation or disease. Humans are better protected from such natural hazards, especially in prosperous societies where the majority live to old age.

8.1.2 Studying ageing cells

All cells undergo some changes with age, though age does not necessarily mean the same thing for the many different types of cell in the bodies of large multicellular animals such as ourselves. Some cells are short-lived and are rapidly replaced by others: for example, in humans this is true of skin cells, cells that line the gut (Chapter 7) and red blood cells. For these cells, ageing occurs over a few weeks; they change in form and function and are then shed or destroyed. Other cells, such as the nerve cells (neurons) in the brain, cannot be replaced after birth, so they tend to be long-lived and brain-ageing occurs over the lifespan of the individual.

One method of studying cells is a technique known as *tissue culture*. Cells are isolated and grown outside the body in containers of nutrient medium. The 'growth potential' of these cells is measured by the number of times the population of cells doubles in number, in other words, by the number of cell divisions. All cultured cells have a period of normal growth (of around 60 doublings) followed by a period of senescence (ageing) when they divide less frequently. In general, the growth potential of cells in laboratory cultures *decreases* slightly with *increasing* age of the donor from whom the original cells came. This is one method of studying cellular age-related changes by comparing the activity of cells taken from individuals of different ages; their appearance and biochemistry can also be investigated

● Suggest one drawback to studying ageing in cells in tissue culture.

■ Tissue culture removes cells from their normal physiological environment and prevents the normal cell-to-cell interactions that would take place in the whole organism — for example, the effects of hormones and nerves are removed.

In comparative studies, it is difficult to know whether the observed differences in cultured cells from donors of different ages are due to intrinsic age-related changes or to differences in the donor's behaviour.

● Why would you have to take this problem into account if you were comparing the activity of muscle cells taken from people of different ages?

■ If the muscle cells of older people differ from those of younger people, is it because of intrinsic ageing processes in the cells, or has lack of activity and a more sedentary lifestyle in the donor brought about changes in their muscle cells?

Despite these and other drawbacks, these methods have identified a number of changes in mammalian cells as they age. The components of cells, the proteins and other molecules as well as the organelles and membranes (Section 3.3), are continuously changing; for example, different amounts of chemicals such as enzymes, hormones and neurotransmitters may be manufactured in response to changing needs. These components are subsequently broken down into smaller constituents for recycling, but, as the cell ages, the rate of *turnover* of essential components declines.

● How might this affect the functioning of the cell?

■ Any component that is defective or damaged remains in place longer, and those in short supply are not replenished as quickly as before; this reduces the efficiency of the cell in performing its normal functions and, potentially, also reduces the efficiency of any organ or tissue of which the cell is a part.

The turnover of proteins in normal cells and body fluids produces a 'marker' of ageing. Proteins are broken down by enzymes into their constituent amino acids (the process is similar to that by which proteins in the diet are digested, as described in Chapter 7), and the amino acids are 'recycled' in the synthesis of new proteins. The efficiency of this recycling decreases with age. A by-product of inefficient protein recycling is granules of a fatty pigment called *lipofuscin* (pronounced 'ly-poh-few-sin'), which start to accumulate in the cell. Lipofuscin is a universal marker of old cells (Figure 8.1). When it is 'fed' to cells in culture it slows their *metabolic activity* — the 'sum total' of chemical interactions taking place in the cell.

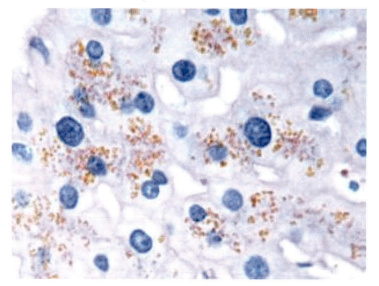

Brown deposits of lipofuscin can be seen in this microscope preparation of cells taken from a 55-year-old woman; a build-up of lipofuscin is a universal marker of 'old' cells. The larger blue circles are the cell nuclei, which have absorbed a biological dye. (The photograph was taken at a magnification of 400.) (Photo: Cellular Pathology, John Radcliffe Hospital, Oxford)

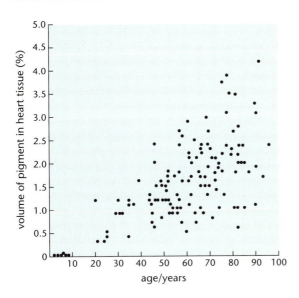

Figure 8.1   *Scatter diagram showing the relationship between age in humans and the concentration of pigment (lipofuscin) in heart muscle cells; notice that the relationship becomes quite weak (the points are more scattered) among the 'oldest old', some of whom have lipofuscin levels similar to those of 20–30-year-olds, while others have levels more than 10 times as great. (Adapted from Strehler, B. L., Mark, D. D., Mildran, A. S. and Gee, M. V., 1959, Rate and magnitude of age pigment accumulation in the human myocardium,* Journal of Gerontology, *14, Figure 2, p. 434)*

● If lipofuscin also has this effect on *living* cells in the body, what are the consequences for cell function as lipofuscin accumulates with ageing?

■ The rate of manufacture and recycling of proteins will further decrease, and there will be a consequent slowing of cell metabolism.

Another noticeable age-related change in mammalian cells is an increase in the number of *lysosomes*, the small intracellular packets of enzymes and other destructive chemicals in the cytosol (Box 3.1 and Figure 3.5). It has been suggested that accumulation of lipofuscin and of lysosomes leads to cell death. There is, however, no good evidence that these are harmful to cells and their appearance could be related to some unknown event, unconnected with age. But some of these 'aged' cells die before the organism dies and, in tissues where cells are not replaced, this leads to diminished functioning of organs. For instance, 50 per cent of nephrons (the filtration units in the kidney) are lost between the ages of 30 and 90 years.

There is considerable evidence that cells are genetically programmed to die *unless* continuously stimulated by chemical signals from other cells; it may turn out to be the failure of these signals in old age that lead to cells 'committing suicide' — a process termed **programmed cell death** (or *apoptosis* — 'appoh-toe-sis'); we will refer to it again at the end of the chapter when we discuss the biological events involved in generating cancer cells.

8.2   The evolution of ageing and death

> Since everything was made for a purpose, everything is necessarily for the best purpose. (Voltaire, 1759)

This optimistic view, expressed by Dr Pangloss in the novel *Candide,* is often accepted by romantics surveying 'wondrous Nature'. It parodies the mistaken belief, in the context of evolution by natural selection, that *every* characteristic of the organisms we see surviving today must be *adaptive*; that is, every characteristic has in some way increased the chance of the organism surviving to leave offspring that in their turn also reproduce. According to this view, surely it must be possible to understand the adaptive value of ageing and death? You should, by now, be able to detect the fallacy in this assumption: some characteristics *are* adaptive in the present environment, but others are deleterious and some are neutral.

As you would expect, there *are* hypotheses that ageing is adaptive and that it evolved through natural selection, but they do not withstand critical examination. Natural selection operates on the *individual* and no hypothesis has been advanced that seriously suggests that it is an advantage to individuals to be dead. There are, however, several hypotheses that ageing evolved through natural selection, but which argue that ageing is deleterious and thus *non-adaptive*.

8.2.1 Is ageing 'non-adaptive'?

At first sight, this appears to be a contradiction: how could natural selection lead to the evolution of a non-adaptive characteristic? You have already met one such hypothesis in Chapter 5 of this book: it states that *late-acting* deleterious genes cannot be eliminated by natural selection.

● How 'late' must the activity of these deleterious genes be in an individual's lifespan, according to this hypothesis?

■ The genes must have a deleterious effect only after some reproductive activity has taken place, thus ensuring that these deleterious genes have had a chance to be passed on to progeny.

Another hypothesis that ageing is non-adaptive and yet evolved through natural selection is based on the fact that many genes have multiple effects — for example, the gene responsible for the disease *phenylketonuria*, PKU (Section 4.9) affects mental function, hair colour and skin tone. If a gene with multiple effects is involved in ageing, it might have favourable effects early in an organism's life but deleterious effects later. Natural selection will favour the spread of such genes because of their beneficial early effects, leading inevitably to the accumulation of genes with deleterious late effects. This hypothesis does not specify which particular genes are likely to be responsible for the process of ageing, but another hypothesis is more specific about the nature of the ageing processes.

The **disposable soma theory** is named after a Western economic phenomenon and the Greek word *soma* meaning 'body'. Motor cars and other machines are typically designed and built to last for a certain length of time. It is possible to make cars that last a very long time, but they are expensive to make and, such are the realities of consumer taste and wealth, have only limited market appeal. Generally, rather little investment is made by machine manufacturers in durability. By analogy, it is suggested that organisms derive little benefit from investing resources in increasing their lifespan beyond a certain point.

Two arguments are involved here. First, the fundamental trade-off between *somatic effort* and *reproductive effort* (discussed in Section 5.5.3), means that somatic effort will never be maximised because to do so might be to pass up the chance to reproduce at all. Thus, some durability must be sacrificed to achieve reproduction. Second, all organisms are subject to accidental death, through a variety of hazards, and so have only a finite expectation of life, even if they do not age. To invest in survival in the expectation of eternal life is inefficient, because the inevitability of eventual death through some kind of accident means that resources that could have been put into reproduction will have been wasted. Thus, the disposable soma theory argues that the *optimal* level of investment in the soma (body) is *less* than would be required for the indefinite survival of the individual. Consequently, organisms show the various manifestations of ageing because they do not invest resources in preventing them from occurring.

These *non-adaptive* explanations of the evolution of ageing are not mutually exclusive. The disposable soma theory is consistent with the basic tenets of *life-history theory* (see Section 5.5.1), and does not present any counter-arguments to the other non-adaptive hypotheses mentioned above. It seems likely that ageing occurs through a combination of harmful genetic effects, the pattern of investment in the soma throughout life, and also to by-products of normal cellular activity. The relative importance of these three factors probably varies greatly from species to species, and between individuals, but there are some aspects of the ageing process that are common to all organisms. These shared cellular signs of ageing are described next.

8.2.2 Is there a maximum lifespan?

> The best of men cannot suspend their fate:
> The good die early and the bad die late.
> (Daniel Defoe, 1661–1731, from 'Character of the
> late Dr S. Annesley', written in 1697)

Death is a separate issue from ageing. It is a matter of common observation that death can occur at any age, but in the UK and other industrialised nations it gradually becomes more likely after about forty years of life and the chance of dying accelerates quite rapidly after the age of seventy (see Figure 5.5). However, this relationship between age and death is not true for all countries and historical periods. In sixteenth century England, and in many parts of the developing world today, it is children under the age of five years who are at the highest risk of dying.[1] Childhood mortality dramatically reduced in developed countries during the twentieth century, and has fallen even in the very low-income group of developing countries since the 1970s, and as a consequence *average* life expectancy has increased.

The events prior to death are clearly a great deal more varied than the events prior to birth. Humans age relatively slowly and the variation between individuals, both in the rate of ageing and the age at death, is huge. But the question remains, if we are not killed by accident or disease, does our life then inevitably terminate after some allotted span? Whether there is an upper limit on human age does not deny that death is inevitable and cannot be prevented by evolution (as Chapter 5 explained), so the first line of Daniel Defoe's assertion is clearly correct.

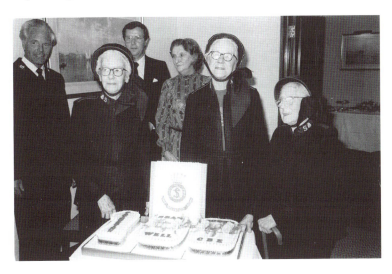

Catherine Branwell-Booth, shown here on her 100th birthday with her two sisters, both in their nineties. All three were officers in the Salvation Army. Is their longevity the result of female biology, of the inheritance of genes that increase lifespan, of companionship and mutual support, or of an abstemious life? (Photo: PA Photo Library)

[1] *World Health and Disease* (Open University Press, 3rd edn 2001) Chapter 6, compares mortality rates and age in a sixteenth-century English parish and in South Africa in 1995 (see Figure 6.3).

Until recently, scientists accepted that each species has an 'in-built' or genetically programmed *maximum* lifespan, which can be estimated by recording the age at which the oldest members of that species die. For humans, this is around 115 years in well-documented cases. However, the idea that there are typical species-specific maximum lifespans has been challenged by experiments on fruit-flies and other invertebrates, which are discussed later in the chapter. The risk of death in these examples does not show an indefinite exponential rise with age, but tends to 'level off' at advanced ages. This finding is important when we consider the *evolutionary* mechanisms underlying ageing, and the relationship between ageing and death, because it suggests that death in old age is not necessarily a genetically programmed event.

8.3   The ageing body

As we get older, our lean body mass reduces and there is also a progressive reduction in the water content of the body. This represents loss from, and consequent decline in functioning of, a variety of organ systems. As you read on, you might like to consider whether all these age-related changes are inevitable.

8.3.1 Functional changes

The major organs in the human body have considerable **reserve capacity** (potential to increase activity in times of need); for example, you could live with only half a kidney functioning instead of two. But there is a marked loss of reserve capacity with age in many organs (see Figure 8.2), which means that an older person may not be able to compensate adequately for some physiological stresses. Notice that the reserve declines at very different rates in different organs.

● What reductions in the efficient functioning of the body are often associated with old age?[2]

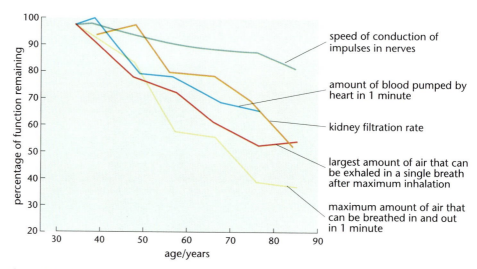

Figure 8.2   *The reserve capacity of some organs declines in humans with increasing age. (Source: Passmore, R. and Robson, J. S., 1980,* A Companion to Medical Studies, Volume 2, Pharmacology, Microbiology, General Pathology and Related Subjects, *2nd edn, Blackwells Scientific Publishing, Oxford; based on data from Shock, N. W. et al., 1957,* Geriatrics, *12(40).)*

[2] *World Health and Disease* (Open University Press, 3rd edn) Chapter 9 reviews the association between age and recent epidemiology of functional restrictions, disability and disease in the UK.

■ The following list is not exhaustive.

Structural problems become more common: for example, muscles are weaker, joints move less freely, bones break more easily and repair less reliably, tooth decay often leads to loss of natural teeth.

Sensory impairments are often reported, such as poorer sight, hearing, sense of balance, smell and taste.

Reduced ability to recall recent and generally trivial events, or to remember 'what I meant to do next' is a problem for some older people.

An increased susceptibility to infectious diseases suggests that there has been some reduction in the efficiency of the immune system (Chapter 6).

Homeostatic mechanisms, such as the ability to maintain a constant temperature in a cold environment, may become less efficient.

After menopause, women lose their ability to conceive a baby without medical intervention.

● Are these changes inevitable? (Think about several elderly people whom you know well.)

■ A striking fact about this list is that (with the exception of menopause) none of these functional losses are inevitable; every old person does not experience all these changes. Nor does an individual who suffers from one impairment necessarily suffer from another.

● What kinds of diseases are more commonly found in older people?

■ The rates of cancers, arthritis and diseases of the cardiovascular and cerebrovascular systems (such as heart attacks and strokes) all increase with age after about forty years, but none of them are exclusively associated with old age.

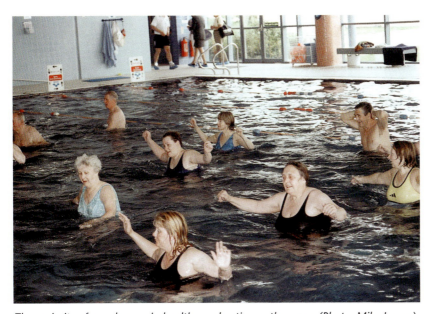

The majority of people remain healthy and active as they age. (Photo: Mike Levers)

The pattern of diseases and disabilities are not the same in men and women as they age; for example, older women are less likely than men to suffer from heart disease but more likely to develop arthritis. These differences are thought to be primarily *sex-related* (i.e. a consequence of different male and female biology) rather than *gender-related* (shaped by the different cultural roles, life experiences and socio-economic position of men and women). In particular, attention has focused on the possible protective effects of female hormones such as oestrogen against known risk factors for heart disease, since the incidence rises quite sharply in women after the menopause.[3]

Later in this chapter we will consider whether any of the bodily signs of ageing listed above can be explained by our knowledge of how cells change with age; and at the end of the chapter we present a case study on the biological changes that occur in cancers. But first, we return to the evolutionary theme by reflecting on a particular aspect of ageing in women — the menopause — which involves particular functional changes in certain parts of the body.

8.3.2 Menopause

Human females are unique among mammals in that they lose the ability to reproduce at menopause, a long time before they die (recall Chapter 2). Various arguments have been put forward to explain the evolution of menopause. Fundamental to these is the fact that, for women, giving birth and feeding babies involves considerable physiological stress that can result in death. Menopause, by 'switching off' reproductive capacity, removes older women from the risks that attend reproduction.

● Suggest an explanation for the menopause as an *adaptive* characteristic in terms of survival of the woman's offspring.

■ Human infants are dependent on their mothers for food, warmth and protection for a large part of their lives. If their mothers did not stop reproducing they would eventually undertake a birth that was so stressful that they would die or would be so severely weakened that they could not continue to care adequately for their existing offspring. Thus menopause favours the survival of existing children, at the expense of potential future children.

Another argument in support of menopause as an adaptive characteristic is that post-menopausal women have a valuable contribution to make to the reproduction of their kin. This can be demonstrated in many primates (monkeys and apes), where infants are cared for not only by their mothers, but also by a variety of relatives, including their siblings, cousins, aunts, uncles and grandparents. There is some evidence that the larger this extended family of care-givers, the higher is the rate of survival of infants born into it. Post-reproductive females may be of special value to the reproductive success of genetically related family members because of their experience. A number of studies of birds and mammals have shown that breeding success increases with age; parents get better at rearing their young at each successive breeding episode.

[3] Sex-specific risk factors in heart disease are discussed in *Dilemmas in UK Health Care* (Open University Press, 2nd edn 1993; 3rd edn 2001), Chapter 10.

These arguments are based on an extension of the theory of natural selection called *kin selection*. According to this hypothesis, genes that cause a female's reproductive activity to be switched off at a certain age will be favoured by natural selection if, as a result of her post-reproductive behaviour, her progeny and those of other close relatives are more likely to survive. Her kin will tend to carry the same genes by descent, so the loss of reproductive potential by post-menopausal females is offset by their contribution to preserving the genes they share with their kin. Thus, the biological changes at menopause are believed to be adaptive, unlike the other age-related changes described above, which are generally accepted to be non-adaptive.[4]

We turn now to take a closer look at some of the reductions in bodily function which commonly (though not inevitably) occur in old age, and investigate whether they are the result of underlying cellular changes.

8.3.3 Muscles, cartilage and bones

Muscular strength

Loss of muscle strength is an irritation to older people, particularly as some deterioration starts to be noticeable from about 45 years of age. Studies indicate that the problem is caused by a loss of muscle *fibres*, rather than by the atrophy (or wasting) that is experienced when muscles are immobilised, in a plaster cast for example. This loss of muscle fibres can probably be explained by a parallel loss of *motor neurons* (the nerves that activate muscles). Muscle fibres that are not activated eventually die. Studies show that between the ages of 30 and 80 years of age, there may be a loss of 30 per cent of muscle fibres. The functional consequence of this loss of strength is that older individuals may become unable to perform some quite ordinary tasks.

● Can you suggest some examples?

■ Opening screw-top bottles and jars or using a screwdriver; opening heavy swing doors; carrying heavy packages; digging the garden.

Many studies show that these changes are not inevitable or irreversible; muscle performance can be improved through exercise at any age.

● Look at Figure 8.3 and suggest what else should be done to ensure the full use of available muscle power.

■ Keep warm! But this is easier said than done for a proportion of older people on low incomes who cannot afford to heat their homes adequately in cold weather.[5]

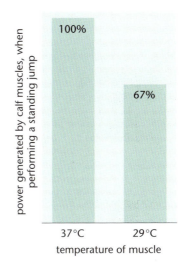

Figure 8.3 *Output of human calf muscles at different temperatures. (Data derived from: Davies, C. T. M. and Young, K., 1983, Effect of temperature on the contractile properties and muscle power of triceps sorae in humans, Journal of Applied Physiology, 55, pp. 191–5)*

---

[4] A sociological analysis of the menopause and how it is experienced by women in the UK occurs in *Birth to Old Age: Health in Transition* (Open University Press, 2nd edn 1995; colour-enhanced 2nd edn 2001), Chapter 9.

[5] The socio-economic circumstances of older people and its effect on housing and heating is referred to in *World Health and Disease* (Open University Press, 3rd edn), Chapter 10; the concept of 'structured dependency' among older people is explored further in *Birth to Old Age: Health in Transition* (Open University Press, 2nd edn 1995; colour-enhanced 2nd edn 2001), Chapters 10 and 11.

Joints

Another sign of advancing age due to reduced muscle power is a deterioration in *gait*, the efficiency with which a person walks or runs. However, factors other than reduced muscle power can contribute to a poor gait.

● Can you suggest other factors?

■ You may have thought of aching joints and stooping posture, or the effects of an injury or an illness that affects muscular coordination.

Not all older people develop these characteristics, but there are changes in cartilage and connective tissue such as tendons that make age an important risk factor in a variety of diseases of the joints and skeleton. In a young, healthy joint where two bones touch, each surface has a covering of *cartilage*, a tissue that is smoother and softer than bone (Figure 8.4). Cartilage gives the joint the ability to articulate (slide one bone over the other) without 'grinding' the bones together, and it absorbs jarring forces. Joints are held together by tough bands of connective tissue called tendons, which are also attached to muscles that bend and flex the joint. The space between the bones is filled with a lubricating fluid (synovial fluid) and the whole joint is encased in a capsule. Joints are not static mechanical structures: cartilage undergoes constant wear and repair; tendons under stress are strengthened by proteins; the fluid within the joint drains and is replenished.

The ability to maintain tissues in the joint alters with age, but it is often difficult to distinguish between intrinsic age-related biological changes, the results of repair following minor injuries, and reactions to persistent mechanical stresses such as poor posture or repetitive actions. The thinning of joint cartilage that occurs with age may be due in part to wear and tear, rather than to any underlying age-related changes in the cells that produce new cartilage. However, one extremely common age-related trait is the appearance of bone cells in cartilage. This is not necessarily associated with any observable disability, but it can make joints less mobile.

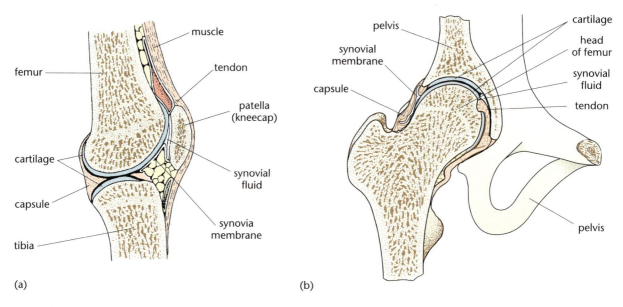

(a)   (b)

Figure 8.4 *Diagram of 'side-on' sections through joints that frequently give problems in elderly people: (a) hinge joint in the knee, and (b) ball-and-socket joint in the hip (part of the pelvis is also shown).*

The deposition of bone in the costal cartilage (which joins the ribs to the breast bone) makes this joint more rigid and restricts movements of the rib cage during breathing. Loss of water from the fibrous cartilage of the shock-absorbing discs between the vertebrae of the backbone is another problem, which can lead to a reduced ability to bear or lift weight.

It has already been observed that the proportion of proteins within cells changes with age, and the same is true for proteins secreted by cells. The amount of a protein called *collagen* in tendons increases with age, making them less elastic. (Incidentally, this change to the proportion of collagen in the skin also makes it wrinkle.) The collagen itself also alters its structure as it ages, becoming more rigid.

None of these changes represent a disability in themselves, but they make the individual more susceptible to diseases of the muscles, joints and skeleton (including arthritis) and less able to recover from accidents and injury. Disorders of the muscles and bones were responsible for approximately 40 per cent of all physical disability in British adults.

Bones and osteoporosis

In Chapter 7, we presented a case study on the evolution of adaptations to certain diets at different latitudes, with consequences for vitamin D synthesis and the absorption of calcium from the diet. Here we return to the subject to analyse why fractures are such a common cause of morbidity in older people.

Although bones are very tough, they are not rigid non-living structures. In healthy bones, new bone material is continually being generated to replace old material, which is continually being broken down. The construction and destruction processes are in equilibrium. However, older bones can become fragile as a consequence of a loss of calcium from them (a condition known as *osteoporosis*, see Figure 8.5) because old bone is being destroyed faster than it can be replaced. The change is observed in all individuals although, as with all other ageing processes, the onset and severity of the loss shows enormous individual variation.

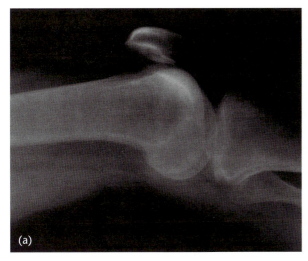
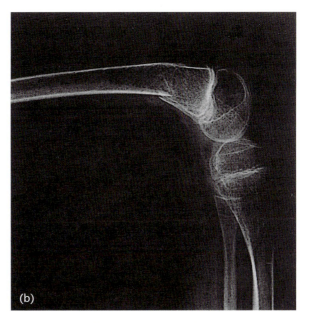

Figure 8.5 *X-ray photographs of human knee joints: (a) healthy young bone has a high density of calcium, which obstructs the transmission of X-rays through the bone so it appears white on the film; (b) this bone from an elderly person with advanced osteoporosis has lost so much calcium that it is almost transparent to X-rays and is prone to fracture. (Sources: (a) Hemel Hempstead General Hospital, Radiography Department; (b) Milton Keynes General Hospital, Radiography Department)*

The underlying factor in osteoporosis seems to be age-associated changes in calcium metabolism (chemical activity involving calcium in the body). Older people absorb less of the calcium that they take in with their diet, due to age-associated changes in the cells lining the gut.

●   Gut lining cells are continuously replaced. What happens to such cells as they get older?

■   As described earlier in this chapter, these cells change gradually in form and function and are eventually shed. Additionally, they divide less frequently as they age, and so they are replaced less often.

In the gut, cells that are replaced every 30 days in young adults are only replaced every 40 days in elderly people. This slowing up of cell division is reflected in how the cells function; the cells lining the gut secrete less mucus and enzymes in old age, which means that the body may digest food less efficiently. As you already know from Chapter 7, vitamin D promotes the absorption of calcium from the food across the gut lining as well as the uptake of calcium in bone. Vitamin D is absorbed by the gut and is converted into an active form in the liver and kidneys. The active form of vitamin D can only be produced if liver and kidney function are intact. As mentioned earlier, *nephrons* (the filtration units of the kidney) are progressively lost from the age of 30 years as cells die and are not replaced; in addition, average liver volume falls by over 30 per cent between the ages of about 25 and 90 years.

●   How are these changes in the kidneys and liver involved in the increase in osteoporosis and the risk of fractures in older people?

■   Reduced function in the kidneys and liver as people age results in a reduction in the amount of vitamin D converted into the active form. This in turn contributes to a reduction in calcium uptake from the diet and its deposition in bone, and hence to the slowing down of new bone growth to replace old bone as it is destroyed.

Changes in calcium metabolism are much more pronounced in women after the menopause than they are in men of the same age. Women in older age groups excrete more calcium in their urine than they take in from their diet, because calcium is withdrawn from their bones as a result of disturbance in the various hormones involved in the normal formation of bone. In some research studies, treatment with oestrogen has had a beneficial effect on calcium balance, and has reduced the rate at which bone density was lost in older women, but the results are contradicted by other studies and so remain controversial. And, unless it is given with another female hormone — progesterone — oestrogen replacement therapy increases the incidence of cancer of the uterus (womb).

The foregoing account should have convinced you that it is because of age-related changes in *cells* that muscles and bones weaken and joints can 'seize up' as we get older, and that these cellular changes are themselves influenced by complex biochemical processes with widespread effects throughout the body. You should also remember that there are a variety of means, principally involving exercise and diet, to reduce the potentially damaging effects of cellular changes in old age.

8.3.4 The senses

Vision

There are many age-associated changes in the eye; perhaps best known is the loss of the ability to change focus. This occurs because the lens grows throughout life, adding fibres of proteins known as *crystallins*. By the time it is 50 to 60 years old it is almost impossible to change the shape of the lens and, although distant objects may be in sharp focus, near objects are usually blurred. There may also be changes in the structure of some crystallins, which can result in the formation of a cataract, an opaque covering of the lens causing blindness. The sensory cells of the eye (called rods and cones) manufacture pigments involved in registering the patterns of light that fall on the eye. Proteins are major constituents of these visual pigments. Lipofuscin can be detected in the rods and cones of children as young as 10 years old; by the age of 24 lipofuscin occupies about 8 per cent of the volume of these cells, rising to over 20 per cent by 80 years of age.

● What might be the possible functional consequences of this accumulation of lipofuscin?

■ As lipofuscin accumulates, the rate of manufacture and recycling of the visual pigments decreases. Any defective or damaged pigment will remain in place longer, making the rods and cones more susceptible to the effects of cumulative damage. This contributes to the deterioration of vision in old age.

Slowing of other metabolic processes will also occur in the presence of high concentrations of lipofuscin, including those that prevent or repair damage from radiation. Our eyes are exposed to the physical effects of sunlight; damage from this source of radiation slowly accumulates as we age.

Hearing

Hearing loss in old age is associated with degeneration of sensory cells in the inner ear and/or the nerves involved in sensitivity to sounds. Some types of hearing loss have a familial tendency and hence probably have a genetic basis.

● Can you suggest an alternative explanation?

■ There could be an environmental effect on hearing that is common to family members, such as living close to a major road or working in the same (noisy) industry such as coal mining or cotton mills.

It is easy to show that hearing is damaged by persistent exposure to loud noises generated by heavy machinery, industrial explosions (e.g. in quarrying) and certain kinds of music, but less obvious that everyday noises (from traffic for example) slowly destroy sensory cells. Comparative studies of people who live in non-industrial societies suggests that high-tone hearing loss (a universal feature of Western societies) is mostly due to the level of 'general background' noise experienced in urban environments. It is difficult to know whether the hearing loss commonly measured in elderly people is the outcome of age-associated changes in sensory cells or the effect of living (or working) for a long time in a noisy environment.

This brief look at some of the changes that can occur as people grow older has revealed some common features. Cells do change with age and so do their protein products. Some cells die before the organism dies. All age-related deficits can be traced back to changed cellular activity, so the next stage in our investigation of the ageing process is to enquire about the mechanisms that bring about cellular ageing.

8.4 Biological mechanisms of cellular ageing

Most biologists view ageing as a *non-adaptive* evolutionary process, as described earlier in this chapter. The tremendous variation in the ways and extent to which different individuals age suggests that numerous mechanisms leading to cellular ageing may be at work simultaneously within the population. These mechanisms range from the effects of lifestyle and environment to the action of genes; we will very briefly review the most important of them. Much of the research into cellular ageing has been carried out on species with very short lifespans, such as fruit-flies and small rodents, in preference to waiting 70–80 years to observe the mechanisms involved in this process in humans.

8.4.1 Lifestyle and cellular ageing

There is evidence that certain aspects of a person's lifestyle can have a considerable effect on his or her lifespan.

● Suggest a number of ways in which lifestyle factors might do this.

■ You might have thought of excessive alcohol consumption damaging the liver, participation in dangerous sports leading to accidental death, or tobacco-related damage to the lungs, heart, blood vessels and other organs, as factors decreasing lifespans; conversely, a 'balanced' diet and a moderate amount of regular exercise might increase one's chances of living to a 'ripe old age'.

Diet is a lifestyle factor that is of particular interest because of evidence from studies on laboratory animals. Rats maintained on a reduced-calorie diet live significantly longer than those allowed to eat as much as they choose.

● Why might these observations have no relevance to humans?

■ Apart from the fact that rats are rats and humans are humans, it is also possible that the laboratory rats that eat as much as they wish are the 'abnormal' group and that a low-calorie diet is nearer to the 'normal' diet of a wild rat.

Scientists are attempting to study the effect of a reduced-calorie diet in non-human primates, but at present there is no evidence that a reduced-calorie diet would lengthen the life of a person who is not already obese. However, it would still be useful to know more about whether, and in what ways, diet might interact with individual genotypes to affect the ageing process, but there is little evidence to date that components of the diet, or any other aspects of lifestyle, *causes* cells to age.

8.4.2 'Wear and tear', toxins and protein turnover

Three other general theories of ageing focus on the cellular level. The first of these emphasises the mechanical aspects of 'wear and tear'. Structures such as teeth, and cartilage at the ends of bones, generally wear out with time. But they out-last many individuals' needs and, with care, they may last a lifetime with almost no signs of mechanical erosion. Although, as mentioned earlier, some cells, such as neurons, cannot be replaced when they die, plenty remain. So mechanical wear and tear resulting from common lifestyles is not a major cause of cellular ageing.

An alternative explanation focuses on the fact that as we get older, the cells of our bodies accumulate *toxins* that are not excreted. The liver is particularly vulnerable as it is the organ with the major role in detoxification (as described in Chapter 7) and it stores toxins that cannot be excreted. Despite the fact that average liver volume falls by over a third during the lifespan, and that old liver cells have increased lipofuscin and other inactive proteins, there is no evidence that liver function is impaired in old livers unless they are damaged by excessive long-term alcohol consumption. It seems unlikely that cell ageing is a result of the accumulation of toxins.

Evidence from a number of species points to a decline in the rate of *protein synthesis* and 'turnover' (i.e. the replacement of 'old' protein molecules by newly synthesised ones) as being a universal characteristic of ageing cells. The accumulation of protein past its 'sell-by' date within the cell may inhibit the production of new protein, while the 'old' protein may be subtly altered and less effective. A reduced-calorie diet *may* lessen these age-associated changes, as well as decreasing the number of proteins that are damaged by reacting with particular sugars. As protein turnover declines, so lipofuscin begins to accumulate, further reducing protein turnover. These processes may be fundamental to ageing, but the cause of this slowing down of cellular metabolism in the first place is unknown.

8.4.3 Genes and cellular ageing

Far more persuasive are theories that focus on the genetic level. Comparative studies of fruit-flies which have been carefully bred to produce strains with either long or short lifespans demonstrate that many genes act together to influence the length of life. However, it is possible for the activity of just *one* gene to be responsible for major age-related changes. There are numerous cases known in a range of organisms where single-gene changes have dramatic effects upon longevity. In the nematode worm (*Caenorhabditis elegans*), for example, a single mutation has been found in a gene named *age-1*, which markedly enhances lifespan (Walker *et al.*, 2000); in the fruit-fly (*Drosophila*), carriers of the aptly named *methusela* gene mutation have a 30 per cent increased lifespan (Lin *et al.*, 1998).

There is evidence that single-gene effects on ageing also occur in humans, from studies of a rare and very distressing group of conditions called the *progerias*. There are several forms of progeria, but they have in common the inheritance of a defective gene which causes the body to age much more rapidly than normal. One such disease is known as *Werner's syndrome*; affected infants develop a senile appearance, diabetes, cataracts and atherosclerosis (vascular degeneration caused by fatty plaques deposited in artery walls, which increase the risk of strokes and heart disease), and many other features of 'normal' old age. The gene that is mutated in this disease encodes a protein that plays an important role in DNA processing (Chapter 4).

● What features of this genetic disease convince you that it must be due to the inheritance of two copies of a recessive allele? (You may want to revise the meaning of 'recessive allele' in Section 4.6.)

■ A gene that causes such dramatic premature ageing would never be passed on to offspring if it were dominant, because affected individuals never reach reproductive age. A dominant gene would therefore be very strongly selected against in the population. But a recessive gene could persist in the population in unaffected 'carriers' (i.e. *heterozygous* individuals who have only one copy of this gene).

Where genes have been identified that influence ageing, the proteins that they encode all function in cellular processes involved either in the maintenance of DNA or in protection of the cell from damage — topics covered in the next section. We turn now to consider general theories explaining the role of DNA in the ageing process.

8.5   DNA and ageing

Three general types of theory have been put forward to explain what happens in the structure (and hence the function) of DNA during ageing. Notice that we have been careful not to imply that these theories offer *causal* explanations — in fact, if there *is* a causal link and not simply an association between two unrelated phenomena, the *direction of causality* is far from clear.[6] For example, in the first of these theories described below, we cannot say whether ageing causes somatic mutation or vice versa.

8.5.1   Somatic mutation theory

Over time, changes called *somatic mutations* occur in the DNA of many body cells (described in Chapters 3 and 4; 'somatic' denotes that the mutation does not affect the germline DNA (Section 3.7) and so is not passed on to the next generation). Most alterations to the sequence of nucleotides in the DNA strand are repaired by special enzymes, but despite this process there is an accumulation of somatic mutations as cells divide and divide again throughout life. However, various experiments suggest that while these changes are not responsible directly for the onset of ageing, they might contribute in some way and they *are* important causes of cancer, as you will see later.

8.5.2   Free radical theory

The structure of DNA and the proteins it encodes can also be altered by the activity of *free radicals*. These are groups of highly reactive atoms, the by-products of normal cellular activity, which are usually very short-lived. They are 'mopped up' by special enzymes, but if they escape deactivation they have the potential to do enormous damage. Free radicals can react with molecules in the cell (the particular chemical process involved is called *oxidation* and was mentioned in Chapter 7), changing the structure of the molecule; as a consequence, this form of damage is often referred to as *oxidative stress*. The changes in long-lasting proteins, like the crystallins of the eye, may be a direct result of free radical damage to the protein, rather than an *indirect* result of damage to the gene that codes for that protein.

There are a number of lines of evidence that fit the notion that free radicals have an important role in ageing. First, human post-mortems show that the brains of older people have more oxidised proteins than are found in younger human brains. Second, experiments on laboratory animals have shown that chemicals that deactivate free radicals improve the performance of old gerbils in memory tests and also lower the levels of oxidised proteins in their brains.

---

[6] Potential problems in determining the 'causal direction' when two factors are associated (i.e. which one causes the other, or is the apparent causal link spurious?) are discussed in *Studying Health and Disease* (Open University Press, 2nd edn 1994; colour-enhanced 2nd edn 2001), Chapter 5.

Third, rodents that exercised to exhaustion were found to have at least trebled their levels of free radicals as well as damaged mitochondria in their cells. Mitochondria are the cell's 'power houses' (Box 3.1); a process takes place in the mitochondria that releases energy by the oxidation of glucose. Prolonged exercise requires an increase in the amount of energy generated in the mitochondria by oxidation; this in turn generates more free radicals, which damage cell function.

Finally, analysis of several genes whose encoded proteins are known to affect cellular ageing (such as *methuselah*) are involved in cellular pathways involved in managing oxidative stress. More recently, scientists have found mice that are defective in a gene (termed *p66shc*), which plays a role in regulating cellular responses to free radicals, can live for a third longer than normal mice (Migliaccio *et al.*, 1999).

The **free radical theory of ageing** is probably the most widely accepted candidate for a *core mechanism* of ageing, i.e. a mechanism that is of universal importance in all animal species. Less than perfect defences against free radical activity would allow wide variation in the damage that ensued, dependent upon the type of molecules attacked and the types of cell that sustained the damage.

8.5.3 Telomere shortening

Telomeres are repeated sequences of nucleotides (the 'building blocks' from which DNA is made; see Figure 3.13), which occur at the very ends of the DNA strands at both ends of every chromosome. They serve to prevent these ends from being eroded when the cell divides. The telomere sequences are a series of repeated nucleotides in the following order — TTAGGG — which are normally present over 1 000 times at the ends of each chromosome. Each 'repeat' of TTAGGG is added to the end of the chromosomes by an enzyme called *telomerase*.

The overall number of these small, repeated telomere sequences decreases with age, suggesting a possible role in cellular ageing. In extreme cases of accelerated ageing — for example in people suffering from Werner's syndrome — the telomere repeats are lost at a very rapid rate, so the telomere regions get progressively shorter over time. A loss of telomeres from the ends of chromosomes could result in genetic damage and possibly cell death.

Scientists have recently shown that by adding extra copies of the gene that encodes the telomerase protein into tissue-cultured cells taken from Werner's syndrome patients, that the cells' life can be extended considerably (Wyllie *et al.*, 2000). This suggests a potential route to therapeutic intervention in this hitherto fatal condition. Whilst telomere length appears to be important in cell death, its relevance to whole body ageing is as yet unclear.

Other processes, as yet unknown, are also likely to be important agents of ageing; individual variation strongly suggests that ageing is a **multifactorial process**, that is, one in which several different causal factors interact. The knowledge of the complete human genome sequence will greatly speed up the identification of genes that exert an influence over longevity.

8.6 Cancer: a case study

In the 1990s, approximately one in five people in industrialised countries died of a cancer, the majority after the age of 65. In this book, we are concentrating on a biological and evolutionary interpretation of human health and disease, which includes ageing and death.[7] The changes in cells and functional abilities described so far in this chapter are not, in themselves, the *ultimate* causes of death. 'Old age' is no longer entered as a cause of death on medical certificates; most deaths among elderly people are attributed to a specific disease, or to a combination of diseases.

Loss of physiological reserves may make older people more susceptible to disease and hence death, but that doesn't explain why certain diseases are so much more prevalent in old age than they are in youth. A partial answer may be that most of the diseases with a high incidence in old age, such as heart disease, strokes, and cancers, have multifactorial causes. Several different factors must interact before the disease develops, and it may take many years before all these factors have coincided in the necessary sequence to produce a disease that leads ultimately to death. We can illustrate this general point by considering cancers, a highly varied group of diseases affecting most parts of the body, which increase in incidence very sharply in old age.

8.6.1 A failure of cell regulation

Medical scientists are beginning to unravel the factors underlying the onset of certain cancers and this increases the chance of future medical control of the disease. In **cancers**, cells that would normally have all the characteristics of a particular cell type (a liver cell, for example), lose their specialised structure and functions and become *undifferentiated*. An undifferentiated cancer cell resembles in many ways the unspecialised cells that existed in the early embryo, before cells differentiated into liver cells, nerve cells, etc. Cancer cells divide repeatedly; the daughter cells are similarly unspecialised and are repeatedly dividing.

A normal cell controls its division such that it divides when *appropriate* for its cell type, and it does so without losing its specialised differentiated 'identity'. For example, you have already seen this process in the lining of the gut, where cells divide repeatedly to replace those shed into the gut contents (Chapter 7).

● Can you think of another example from Chapter 6?

■ In the immune response, activated white cells divide many times to produce a greatly expanded *clone* of identical cells, all adapted to recognise and counteract a specific antigen (for example, an invading pathogen).

What triggers the transformation of a normal cell into a cancerous (or *malignant*) one? In normal situations, the cell's response is controlled by both *positive* factors that stimulate division and *negative* factors that serve to protect the cell from undertaking inappropriate division (e.g. when its DNA is damaged, or before it has finished copying its chromosomes, or when it is not supposed to!). A cancer cell is one in which this regulating process has gone awry and cellular division occurs in an uncontrolled manner. The underlying cause is genetic damage in the DNA of the cancerous cell.

The progression from a normal cell to a cancer cell is a *multistage process*, by which we mean that it involves several cellular changes and that these have to occur sequentially (see Figure 8.6). The pathways by which cancerous cells arise are immensely complicated and are still poorly understood, but we can group together certain types of genes that are involved.

[7] The sociological, personal and ethical aspects of ageing and dying are discussed in *Birth to Old Age: Health in Transition* (Open University Press, 2nd edn 1995; colour-enhanced 2nd edn 2001).

Genes that send positive signals for cancer cells to divide are termed **oncogenes** (*onco* comes from the Greek word meaning 'a lump'). Most of the known oncogenes are variants of normal genes that code for proteins involved in cell division. When a cell becomes cancerous, the normal gene is altered or mutated in some way, causing the protein to become constantly active. Over 50 oncogenes have been identified, and several must be activated before they cause a normal cell to become cancerous. Mutated oncogenes promote a rapid increase in cell numbers (Figure 8.6), but before a cell can become cancerous, the *negative* control pathway must also be disrupted.

The genes in the negative pathways are termed *anti-oncogenes* or **tumour suppressor** genes and these send signals to halt cell division or to promote differentiation into the appropriate cell type. (It should be noted that their role is crucial in the *normal* development of cells; tumour suppressor genes are activated repeatedly throughout the life of the cell, not only when oncogenes are expressed.) If a cell attempts to divide inappropriately or has major DNA damage, the balance of signals within a cell will activate a mechanism that causes the cell to 'commit suicide', a process mentioned earlier called programmed cell death (or apoptosis).

Programmed cell death acts as an in-built quality control mechanism whereby the body disposes of cells that have sustained some irreparable DNA damage and which might potentially become cancerous. Thus, a cancer cell is one that has been affected by the positive activity of oncogenes, and has escaped the biological control mechanisms evolved to stop division (tumour suppressors) and to eliminate damaged cells (apoptosis).

● How does the description of normal processes that protect us against the formation of cancer cells, and the model proposed for how they 'escape' from these constraints, resemble the evolutionary process of natural selection?

■ Normal cellular responses such as apoptosis and tumour suppression remove (i.e. select against) most pre-cancerous cells, leaving only those that have in some way or another evolved a suitable avoidance mechanism (the best adapted to survival). These cells are at an advantage and as they proliferate they

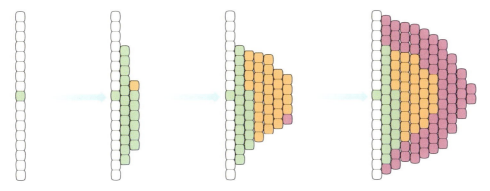

Figure 8.6 *Cancer is a multistage process. Here, a cell (green) undergoes a mutation event to give rise to a new population of cells that are less differentiated than the normal cells (cream) around them. These mutant cells divide and subsequently a second mutation arises (orange) and then a third one (purple). The process continues until a mass of undifferentiated and rapidly growing cells produces a malignant tumour (or neoplasm in medical jargon). These cells will continue to divide rapidly and some will break away from the original mass to form secondary tumours (metastases) around the body.*

accumulate more genetic mutations and undergo more rounds of selection in which only the best adapted survive. Eventually, a cell arises that has the ability to evade all the body's natural defences and is able to proliferate into a tumour. (You met an example with a similar series of steps in Chapter 5, where we discussed the evolution of antibiotic-resistant bacteria.)

An ability to detect failed control mechanisms involved in a particular individual's disease may lead to improved therapy and even prevention of some cancers. Knowledge of every human gene will greatly increase our ability to identify and detect these changes. But an underlying question remains: what causes the increased incidence of cancer with *age*? Could it be accumulated damage to the DNA from free radicals, radiation or chemical toxins in the environment, or part of a genetically programmed process of ageing? All of these theories may be accurate, since the development of cancer is accepted to be multifactorial in its origin.

The ability to correct 'errors' in DNA caused by chemical carcinogens (cancer-causing agents) or radiation appears to decline with age. Moreover, small errors in the replication of DNA occur each time a cell divides and a new set of DNA molecules is synthesised (Chapter 4) so, as a person ages, more cell divisions will have occurred and more uncorrected errors will have accumulated. The chance of damaged DNA leading to *activated* oncogenes and *inactivated* suppressor genes, and hence to cancer, is therefore likely to increase with increasing age. This is further supported by the observation that individuals who inherit a genetic predisposition to colon cancer also inherit a defective DNA repair gene.

● What effect will this have?

■ The somatic cells within an individual who inherits a defective DNA repair gene will have an intrinsically higher mutation rate than normal cells, and hence will accumulate errors at a faster rate; this is likely to lead eventually to the development of cancerous cells earlier in life.

8.6.2 Cancer and the body

Cancer cells can 'break away' from the original mass (the primary tumour), and travel around the body in the bloodstream and lymphatic circulation (Figures 3.21 and 6.9), eventually settling in a distant site to multiply into secondary tumours (or *metastases*).

● In what ways do you think cancer cells might damage the body?

■ Primary or secondary tumours in organs (such as the liver), use nutrients and oxygen, but do not contribute to the organ function. As cell numbers increase, they may hinder normal functioning of other cells and organs by, for instance, exerting pressure on nearby tissues, distorting them or blocking their blood supply, or interfering with the nerves controlling their function. The cells may also undergo further mutations to 'adapt' to their new secondary sites.

Cancer cells may also produce chemicals that disrupt the normal working of the body, or weaken bones by infiltrating them; tumours set off inflammatory reactions (Chapter 6) and can cause severe pain. Cancers are extremely variable in their progress and in their effects, because the original cancer may have arisen in almost any part of the body and the secondary tumours can be highly variable in their location. Thus, lung cancer is a very different condition from (say) breast cancer or leukaemia (cancer of the white cells in the bloodstream). If a cancer leads to death, it may be from multiple organ failures and generalised breakdown of the body's biochemistry and ability to maintain homeostasis.

It is important to end this section by reminding you that most cancers are now medically treatable with high or increasing success rates (e.g. childhood leukaemia, testicular cancer), and the incidence of many cancers in the UK is steadily falling (e.g. stomach cancer).[8] Although some cancers are rising (e.g. prostate cancer), the potential for new genetic therapies to intervene in malignant diseases is envisaged to be one of the major areas of rapid medical advance in the twenty-first century.

8.7 Conclusion

Death is inevitable, but in prosperous, industrialised human societies ageing presents a formidable challenge to health services because the proportion of the population in the oldest age groups is rising. In evolutionary terms, the manifestations of ageing (with the exception of menopause) are not adaptive processes. Currently, medical science does not understand the underlying mechanisms sufficiently to alter the progress of biological ageing in individuals; doctors can treat the diseases of old age, but they cannot stop people from getting old. If such knowledge becomes available through biomedical research, it will raise important ethical questions about the extent to which humans are justified in 'tinkering with nature'.

However, we do not have to wait for a breakthrough in research into ageing before addressing the ethics of altering human biology in profound ways. The debate has become increasingly heated since the 1990s as a result of progress in other areas of medical science — particularly in genetics and transplant surgery. The next chapter will describe some ways in which medical science is, or may soon become, able to change the quantity and quality of individuals' lives, which have far-reaching ethical and social consequences.

---

[8] Cancer rates in the UK are discussed in *World Health and Disease* (Open University Press, 3rd edn 2001), Chapter 9. Cancer screening is discussed in *Dilemmas in UK Health Care* (Open University Press, 3rd edn 2001), Chapter 9.

OBJECTIVES FOR CHAPTER 8

When you have studied this chapter, you should be able to:

8.1 Define and use, or recognise definitions and applications of, each of the terms printed in **bold** in the text.

8.2 Discuss alternative hypotheses about the evolution of ageing — including the menopause — distinguishing between views of ageing as adaptive or non-adaptive.

8.3 Describe the main age-related changes in the human body and in ageing cells.

8.4 Review the major biological theories about core mechanisms that may be involved in causing age-related changes in DNA, cells, tissues and organs.

8.5 Discuss cancer as an example of a disease with a multifactorial origin, which develops through a multistage process at the cellular and genetic level.

QUESTIONS FOR CHAPTER 8

1 (*Objective 8.2*)

It has been suggested that ageing and death are adaptive because they prevent overcrowding and consequent depletion of resources. What is the fundamental flaw in this argument?

2 (*Objective 8.3*)

Collagen is a fibrous protein that is an important constituent of tendons and hence joints. It is also found in many other tissues including the lens of the eye, skin and arteries. In all these tissues collagen becomes more rigid with age. Briefly summarise the age-related changes in these tissues and consequent effects on health in old age.

3 (*Objective 8.4*)

Outline how the biological mechanisms of cellular ageing described in this chapter could lead to cell damage and death.

4 (*Objective 8.5*)

Cancer is a multistage process. Outline the types of cellular processes that are affected when a normal cell becomes cancerous. Then look at Figure 8.6. If a person inherited the second DNA mutation which converts the green cell into the orange cell, what would you predict would be the effect upon their risk of cancer?

CHAPTER 9

Tinkering with nature

Study notes for OU students

This chapter builds on the discussion of the structure and function of DNA and cell membranes (Chapter 3), the contribution of human genes to disease (Chapter 4) and the functioning of the immune system (Chapter 6). The discussion of development in early embryonic life, which begins here, is extended in *Birth to Old Age: Health in Transition* (Open University Press, second edition 1995; colour-enhanced second edition 2001), Chapter 3. During this chapter you will be asked to read three short articles: 'One parent's reflection on genetic counselling' by Ruth McGowan (in Section 9.4.1); 'The shadow of genetic injustice' by Benno Müller-Hill (in Section 9.7.2); and 'Good gene, bad gene' by James Watson (in Section 9.9). All three articles are in *Health and Disease: A Reader* (Open University Press, third edition 2001). The audiotape 'Tinkering with nature' illustrates the ethical aspects of genetic research discussed in Section 9.7. The TV programme 'Bloodlines: A family legacy', which you watched during Chapters 3 and 4, also provides relevant background material for the chapter and the audiotape.

9.1   Introduction

At this point in the book, our focus shifts gradually from the present to the near future, as we speculate about the possible impact of medical science on human biology and even on the evolution of the human species in generations to come. In biological terms, the human species has become hugely successful in the last 300 years, increasing with breathtaking speed from a global population of about 600 million in 1700 to 6 billion (6 thousand million) by the end of the twentieth century. The reasons underlying this population explosion are discussed elsewhere,[1] but the central point is that the contribution of cultural evolution, such as the advent of agriculture, industrial practices and sanitation, have far outweighed the contribution of medical science to the dramatic increase in human survival.

However, the balance is tilting as we enter the twenty-first century. The power of cultural change to improve human health may be diminishing, as industrial development and urbanisation reach more and more of the globe. Indeed, some would claim that 'modern culture' is having the reverse effect by inflicting new diseases and exacerbating old ones — a view we debate in the final two chapters of this book. Medical science rather than cultural change is now expected to provide solutions to many hitherto intractable human diseases, particularly in Western industrialised nations. The significant increase in life expectancy in the developed world has brought with it an epidemic of degenerative diseases, which reduce the quality of the 'added' years and put severe pressure on the ability of health services to meet demand.

Chronic conditions affecting children and young adults, such as diabetes, cystic fibrosis, AIDS and multiple sclerosis, have achieved heightened public attention because they have defied all attempts at cure. As we enter into a new millennium, the opportunities for medical science to affect the future health not only of

---

[1] See *World Health and Disease* (Open University Press, 3rd edn 2001), Chapters 5 and 6, particularly Figure 5.2 for global population estimates from 40 000 BC to AD 2025.

individuals, but of the human species, are expanding at a seemingly unstoppable pace. News of 'breakthroughs' is reported daily, generating not only hope that suffering may be alleviated and lives saved, but also anxiety about the ethical and practical implications of 'tinkering with nature'.

● Think about recent media coverage of biomedical breakthroughs. Which have caused controversy about the ethics of 'tinkering with nature'?

■ Many of the issues you are likely to have thought of involve new developments in genetics, and the ability to manipulate animals by inserting new genes into their genomes, or by generating identical copies — or 'clones' — of animals from adult cells. In particular, you may have recalled the arrival in 1997 of 'Dolly the sheep' (a clone from an adult sheep cell), which raised the possibility of similar experiments with humans. (We discuss the technology and the ethical concerns posed by all of these issues later in the chapter.) You may also have thought of:

- The completion of the Human Genome Project and an almost daily announcement of the discovery of genes for this disorder or that characteristic;
- The patenting of DNA sequences and diagnostic tests by commercial companies;
- Genetic modification of our foodstuffs;
- The use of animals to grow organs for human transplantation;
- The use of human fetal cells in medical therapies.

In this chapter, we will at least touch on these subjects and the ethical dilemmas they raise, but we will also focus on the *techniques* for manipulating human cells, organs and genes. And, as you might expect in a book with an evolutionary perspective on human health and disease, we ask whether by altering human genes, medical science can alter human evolution? The potential benefits to an individual with a genetically determined disorder are enormous and yet many scientists and lay people question where we should draw the line. It is difficult, even for biologists who work outside the rapidly advancing field of genetics, to discriminate between genuine scientific potential and 'media hype'. The extraordinary pace at which new knowledge about human genes has been acquired has astounded even those performing the research, and as a result even the scientific 'elite' is struggling to grasp the implications for human health and human ethics.

Although the main focus of this chapter is on genetics, the very newness of the biology involved in recent developments carries with it the shock of the unexpected, so we start with a brief look at a more familiar example of 'tinkering with nature' — medical techniques involving the exchange of tissues and organs from the dead to the living. Here, you are on biologically familiar ground prepared in preceding chapters, which nonetheless sharply illustrates the debate about where to draw the line between legitimate medical science and unacceptable interference with human biology. Notice that 'the line' shifts as a technique becomes more widespread. We will follow the transplantation storyline right up to current advances and the issues they raise. You will see how, as we approach the areas where research and practice merge, moral and even scientific certainty is left behind, and a plethora of new legislative and regulatory bodies are at their most active.

9.2   Transplants and implants

The transfusion of blood from person to person has become so commonplace in medicine that, for most people in the industrialised world, it would not be considered as interfering with natural biology. We have forgotten the controversy that blood transfusion caused when experiments began in the seventeenth century, and few but Jehovah's Witnesses today believe it is forbidden by God.[2]

The willingness of the majority of the population to accept several pints of another person's blood into their circulation on the advice of a doctor seems a little strange in the context of heated debates about some other types of transplant. Blood may be viewed more like a 'medicinal fluid' which is freely given by one living person to another, whereas the removal of organs from recently dead people for transplantation into a living body has aroused much anxiety about the ethics of 'spare-part surgery'. As you will see, this level of anxiety increases still further when we consider the use of fetal cells, which in themselves have the biological capacity to grow into human beings.

9.2.1   Organ transplants

The ethical debate over organ transplantation began in December 1967, with the news that a South African surgeon, Christiaan Barnard, had transplanted the first human heart from a recently dead person into a man with chronic heart disease. This first recipient, Lewis Washkansky, died 18 days later and the failure of this and so many of the pioneering heart transplants over the next few years led to the practice being abandoned for about a decade. Then, in the 1980s, advances in medical science led to **organ transplantation** programmes being established in most industrialised countries, with relatively high rates of success. The breakthrough was due to a combination of progress in different fields: advances in surgical techniques and intensive post-operative care; the development of new drugs that suppress the recipient's immune system so that it does not 'reject' the graft (as described in Section 6.4.1); and techniques for 'tissue-typing' organ-donors and matching them with suitable recipients.

● Why is 'matching' necessary? (Think back to Chapter 6.)

■ The donor and recipient are genetically different (except in the rare case of identical twins), so the pattern of proteins and carbohydrates on the surface membrane of their cells differs. Unless it is totally suppressed with drugs, the immune system of the recipient will respond to these *epitopes* by attacking the cells of the graft as though they were a mass of invading organisms. Matching the donor and recipient to minimise the degree of genetic difference between them reduces the severity of the immune response and the chance of *graft rejection*. It also reduces the need to suppress the immune system with drugs, which inevitably leaves the patient prone to infection. You may also have thought about matching for size: an adult heart is not suitable for transplanting into a baby and vice versa.

[2] The medical history of blood, including transfusion, is discussed in *Medical Knowledge: Doubt and Certainty* (Open University Press, 2nd edn 1994; colour-enhanced 2nd edn 2001), Chapter 5.

Single-organ transplants are now routine practice in industrialised countries; among the most numerous and successful are kidney grafts, of which about 1 500 are performed in the UK annually. A similar number of Britons have their sight restored each year by a simple operation to transplant a healthy cornea (lens) into the eye. (The cornea has no blood supply and is beyond the reach of the immune system, so there is no need to match donor and recipient.)

Despite these successes, the number of organs available for transplantation is limited by the number of donors for whom permission can be obtained to remove their organs after death. Demand outstrips supply: in spring 2001, over 5 600 people were on the UK national transplant waiting list and the number of donors was declining. In October 2000, a computerised national register of organ donors — the NHS Organ Donor Register — was launched; it can be accessed 24 hours a day to see whether an individual has registered a willingness to be an organ donor.

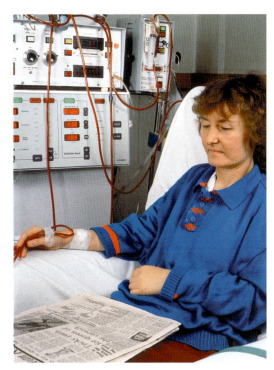

The frequency and success of organ transplant operations has not eliminated ethical concerns; for example, whole organs such as a heart or a kidney are mainly given to children and adults who are below retirement age.

● What *medical* reasons might there be for the majority of organ transplants to be performed on these age groups? What *non*-medical considerations might also be taken into account when selecting suitable candidates for transplantation?

■ The principal medical consideration is whether very young or very old patients could withstand such major surgery. Social reasons may also influence selection of recipients: the shortage of organs donated for transplantation and the high cost of major surgery may tilt the choice towards children and adults who could expect a significant number of extra years of life from the operation; younger adults are also likely to have dependants.[3]

The shortage of donor human kidneys can mean many years of dialysis treatment, in which the person's blood is fed through a dialysis machine several times a week to remove the toxic waste that would normally be filtered out by healthy kidneys. (Photo: Simon Fraser/Science Photo Library)

Concern that some patients are being passed over in the competition for organs has been less of an issue than the fear that pressure may be put on the relatives of a dying person to donate his or her organs, so that someone else can live. There have also been a very few cases of kidneys being sold for cash by healthy but impoverished donors. The need for 'rationing' underlines the extreme shortage of organs for transplantation and has forced medical science to turn to other sources of organs such as donor animals.

[3] Concern that people may be discriminated against in their access to health services on the grounds of age are discussed in *Birth to Old Age: Health in Transition* (Open University Press, 2nd edn 1995; colour-enhanced 2nd edn 2001), Chapter 10, which also refers to an article on this subject by Ann Bowling in *Health and Disease: A Reader* (Open University Press, 3rd edn 2001). Dilemmas in the rationing of scarce health service resources are the subject of Chapter 2 in *Dilemmas in UK Health Care* (Open University Press, 3rd edn 2001).

9.2.2 Organs from animals

The *origin* of transplanted organs and tissues is yet another area of contention. Most people would sanction the properly negotiated use of an organ from an adult human donor, but some would draw the line at giving a person the heart and lungs of a pig. Yet the shortage of human donors means that many potential transplant-recipients will die waiting, *unless* doctors develop ways of using the organs of other species. In fact, organs from chimpanzees, baboons and pigs have been transplanted into humans for over 40 years — a technique called **xenotransplantation** (from the Greek 'xeno' meaning 'foreign'). These experiments were largely unsuccessful because they either resulted in graft rejection by the recipient's immune system, or because the recipient could not cope with infection after treatment with drugs to suppress the immune system in an attempt to preserve the graft.

Then, in the late 1990s, genetically modified (GM) pigs were developed as a potential source of donor organs. The genetic make-up of these pigs was altered to make it less likely that the donated organ will be rejected, because its antigens appear 'less foreign' to the human immune system.

● Setting aside ethical objections for a moment, can you identify a potential biological risk associated with pig-to-human organ transplants? (Think back to Chapter 5.)

■ Concern has been raised among scientists as to whether there is a risk of transfer of pig viruses to the organ recipients, but as yet this is an unknown factor.

The creation of GM pigs as a source of human donor organs is morally reprehensible to some people — perhaps the majority in the UK in 2000. However, 100 breeding sows could meet the entire UK shortfall in kidneys for transplantation, ending long waits on dialysis and solving rationing dilemmas about allocating organs. A UK survey of people who had suffered a renal failure showed that 78 per cent would accept a pig kidney for their transplant organ (Ward, 1997). Pig-derived tissues are already used for skin grafts, and for pancreas, spleen and liver implants, and the 'humanised' pigs could have a major impact on renal patient care. These are compelling reasons for continuing research on these animals.

As time passes, the use of pig organs may become more accepted — just as human heart transplants did in the 1980s after initial outcries against them as being 'unnatural'. In the end, the efficacy (how effective it is therapeutically) of using pig organs will be judged through the usual rounds of clinical trials.[4] Such trials are carefully monitored and overseen by a scientific and medical watchdog called the UK Xenotransplantation Interim Regulatory Authority, which makes recommendations on the feasibility and safety of the organs.

9.2.3 Cell therapies

Instead of using surgery to transplant whole organs or tissues, techniques have been developed in which *cells* are transferred between individuals. These **cell therapies** have varying degrees of success depending on the origin of the cells, and they have also aroused very different levels of ethical concern.

---

[4] The design and interpretation of clinical trials are discussed in detail in *Studying Health and Disease* (Open University Press, 2nd edn 1994; colour-enhanced 2nd edn 2001), Chapter 8.

Adult bone marrow stem cells

Bone marrow transplants, rather like organ transplants, have become routine medical procedures. It is now common practice to replace a person's bone marrow by donated tissue after the patient's own bone marrow has been destroyed by chemotherapy or radiotherapy to treat certain types of cancer. The cells that are transferred are called *adult bone marrow stem cells* and they divide repeatedly to form all the white cells and red blood cells in the body. (These stem cells were mentioned in Section 6.5.4.)

Sometimes these cells are removed from a patient's own bone marrow prior to treatment for leukaemia, stored at very low temperatures, and transferred back after the toxic therapy has been completed. This avoids the need for drugs that suppress the immune system because the cells are perfectly 'matched', coming from the same individual. (This also a possible route for *gene therapy*, which we shall discuss later in this chapter.)

In most cases, however, the bone marrow transplant is from a closely related donor. This means that the recipient's immune system must first be suppressed or destroyed, to prevent the donated stem cells from being attacked as 'non-self'. But the very property that makes these stem cells so powerful therapeutically, also causes a major problem. The transplanted stem cells *develop into* a functioning immune system, repopulating and replacing the patient's white cells, which were destroyed by medical treatment.

● What threat does this 'new' immune system pose to the patient?

■ The new white cells attack the body of the person who received the graft, because the patient's tissues and organs are recognised as 'non-self' by the donated cells. (If untreated, this condition is known as *graft-versus-host disease* and can be fatal.)

Fetal cell implants

The rejection problem can be overcome by a controversial technique, based on the use of *fetal cell implants* taken from the organs of aborted fetuses. The medical benefits of using fetal cell implants in non-related individuals to compensate for cellular deficiencies are very wide-ranging and depend on the very immaturity of these cells. Fetal cells have not yet developed the ability to distinguish between 'self' and 'non-self' so they become *tolerant* of their new host (*self-tolerance* was discussed in Chapter 6). The fetal graft survives but does not attack the patient's tissues.

In the late 1980s, the first implants of fetal cells taken from the brains of aborted fetuses were made into the brains of people suffering from Parkinson's disease — a progressive deterioration of coordinated muscle movements, caused by the loss of certain cells from a particular region of the brain. Cells taken from the corresponding region in the *fetal* brain were able to grow and multiply in the patient's brain because the immune system of the recipient does not recognise fetal cells as 'foreign'. The effectiveness of this treatment has been highly variable, ranging from complete remission of symptoms in a minority of patients, to disastrous side-effects resulting from the continued growth of fetal cells in the patient's brain. However, since degenerative diseases (such as Alzheimer's disease) are an increasing health problem in the developed world, much research is being pursued along this avenue.

The use of cells from fetal organs for therapeutic purposes raises some specific ethical concerns. Organs for transplantation have been removed, with parental permission, soon after the death of very young babies without public objection, but there has been a furore when the origin of the donated tissue is an aborted fetus. (Cells can be kept alive for a time after removal from a recently aborted fetus, just as an organ can be kept alive temporarily after removal from a person soon after death.) But this source of transplant material opens up the question of how these cells are obtained. Fears have been expressed that abortion clinics could turn into centres that serve as 'factory farms' for fetal transplant material.

Fetal stem cells

Another medical breakthrough occurred in 1999, which may obviate the need to use implants taken from fetal organs. This technique generated a new and potentially inexhaustible supply of **fetal stem cells** — the forerunners of the adult bone marrow stem cells we described earlier.

We mentioned earlier that fetal cells can be grown for limited lengths of time outside the body. Fetal *stem* cells, rather like bone marrow stem cells, can continue dividing *indefinitely* in the laboratory. They are *undifferentiated*, i.e. unspecialised, and given appropriate chemical signals, are capable of differentiating to form *every cell type* that exists within the human body. For this reason, fetal stem cells are referred to as **totipotent** cells ('all potentialities'). This property means that they have the potential to be used for direct transplantation into patients, as already discussed for Parkinson's disease, but more importantly, they might allow the development of replacement tissues grown in the laboratory.

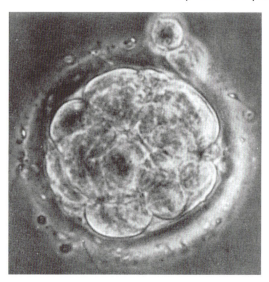

A very early stage in the development of a human embryo growing in a laboratory; this ball of cells formed by repeated divisions since the egg was fertilised 3 days ago. (Photo: Courtesy of Professor R. G. Edwards)

Fetal stem cells were originally isolated from aborted human fetuses and from 'extra' embryos generated during ***in vitro fertilisation*** (IVF) programmes. ('*In vitro*' literally means 'in glass', but conventionally refers to experiments in laboratories, e.g. in test-tubes or tissue-culture vessels.) In human IVF programmes, eggs are removed from women who cannot conceive without this intervention and fertilised in tissue cultures, usually with her partner's sperm. The cell divides to form a tiny ball of cells which is transplanted back into the woman's uterus before it reaches the 14-day stage, which is the legal limit in the UK for keeping human embryos outside the body. Usually, a larger number of embryos are generated than is safe to put back into the woman. These 'extra' embryos have either been discarded or 'deep frozen' for possible future re-implantation. In 2001, the UK government passed legislation allowing licensed research institutes to conduct experiments on these embryos within the existing 14-day limit.

The use of aborted fetuses or 'spare' embryos obviously raises similar ethical dilemmas to those we discussed earlier, but these debates were overtaken at the end of 2000 by news of another scientific breakthrough. It was discovered that fetal stem cells could easily be extracted from blood in the umbilical cord attaching newborn babies to the placenta. Millions of these totipotent cells can be obtained from a single umbilical cord, which would otherwise be incinerated.

By 2001, private companies were offering parents a new service: for a fee, they could have a 'named' sample of their newborn baby's fetal stem cells deep-frozen and stored, so that — if the need ever arose — the cells could be re-introduced into the donor in adult life, for example to repopulate his or her bone marrow after treatment for cancer. This creates a new ethical dilemma: is it morally acceptable for stocks of fetal stem cells to be held in storage 'just in case' they are needed by their donors in 20 years' time, when people for whom this technology came too late are currently dying for lack of them? Or will a new 'gift relationship' emerge, in which new parents are willing to donate some of their baby's fetal stem cells for the 'common good'?

The continual advance of medical research at the start of the twenty-first century is testing the ethical boundaries almost daily. Later in this chapter, you will see that the story of cell therapy is not yet complete, as the creation of 'Dolly the sheep' opened new avenues to researchers. The issues raised by the use of fetal cells are not only discussed in the media, but between medical researchers and ethicists and by governments. You will see examples of ethical debates leading to new legislation in the following section.

9.3   Reproductive issues

In 1990, the growing complexity of the ethical issues raised by scientific progress in fetal research led to the setting up, by the UK government, of the Human Fertilisation and Embryology Authority (HFEA), a panel of experts in human biology, medicine, ethics, religion and the law, with lay representatives. The HFEA licences institutes conducting fetal research and IVF programmes and advises government on changes to legislation in this area. Their contribution to debates in the UK is evident in the following discussion of egg donation.

9.3.1 Fetal egg donation

The ovaries develop quite early in fetal life and contain millions of immature eggs. If these eggs were recovered from aborted fetuses and 'matured' by culturing in the laboratory, this would solve the considerable shortage of donated eggs for infertility treatment.

● What ethical issues does the use of fetal eggs raise, over and above those already discussed in relation to fetal stem cells or implants?

■ There are three main ethical issues. First, there is the question of consent: in removing the egg from a fetus to use in infertility treatment the germline is being 'donated' from an individual who cannot consent to this use of her eggs. Second, the fetal egg contains germline DNA from the man and woman who created that fetus, so should *they* have some say in what use is made of their genes? Third, what psychological consequences might there be for a child who discovers that its biological 'mother' was an aborted fetus?

Similar issues are raised by the potential use of eggs taken from women and girls soon after death, although in theory an adult female could carry a donor card that allowed this use of her eggs, just as she can currently sanction the donation of certain organs after her death. There are also *biological* concerns, which were addressed in a public consultation document by the HFEA:

> … eggs from an aborted fetus have not been subjected to the [selection] pressures which govern survival and normal development to adulthood. This raises questions about the degree of risk of abnormality, at present unquantifiable, in embryos produced using such tissue. This might be seen as breaking a

natural law of biology. A further consideration is that miscarriage is frequently due to chromosomal defects in the fetus. Unless it is possible to test a fetus which is the result of miscarriage for such abnormalities, it may seem inadvisable to consider using ovarian tissue from miscarried fetuses for subsequent fertilisation and treatment because of the risk of transmitting genetic abnormality. (Human Fertilisation and Embryology Authority, 1994, p. 6)

In April 1994, an amendment to the Criminal Justice Act was passed which made it a criminal offence in the UK to use eggs from an aborted fetus for subsequent transplantation into infertile women.

Similar debates have occurred in relation to IVF and reproductive biology. It wasn't until 2000 that the HFEA permitted the use of frozen *eggs* (as opposed to frozen embryos) to be used in IVF treatment, for example eggs that had been removed from women before undergoing chemotherapy. As reproductive technologies become more common and successful, new ethical issues constantly arise. For example, it is possible to find advertisements from young women offering their eggs for sale on the Internet, accompanied by a complete family medical record alongside photographs, body measurements and exam grades.

9.3.2 Dolly the sheep and reproductive cloning

In 1997, a sheep called Dolly dominated the world's headlines.

It was supposed to be impossible. When [scientists] cloned an adult sheep to recreate a lamb with no father, they did not merely stun a world unprepared to contemplate human virgin births. They also startled a generation of researchers who had grown to believe…that cells from adult animals cannot be reprogrammed to make a whole new body. (Tim Beardsley, *Scientific American*, May 1997, p. 10)

To understand why the birth of Dolly caused a fuss even among the scientific community, we must first note some important aspects of early embryonic life in the stages just after fertilisation.[5] The ball of cells which has formed by 7 days after the egg was fertilised, separates into two populations: one group of cells goes on to form the new embryo, while the remainder implants in the wall of the uterus and forms support tissues such as the placenta. At this very early stage, all these cells are totipotent and they will only become specialised as development proceeds. From about 12 weeks onwards, the cells start to differentiate into the new organs and tissues of the baby. However, a population of fetal stem cells persists to replenish other cells as they die or are lost from the body, and these later become the adult bone marrow stem cells referred to earlier.

As described in Chapter 4, most cells in the body from birth onwards — the *somatic* cells — contain a complete set of genetic instructions to make a complete animal but, until 1987, scientists believed that the DNA in somatic cells in adult animals had undergone irreversible modifications or mutations associated with ageing (Section 8.5) such that it was impossible to use these cells as a starting point to produce a complete healthy animal. The birth of Dolly overturned this concept.

[5] Growth and development from single-cell stage, to embryo implanted in the uterus, and fetal development to a full-term baby nine months later is described in *Birth to Old Age: Health in Transition* (Open University Press, 2nd edn 1995; colour-enhanced 2nd edn 2001), Chapter 3; Figure 3.2 is particularly relevant here.

Dolly was created by taking the nucleus (containing all the genetic material) from a single somatic cell of an *adult* sheep and transferring it into an unfertilised sheep egg from which the donor's nucleus had been removed. The new cell 'engineered' by this process then divided as though it was a fertilised egg, and developed along the same pathway as 'normal' sheep embryos.

● How does the genetic material in the embryo from which Dolly developed differ from that in an embryo arising from sexual reproduction? (*Hint*: Somatic cells in sheep have 54 chromosomes.)

■ All Dolly's genes came from a single parent — in this case the adult sheep who 'donated' a new nucleus containing 54 chromosomes to the 'empty' egg cell. In normal sheep embryos, half the genes are inherited from each parent, transmitted in the 27 chromosomes in the egg and 27 in the sperm.

Thus, the 'nuclear transfer' converted the genetic material from one adult sheep cell into a new embryo, which was then implanted into the uterus of a *surrogate* ewe ('surrogate' means 'to stand in place of' — in this case it was an unrelated sheep). There, Dolly developed normally and was born naturally. This technique is called **reproductive cloning**, and has subsequently been used to generate cows, mice and monkeys, all from DNA taken from adult cells.

It is important to emphasise that in all these experiments, although thousands of cloned embryos have been created, the 'success' rate in producing healthy animals has been very low. Either the early embryos do not implant in the surrogate mother (a problem with human IVF programmes too), or the resulting fetus aborts or develops with serious abnormalities. In some cases, cloned animals have died soon after birth.

It is not immediately obvious why so much costly research has gone into reproductive cloning, until you consider the potential agricultural or pharmaceutical uses of cloned animals. Many genetically modified (GM) animals are currently being

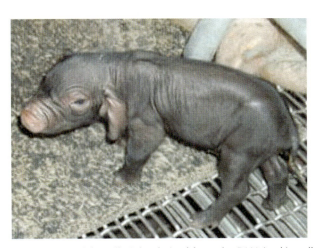 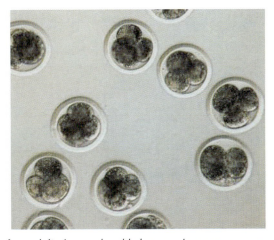

(Left) Xena, a 'cloned' piglet derived from the DNA in skin cells of an adult pig, was heralded as opening new avenues for improving livestock and producing organs for human transplantation. (Photo: Press Association) (right) 40-hour-old pig embryos, one of which gave rise to Xena, ready for re-implantation into a surrogate sow, created by a research team in Japan. The embryos were made by the insertion of pig DNA from adult skin cells into pig eggs which had been stripped of their own genetic material. (Photo: Press Association)

developed by introducing genes from one species into another. For example, transferring a human gene to a cow or sheep may induce the animal to secrete a human protein in its milk, which can be harvested for therapeutic use; blood clotting factors, human insulin and various enzymes are among the proteins already in production. GM animals may also become sources of transplant organs, as described earlier for 'humanised' pigs. (Near the end of the chapter, in Section 9.8.2, we describe these GM techniques in more detail; for the moment we are focusing on the rationale for reproductive cloning.)

● Can you suggest why it would be advantageous to be able to 'clone' a GM animal created for one of the purposes outlined above?

■ The production of identical clones of a GM animal would be of great commercial benefit, since a herd could be built up rapidly from a single GM 'parent' and be maintained over many years; this pure-bred line of animals would yield a consistent 'product' since they are genetically identical.

Before the end of 1997, the research institute that produced Dolly earlier in the year, announced the birth of Polly — a GM sheep who secreted a human blood clotting factor in her milk. A sheep cell had first been genetically modified to carry the human Factor IX gene, before its nucleus was used for reproductive cloning to create Polly. The intention is that Factor IX extracted from her milk will be used therapeutically to treat haemophilia.

● Can you suggest an advantage of such a source of clotting factors, which have hitherto been extracted from donated human blood?

■ In the past, people with haemophilia have become infected with viruses (including HIV and hepatitis C) transferred from infected blood donors in the clotting factors they have to inject every day to stay alive.[6]

The advent of limited reproductive cloning successes in animals has inevitably led to discussion of its use in humans. Circumstances where an ethical case could be made in support of reproductive cloning of a new individual from an adult human cell have been widely debated, primarily to assist infertile couples. In the UK, the question was examined in a joint study by the HFEA and the Human Genetics Advisory Commission (established in 1996 to examine issues related to genetic screening). In 1998 they expressed an opinion that although the Human Fertilisation and Embryology Act (1990) covered most of the issues relating to the cloning of humans, new legislation might be required explicitly to ban it. They also suggested that research into its potential medical applications be examined and, as we mentioned earlier in relation to embryo research, an amendment to the 1990 Act was passed in 2001, which allowed some limited research in this field to take place.

This snapshot of a few key issues in the debate about transplantation of biological material from person to person (and between animals and humans) illustrates the extent to which cultural and social factors influence whether we consider a procedure to be 'standard medical practice' or 'tinkering with nature'. Concerns have focused on the *extent* of the interference with human biology and the biology of other species, the *origins* of the material transferred, the issue of informed consent, and

[6] Further discussion of HIV infection among people with haemophilia occurs in the HIV/AIDS case study in *Experiencing and Explaining Disease* (Open University Press, 2nd edn 1996; colour-enhanced 2nd edn 2001), Chapter 4.

possible psychological damage to those concerned. All these considerations are evident in the rest of this chapter, where we discuss the medical potential and ethical consequences of research on human genes.

The twenty-first century started with the completion of the first draft of the complete sequence of the human genome (Section 3.4.4). Coupled with new techniques for intervening in genetic disorders, such as mass genetic screening, gene therapy and genetic manipulation, these are among the most fraught areas of debate in modern biology and medical science. Such revolutionary techniques bring with them profound social and ethical dilemmas, since they open up the possibility of redirecting our future evolution.

9.4 Personal decisions in genetic disorders

We begin with the most familiar aspect of medical genetics by looking at genetic disorders from the perspective of affected families. What are the choices available to families where there is either a known history of predisposition to a genetic disorder, or alternatively an affected child is born where there is no previous family history? The dilemmas involved are different in the situations discussed below: prenatal diagnosis, carrier testing and pre-symptomatic diagnostic testing. In addition there is the most pressing question following a positive test for a genetic disorder — is there an effective treatment?

In the past, human pedigrees (family trees) and family histories often played an important role in marriage contracts, particularly in terms of their financial aspects. Today they are often the first step in investigating a genetic disorder.

9.4.1 Genetic counselling and prenatal diagnosis

Almost 85 per cent of all new cases of cystic fibrosis (CF) are diagnosed in families with no apparent family history of the disease. This is because (as Section 4.7.4 showed) cystic fibrosis is a *recessive disorder* and the disease phenotype only occurs when two mutant alleles come together in the same individual — a comparatively rare event even for CF, the commonest genetic disorder in European and North American populations and their descendents in Australia and New Zealand. When a baby affected by a genetic disorder is born 'out of the blue', the parents usually undergo **genetic counselling** to explore the choices that affect them and their future children.

Genetic counselling involves communicating information about the disorder, the risks of occurrence and the psychological and practical implications of raising an affected child. Many European countries and the USA have evolved a system of regional genetic counselling centres to provide a specialist service; in the UK genetic counselling is within the framework of the National Health Service (NHS). The role of the counsellor is not to be *directive*, but rather to ensure that couples have sufficient information on which to base a decision. (Open University students may wish to read an article by Ruth McGowan at this point, 'Beyond the disorder: One parent's reflection on genetic counselling', which appears in *Health and Disease: A Reader* (Open University Press, 3rd edn 2001). The author describes her experiences after discovering that two of her three sons had inherited a genetic disorder — adrenoleukodystrophy — which carries a high risk of premature death.[7])

[7] This Reader article is referred to again in the notes associated with an audiotape entitled 'Tinkering with nature', recorded for Open University students studying this book.

Many of the experiences described by Ruth McGowan also occur in families affected by cystic fibrosis. Figure 9.1 shows the family tree of an imaginary family in which both parents are carriers of the *CF* allele. The woman is pregnant and the couple are concerned about the health of their second child, since the first has cystic fibrosis. At present, the only help such couples can be offered is genetic counselling and **prenatal diagnosis** (genetic testing of the fetus before birth) to see if it carries two copies of the recessive *CF* allele. If it does, then an induced abortion is the only currently available alternative (in 2000) to proceeding with the pregnancy and raising a second affected child. Although improvements in treatment have extended the predicted life expectancy of a child born with cystic fibrosis in 2000 to over forty years, there is as yet no cure.

● Since cystic fibrosis is an inherited disorder caused by two copies of a recessive allele, what is the risk of the unborn child indicated by a question mark in Figure 9.1 being affected? (You may need to refer back to the text and Figure 4.16, where a similar situation is considered.)

■ The risk is one-quarter, or 1 in 4.

An important point to bear in mind when assessing risks is that the outcome of any fertilisation is *independent* of any other. So, even though the first child of the partners shown in Figure 9.1 is affected by cystic fibrosis, the chance of the second child being affected is not reduced — it is still 1 in 4. You might like to reflect on what risk you might be prepared to take in these circumstances, and what decision you might make if the risk seemed unacceptably high.

Genetic testing can also occur *before* a couple choose to have a baby. **Carrier testing** is conducted before conception to determine whether or not an individual is a 'carrier' for a genetic disorder.

● What is the genotype and the phenotype of a carrier of a recessive genetic disorder such as cystic fibrosis?

■ The genotype is heterozygous, i.e. the person has a normal dominant gene and a recessive disease allele; the phenotype is 'normal' for this particular characteristic because the dominant gene codes for the normal protein.

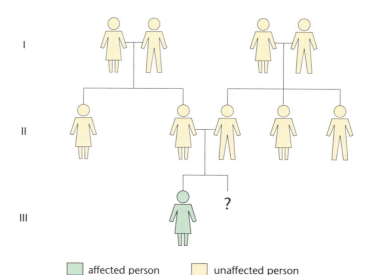

Figure 9.1 *A family history of cystic fibrosis.*

☐ affected person   ☐ unaffected person

If both prospective parents are found to be carriers, genetic counsellors can offer information on the options available to couples who consider the risk of having an affected child to be too high, such as contraception, adoption, artificial insemination by donor (which ensures that the affected allele is not transmitted by the father), or prenatal diagnosis of the fetus with the option of termination.

Where they are possible, prenatal diagnosis and carrier testing have removed from genetic counselling much of the uncertainty about the risks of some genetic disorders. However, it must be stressed that genetic testing cannot rule out all possible birth defects (some are not genetic in origin), nor even all genetic disorders, because suitable tests do not yet exist to detect them. Nor is it foolproof even for those disorders that it can generally detect (a point we return to later).

A number of techniques are available for diagnosing disorders early in pregnancy and are listed in Table 9.1 (and described in more detail below), with some indications of the conditions they can be used to detect. Note that some conditions, for example spina bifida, or not due to mutated genes.

Of the techniques for prenatal diagnosis shown in Table 9.1, only *ultrasound scanning* is non-invasive with no

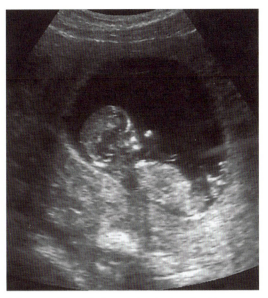

A fetus at 12 weeks' gestation is visualised by ultrasound scanning to check that it is the correct 'size for date'; this technique is also essential to guide the devices used in amniocentesis and chorionic villi sampling to collect samples of fetal cells and fluids. (Photo: Milton Keynes Hospital)

known risk to the mother or fetus; it involves 'bouncing' very high frequency sound waves off the fetus, which are reflected back into a receiver and converted into visual images.[8] It can reveal the outline of fetal organs and bones, and detect important 'spaces' such as the chambers in the heart and the fluid in the bladder.

Fetoscopy has the advantage that the fetus can be visualised directly by inserting a very fine optic telescope (fetoscope) through the abdominal wall into the uterine cavity. Using this method it is also possible to insert a hypodermic needle into the umbilical cord and withdraw blood and skin samples for genetic analysis.

Table 9.1   Techniques for prenatal diagnosis of fetal abnormalities.

Technique	Abnormalities detected
ultrasound scanning	organ abnormalities of nervous system, kidneys, heart, gut and limbs
fetoscopy	organ and limb abnormalities, skin disorders, blood disorders
amniocentesis (cells)	chromosomal disorders (e.g. Down's syndrome) metabolic disorders (e.g. PKU) DNA studies (many genetic disorders)
amniocentesis (fluid)	certain fetal protein levels (which may indicate disorders, e.g. spina bifida)
chorionic villi sampling, or chorion biopsy	chromosomal disorders (e.g. Down's syndrome) metabolic disorders (e.g. PKU) DNA studies (many genetic disorders)

[8] The use of ultrasound as a routine screening technique during pregnancy in the UK is discussed in *Birth to Old Age: Health in Transition* (Open University Press, 2nd edn 1995; colour-enhanced 2nd edn 2001), Chapter 3.

Amniocentesis involves the removal of a small amount of amniotic fluid with a hypodermic syringe (Figure 9.2). The fluid bathes the developing fetus during pregnancy and contains cells sloughed from the fetus. The fluid can be analysed for its protein content, which may be abnormal in *spina bifida* and other neural-tube defects.[9] The cells can be grown as a cell culture in the laboratory, which (after several weeks) can be examined with a microscope (e.g. to count the number of chromosomes), or subjected to biochemical tests, or the DNA can be analysed for certain genetic abnormalities. This form of prenatal diagnosis is mainly offered to women over the age of 35 years, who are at increased risk of having a child affected by Down's syndrome (look back at Figure 4.20), or women with a family history of a genetic disorder or a neural-tube defect.

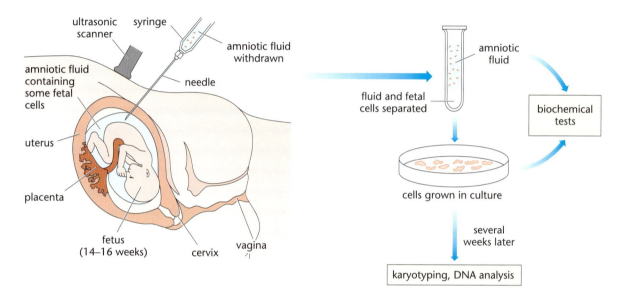

Figure 9.2   *Diagram illustrating the technique of amniocentesis used for prenatal diagnosis.*

Another approach is *chorionic villi sampling* (or *CVS*) (Figure 9.3), also known as chorion biopsy. Most of the placenta is *fetal* tissue, derived by cell division from the original fertilised egg, so it is genetically identical to the cells of the fetus; small samples of the highly frilled surface of the placenta (called the chorionic villi, rather like the gut villi you saw in Figure 7.2) are removed via a small tube inserted through the vagina of the mother. This technique has the advantage of yielding a greater amount of DNA than is obtainable by culturing the relatively few cells in a sample of amniotic fluid.

These sampling techniques for prenatal diagnosis are associated with a small increase in the risk of spontaneous abortion, compared with the risk in pregnancies not screened by these methods, so they raise the acute personal dilemma of whether or not to have a test and, if it detects an abnormality, whether or not to have an induced abortion. We return to the ethical considerations later in the chapter; here we focus on the analysis of DNA obtained by these methods.

[9] Neural-tube defects are the subject of a case study in *Studying Health and Disease* (Open University Press, 2nd edn 1994; colour-enhanced 2nd edn 2001), Chapter 8, and are the subject of a collection of research reports and correspondence from medical journals entitled 'Ethical dilemmas in evaluation', which can be found in *Health and Disease: A Reader* (Open University Press, 2nd edn 1995; 3rd edn 2001).

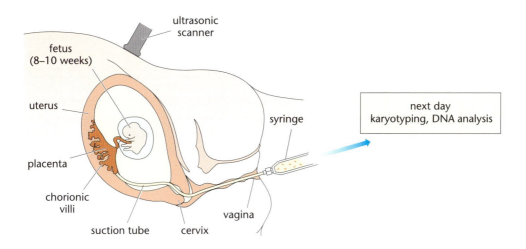

Figure 9.3 *Diagram illustrating the technique of chorionic villi sampling used for prenatal diagnosis.*

DNA analysis in prenatal diagnosis

Following the extraction of DNA from fetal cells in the laboratory, powerful techniques can enable the detection of certain mutations involved in genetic disorders, often involving only a single nucleotide change. The methods for detecting mutations are expanding rapidly, with the result that the number of disorders that can be diagnosed prenatally is increasing almost weekly. However, for each disorder a number of technical problems have to be overcome.

First, the techniques of DNA analysis rely on the ability to identify the gene involved in the disorder as a specific piece of DNA. Identifying such a gene is becoming much easier due to the availability of the complete DNA sequence of the human genome — three billion nucleotides of it! In most cases, once a precise genetic cause is known, a simple test can be performed to detect the presence or absence of the 'disease gene', or more correctly the **disease allele**. This is a shorthand term for a variant sequence of DNA produced by mutation, which is associated with a particular genetic disorder. By the year 2000, disease alleles had been identified in over 3 000 disorders and laboratory DNA tests were routinely available for over 400 of them, including those causing cystic fibrosis, Huntington's disease, sickle-cell disease and Tay–Sach's disease.

Although we have been referring to 'the' disease allele involved in a certain genetic disorder, there is considerable variation between the alleles inherited by affected individuals. For example, 70 per cent of people carrying a cystic fibrosis allele have an identical DNA mutation, which can be readily detected (see Figure 9.4 overleaf). Thirty alternative mutations (changes at different DNA positions within the *CFTR* gene, each of which causes the protein to be defective) account for another 20 per cent, and the remaining 10 per cent have been found to have one of over 800 different mutations (and more are still being found). So, to be absolutely certain of a CF diagnosis would require over 800 tests to be performed on each individual, which is beyond the current practicalities of genetic testing.

Routine screening uses tests for the most common mutations. Newer techniques are expanding the ability to detect novel mutations that cause disease, so in time the degree of certainty of prenatal diagnosis from DNA analysis will be near to 100 per cent for each genetic disorder.

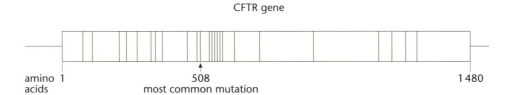

CFTR gene

amino 1
acids

508
most common mutation

1 480

Figure 9.4 *Schematic representation of the cystic fibrosis gene (CFTR), with the positions of the 24 most common mutations that cause cystic fibrosis (CF) marked as vertical black bars along the length of the gene. The numbers refer to the amino acids coded for by the CFTR gene, when the DNA code is translated into a functional protein, starting at amino acid number 1 on the left and extending to amino acid number 1 480 on the right. The most common mutation results in a deletion of the single amino acid numbered 508.*

As more prenatal testing is performed, there is a concern that an increase in abortions will follow. However, supporters of prenatal diagnosis point out that as the accuracy of the tests improve, it should lead to a *reduction* in the number of abortions.

● Can you explain why this might come about?

■ Where the accuracy of tests is less than 100 per cent (as is currently the case), some *normal* pregnancies are terminated because the *estimated risk* of the fetus being affected is higher than the parents can endure. With accurate diagnosis, these fetuses could be saved.

To others, selective abortion of affected fetuses is morally objectionable, especially when the disease might not be life threatening, as in many individuals with Down's syndrome. We will return to these issues later in the chapter.

9.4.2 Huntington's disease: to know or not to know?

Genetic testing for a few 'late-acting' disorders generally takes place in adults rather than prenatally or in newborn babies and infants, because the individual may not realise that they have inherited a disease allele until its effects begin to cause symptoms later in life. The best known example is *Huntington's disease*. Consider the family tree in Figure 9.5.

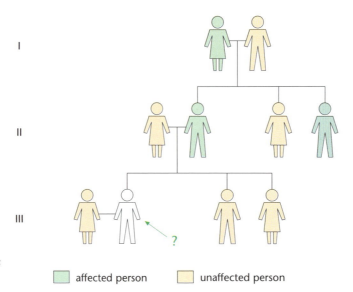

I

II

III

?

Figure 9.5 *Huntington's disease family tree.*

affected person   unaffected person

● Huntington's disease is a dominant disorder. What is the chance that the highlighted individual in generation III has inherited the *HD* gene?

■ There is a 50 per cent chance (1 in 2) that he (and his brother and sister) has inherited the disease allele from his father.

As soon as the first diagnosis of Huntington's disease occurs in a family, close family members of the affected person are generally contacted and offered genetic counselling to help them consider its implications for them. One key element in this process is to try to draw up family trees, to trace the inheritance pattern and so that other potentially affected relatives can be identified. Often the genetic link to the past is lost due to the break-up or movement of families (possibly caused by the disease itself), or by the lack of medical records for earlier generations. But where individuals can be traced, they are faced with a profound dilemma. **Pre-symptomatic diagnostic testing**, where a diagnosis can be made before the development of the disease, leads to the difficult choice of whether to take a test that will reveals one's own fate. It also poses the question of who else has the right to know.

Before the allele involved in Huntington's disease was identified and its nucleotide sequence was worked out (in 1993), family members could only be given personal risk estimates based upon the chances of inheriting the affected gene. Once the gene was isolated, a reliable genetic test soon followed, which enabled diagnostic testing to become a reality. As part of the counselling process, members of families such as the one in Figure 9.5, can now be offered a test that will tell them with absolute certainty whether they will develop a progressive, ultimately fatal disease, later in life. By choosing not to take the test, *unaffected* individuals may live with needless anxiety about their fate, but some have preferred this uncertainty rather than taking the chance that they would have to live with the knowledge of future disease.

● What does the DNA test for Huntington's disease identify? (You might want to look back at Section 4.10.2.)

■ The test directly measures the increase in the number of CAG triplets within the gene. This increased number of triplets gives rise to a neurotoxic protein that leads to progressive neuro-degeneration.

Diagnostic tests such as those for Huntington's disease present acutely difficult personal dilemmas, especially in the case of genetic disorders for which no cure is available. These tests also raise issues about the availability of life insurance for affected people, as well as questions involving pensions, health care and whether to tell their employer; these are not short-term problems — the individuals concerned may have 20 or 30 years of healthy life in front of them before the disease develops. We will return to these wider social issues later in the chapter.

As knowledge accumulates about the nature and function of human genes and their numerous alternative alleles, the more affluent populations of the industrialised world will be faced with ever-increasing information about their personal risk factors. As you will see in Section 9.6, this opens the possibility of mass genetic *screening* for genes that predispose individuals to develop multifactorial diseases such as cancers, respiratory disorders, high blood pressure and heart disease. This raises a new set of dilemmas, where personal choices in lifestyle or behaviour *might* influence when — or even *if* — the disease develops. But before we examine these issues, we need to look in more detail at the source of all this new knowledge about human genetics.

9.5   The Human Genome Project

We have so far discussed DNA testing without mentioning the many years of medical research that led to the discovery of the genes involved. In June 2000, scientists on both sides of the Atlantic announced simultaneously that they had completed the first draft of the human genome sequence, that is the complete sequence of 3 billion bases (A, C, G and T) along the DNA strands of all 23 pairs of chromosomes in the human genome. The research was finally published in the scientific press in spring 2001 and has been hailed as one of the greatest of all scientific achievements.

Knowledge of the human DNA sequence will speed up the search for new disease alleles and open up possible routes for therapy and intervention. The first impact will most likely be felt through an increased number of tests for genetic disorders based on direct identification of mutated DNA sequences, but we can also expect to see more tests becoming available which detect 'high risk' or 'susceptibility alleles' in the development of common multifactorial diseases, such as cancers and cardiovascular diseases. In addition, the improvements in technology that have occurred as part of the requirements to sequence the human genome, are likely to lead to the ability to perform many hundreds of genetic tests simultaneously on a very small DNA sample.

In identifying disease genes and developing genetic tests, scientists have also opened up new areas of ethical concern. As commercial interests in human genetics have increased, the overlap between public and commercially funded research has raised issues as to who owns the human DNA sequence and who can use some DNA tests.

9.5.1   Who owns human DNA sequences?

The human genome itself must be freely available to all humankind.

(Bruce Alberts (president of the US National Academy of Sciences) and Sir Aaron Klug (president of the Royal Society of London), 2000)

In the year leading up to the completion of the human genome sequence, a heated debate developed between the publicly and the privately funded scientists over the right to 'own' the completed product.

Central to the debate was a public and political outcry that no-one could actually 'own' the DNA sequence that carries the genetic code for a human being. However, the long-awaited public declaration that the first stage of the sequencing project was complete was a joint announcement between the public and private laboratories, and on its publication at the beginning of 2001, access to the human genome sequence became freely available to everyone on the Internet. It remains to be seen, however, what rights or ownership claims have been filed as patent applications. Issues of ownership have also arisen for specific genetic tests.

Research into medical genetics is an expensive business and, although it has become much easier because of the availability of the complete human DNA sequence, the identification of disease genes still requires input from families and affected individuals (sometimes many thousands of people). Many of the currently available genetic tests have resulted from large international collaborations between research laboratories in the public sector (i.e. funded by governments, universities, charities), which were also supported by the donation of tissues, DNA samples and often money raised by disease-affected families. While public funds still support a large amount of this work, in recent years commercial interests have become involved, tempted by the opportunities to market 'pay-to-test' kits and the rights to sell information to pharmaceutical companies about specific disease genes or therapeutic proteins encoded by human genes.

There is some justification to the claim that patents are necessary to protect the massive financial investment made by private companies to bring a pharmaceutical product to market, but the application of patents to genetic tests is more controversial. Concerns have centred on restrictions on the availability of the tests themselves, either through monopolistic licensing agreements or the charging of high fees or royalties. Any limited or restrictive testing agreements constrain the dissemination of diagnostic skills and reduce the number of suitably trained individuals who can assist in the diagnostic process (such as clinicians, geneticists and counsellors), and might also hinder the development of national genetic screening programmes.

For example, much of the research work that led to the isolation of genes that predispose women to breast and ovarian cancer was performed within the public sector using DNA samples donated by affected individuals and their families. However, the DNA sequences of these genes were patented by a private company, which owns licences on genetic tests to detect the mutations in these genes, which account for between 5 and 10 per cent of such cancers. The gene test charge in 2000 was US$2 500, a price that has had an impact on the availability of these tests in public health programmes. On the positive side, the mass production of standardised genetic tests with a high level of quality assurance can supply well-costed diagnostic kits. For example, a laboratory performing over 5 000 tests a year for the most common mutations leading to cystic fibrosis can purchase a kit for £12 per test, including royalties and licence fees (at 2001 prices).

9.6   Population screening for genetic disorders

As more is discovered about human genes, difficult choices will become common for families and individuals. So far we have considered the implications of examining relatives within an affected family for the presence or absence of particular disease alleles, and discussed the role of the genetic counsellor. Next, we broaden the focus to discuss the implications of searching for disease alleles within whole populations.

Genetic counselling and prenatal DNA analysis are available for those families with a *known* risk of having a child with a genetic disorder, or of developing a late-acting disorder such as Huntington's disease. This is quite distinct from **population genetic screening**, the search in a population of apparently unaffected individuals for people with certain genotypes that are associated with a particular disease. Screening tests are carried out proactively, rather than retrospectively as a result of a patient's symptoms.

●   What advantages might there be in conducting genetic screening of the whole population, or at least a defined population group?

■   Individuals with *treatable* or *avoidable* conditions who do not yet know that they have an increased risk of developing a disease, could be identified early so that treatment or behavioural changes can start before symptoms develop. Individuals or couples at increased risk of having children affected with severe genetic diseases can be warned in advance, instead of finding this out only when the first affected child is born.

Some see genetic screening of the population as an important public health activity because the incidence of certain genetic disorders would fall and the adverse effects of others could be reduced, but critics believe that the outcomes may have more sinister implications. **Screening programmes** (whether based on genetic or any other type of test) must fulfil several basic criteria (Box 9.1).

Box 9.1   Basic criteria for health screening programmes

- The disorder being screened for must be an important health problem, i.e. it affects many people, or has very damaging or life-threatening effects on a few;

- The disorder must either be treatable, or its detection must generate information that could prevent others from being affected;

- The screening test must be inexpensive, or at least cost-effective;

- It must also be reliable (it gives the same results if repeated) and valid (it genuinely detects what it claims to detect) and does not 'miss' cases;

- The form of the test must be safe and acceptable to the people screened.

Inherited disorders meet the first criterion in that they are undoubtedly important health problems; for example, in the UK and most other developed countries they account for over a third of all deaths in infancy. Some of these conditions are treatable if detected early enough. Genetic screening could be defended, even when the condition itself is untreatable, on the grounds that early identification leads to prompt genetic counselling and reduces the number of abortions and affected children born 'out of the blue'. A number of screening programmes have been set up for specific genetic disorders in order to achieve these aims.

9.6.1 Screening for phenylketonuria

Genetic screening began uncontroversially in the 1970s with population screening of newborn babies — **newborn screening** — to identify those with genetic diseases for which early treatment could prevent, or alleviate the symptoms. Phenylketonuria (PKU, discussed in Section 4.9) was the first genetic disease for which mass screening was conducted, by analysing blood samples taken from a needle-prick in the baby's heel. An inexpensive and definitive test is available and, if dietary control for those affected begins soon after birth and is maintained, growth and development proceed normally and mental impairment is prevented.

PKU is a recessive disorder occurring in Northern European populations in about 1 in 15 000 live births. Before the introduction of screening, it was estimated that the disorder accounted for about 1 per cent of severe mental retardation. Newborn screening has virtually eliminated this. However, the 'heel-prick' test only detects the presence of the PKU alleles *indirectly*; it detects raised levels of the amino acid phenylalanine in the baby's blood, which occur as a result of the defective alleles. There are six known causes for raised phenylalanine in the blood, only one of which is due to PKU.

● What does this suggest about the detection of PKU by this test?

■ A baby born with raised phenylalanine may not in fact have inherited the alleles involved in PKU, and hence may be wrongly diagnosed.

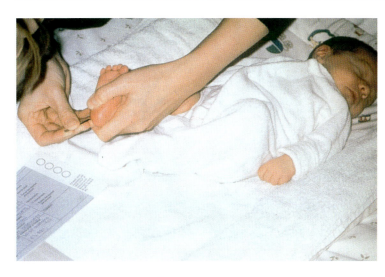

All newborn babies in the UK have been screened for phenylketonuria (PKU) since the 1970s; if untreated, this genetic disorder leads to severe mental retardation, but it can be controlled by a carefully regulated diet. (Photo: Science Photo Library)

Such a baby would be a **false positive**, i.e. falsely identified as being positive for the screened defect. Many babies have moderately raised phenylalanine which does not lead to clinical symptoms. Another group has high blood levels of phenylalanine which persist for only a short time and then spontaneously return to normal. Thus, babies identified as having raised phenylalanine are given more detailed tests to ensure that treatment for PKU is only administered when necessary, since a phenylalanine-restricted diet may be harmful. The screening programmes for detection of babies with raised phenylalanine have also provided information on the general frequency of other genes involved in this condition.

9.6.2 Screening for cystic fibrosis

Uncertainty about the advantages of population screening are well illustrated by cystic fibrosis. When the *CFTR* gene was identified in 1989, mass screening for its mutant alleles in European populations became a possibility. Over the following years, however, over 800 different mutations were identified in the same gene, all of which can cause the disease. In principle, the tests themselves are straightforward. The samples of DNA for screening are simple to extract from cells collected from a 'rinse-and-spit' mouthwash, a non-invasive procedure that most people find acceptable.

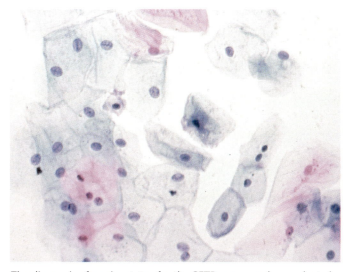

The detection of *CFTR* mutations would enable a man and a woman, who each know that they are carriers, to recognise their risk of having an affected child together, and to seek counselling. However, with so many mutations to detect, this presents the practical problem of how to test for them all in a population of millions of people, and a financial problem of how much it will cost and whether this is the most cost-effective use of public funding (a point we consider below). Moreover, some mutations involved in cystic fibrosis might still escape detection. Screening for the most common mutations

The diagnosis of carrier status for the CFTR *gene can be conducted on the DNA in cheek cells like these, collected from a 'rinse-and-spit' mouthwash. (The cells shown here have been stained to reveal their nuclei.) (Photo: Mike Stewart/The Open University)*

would mean that only about 75 per cent of at-risk couples would be identified, even if *everyone* were screened. This number could be increased to almost 85 per cent by screening for the next most common mutations (at increased cost), but the *undetected* cases of the carrier state are **false negatives**, since these individuals have the mutant allele but would be falsely reassured by the negative test result.

Problems with the accuracy of the screening test, as well as ethical considerations (discussed later), have fuelled the debate as to whether population genetic screening for cystic fibrosis should be implemented. A number of pilot antenatal screening programmes in the UK have found a high uptake (over 70 per cent) when the tests were offered. Most carrier couples accepted prenatal diagnosis and chose not to proceed with affected pregnancies in the majority of cases.

As newer and more sensitive techniques are developed to detect gene mutations, so the number of genetic disorders subjected to population screening is likely to increase. Discussions and decisions on the issues surrounding population screening for certain genes may involve us all in the near future. They raise lots of questions and no easy answers.

9.6.3 Economic analysis of genetic screening

Consider the apparently uncontroversial example of population screening for PKU. Is screening all newborn babies financially 'worthwhile' or, put in the jargon of market economics, is it cost-effective compared with *not* screening?

● What cost factors need to be taken into account in comparing screening with not screening?

■ The direct cost of the screening test for all babies and the dietary treatment of those found to have raised levels of phenylalanine, versus the cost of treating and caring for individuals who were not detected early and who suffered brain damage and other defects during infancy.

In the UK, where newborn PKU screening covers almost all the population, the financial benefits of screening outweigh the costs by over fourfold. In 1995 prices, the costs of screening 100 000 newborns was estimated at £795 000, whereas the 'saving' in health care costs was over £3 million (HTA, 1997). While lifelong treatment is not necessary (because the adult brain seems to be resistant to the abnormal level of phenylalanine found in someone with PKU), failure to detect an affected baby means that it will almost certainly have to be institutionalised for the rest of its life (on average 45 years). So, when reduced to economic values, the question could be asked 'Is it better to spend the money on testing now, or four times that sum later?'

An economic case can also be made for the antenatal screening of cystic fibrosis in the UK. To detect a single affected fetus through mass population screening programmes costs about £50 000, compared to a conservative estimate of £165 000 for lifelong care (1995 prices). As the long-term prognosis for children with cystic fibrosis born today is improving, with life expectancy now exceeding 40 years, the cost of care will increase still further. However, this cost could only be 'saved' by aborting affected fetuses, since there is still no cure for CF. This fact changes the issue of 'cost' fundamentally, where the condition is one with a rising life expectancy and some hope for the future of radical new treatments that alter affected genes.

The examples of genetic screening programmes for PKU and CF illustrate the complexity of cost–benefit analyses. And it is important to note that the calculations are solely based on *medical* costs. They ignore the financial and personal cost to affected families, and the financial and personal *contribution* to society made by a person who has a genetic disorder, some of whom are able to work and generate direct income for the state, as well as contribute in many other ways. But what if the unmeasured humanitarian benefits, such as the 'saving' in personal anguish, are large relative to the saving in financial costs? Would you cancel a screening programme that cost £25 000, but saved in total only £15 000 in medical expenditure? Should health-care decision-making also take account of the humanitarian benefits?

Population screening would inevitably result in an increase in abortion of affected fetuses and a decrease in the number of affected people in the population. Society has to consider what it would lose by such a strategy as well as what it might gain. In December 1993, the Nuffield Council on Bioethics published a report, *Genetic Screening: Ethical Issues*, in which the authors expressed concern that cost-effectiveness calculations might carry too much weight in decisions to implement population genetic screening:

> The public health definition of 'success' or 'failure' of a programme may be in danger of turning on too narrow a calculation of costs and benefits. Benefits must not be calculated in purely financial terms of preventing the birth of individuals who may have higher than average health care needs and costs. The benefits should be seen as enabling individuals to take account of the information for their own lives and empowering prospective parents to make informed choices about having children. (Nuffield Council on Bioethics, 1993, p. 80)

9.6.4 Effects of genetic screening on the incidence of disease

A number of important questions arise from the prospect of population genetic screening increasing in the future. For those genetic disorders where a reliable test already exists, what effect will population screening have on the *incidence* of the disease (i.e. the number of new cases per year) and on the frequency of the abnormal allele in the population, and what are the social consequences of screening?

The impact of genetic screening (together with counselling and selective abortion) in lowering the incidence of diseases can be dramatic, as the following examples demonstrate. Children with Tay–Sachs disease develop paralysis, dementia and blindness and usually die before their third birthday. There is no known cure. Population screening has been carried out on a massive scale in North America since 1969 in the Ashkenazi Jewish populations, in which between 3 and 5 per cent carry the gene, compared with 0.5 per cent in non-Jewish populations.[10] Screening followed by prenatal diagnosis of fetuses where both parents are carriers, has already lowered the incidence of the disease in these populations by about 80 per cent.

Thalassaemia, similar in many respects to sickle-cell disease, is a disorder of haemoglobin synthesis which affects the functioning of the red cells, causing

---

[10] Ashkenazi Jews are mainly of Central and Eastern European descent, including some who migrated to North and South America, South Africa and Australia.

anaemia. Like sickle-cell disease, it confers some resistance to malaria.[11] In the 1970s and 1980s in a large-scale screening programme, prevention of *thalassaemia* by carrier detection and prenatal diagnosis brought about large reductions in the incidence of the disease in heavily affected areas such as Cyprus, Greece and parts of Italy (see Figure 9.6). In these countries, screening was often premarital, being tied into the religious structures. However, different communities responded differently to the availability of genetic screening.

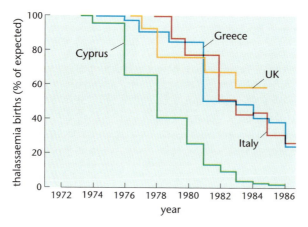

Figure 9.6   *Results of thalassaemia control programmes in Europe. UK data relate to Cypriot families living in the UK. (Data from Modell, B., Kuliev, A. M. and Wagner, M., 1991,* Community Genetics Services in Europe, *WHO Regional Publications, European series no. 38, WHO Regional Office for Europe, Copenhagen)*

● What does Figure 9.6 reveal about the trend in thalassaemia in Cypriot families in the UK and in Cyprus during this period?

■ Population screening reduced the incidence of thalassaemia by almost 100 per cent in Cyprus, but only by about 40 percentage points (from 100 down to 60 per cent) in the UK.

● Can you suggest a reason for the much lower success in the UK?

■ It is likely to be due mainly to the problem of offering a screeing service to high-risk families who are scattered among a host community at low risk. Few of those at high risk realise that they could be screened.

Screening within the UK has had variable results. By the mid 1990s, prevention of thalassaemia by carrier detection and prenatal diagnosis in Asian communities in the UK reduced the incidence of the disease by only 2 per cent, even though about 60 per cent of Asian at-risk couples accepted fetal diagnosis. One reason for this appears to be that many couples at risk of conceiving an affected child are identified too late in pregnancy for prenatal diagnosis to be acceptable to them (Modell, 1997). This highlights the difference in effectiveness between pre-conception screening with early counselling about risks, and prenatal diagnosis occurring later

[11] The biological features of thalassaemia are illustrated in the Open University TV programme 'Bloodlines: A family legacy' associated with Chapters 3 and 4 of this book; the issues raised by genetic counselling in families and communities affected by thalassaemia are the subject of the audiotape 'Tinkering with nature'.

in pregnancy. An additional factor in uptake of screening is the level of knowledge within the various at-risk communities themselves. Whereas much of the intensive Cypriot educational campaigns have carried over into these communities in the UK, there have been no similar programmes in countries such as India and Pakistan to raise community awareness in the UK. Most UK regions have had inadequate screening programmes aimed at the Asian communities, although recent studies suggest they can be implemented successfully (Modell, 1998).

However, even if prenatal diagnosis and selective abortion were widely practised, would the frequency of a disease *allele* in the population (as distinct from the frequency of the *disease*) be reduced? For diseases due to inheritance of a single *dominant* allele, mass prenatal detection of the allele followed by selective abortion would gradually eliminate the allele from the population. But most genetic diseases are due to inheritance of two *recessive* alleles.

● In recessive disorders, what effect might prenatal diagnosis and selective abortion have on the frequency of the allele in the population?

■ Very little effect, since only *homozygous* fetuses would be aborted because only they will develop the disease. Heterozygous fetuses (carriers of a single disease allele) would be born with about the same frequency as before.

Indeed, couples in which *both* partners carry the recessive allele may have *more* heterozygous children to replace the affected homozygous fetuses lost through abortion, so the number of disease alleles in the population could potentially increase. However, a primary goal of screening and counselling is to prevent disease, not to reduce the number of carriers. Prior to the availability of genetic screening, such couples might have limited their family after the birth of the first affected child. So the overall outcome of genetic screening on the frequency of the allele will depend on how many children carrier-couples choose to have. Acceptability of genetic risk and abortion varies greatly between ethnic groups; this is but one of several important features that must be taken into account when planning a population screening programme.

The genetic screening programmes for Tay–Sachs disease and thalassaemia were well planned and provided genetic counselling; neither were compulsory and both succeeded in reducing the incidence of the disease. The importance of these features can be seen in the comparison carried out by Modell (1983) between these two programmes and the detection of carriers of sickle-cell disease in the black American population of the USA, where the programme has had little effect on the incidence of the disease. The aim of the American screening programme was to identify partners at risk of having children with sickle-cell disease, but there is no successful treatment for the condition and prenatal diagnosis was not offered, so the only preventive measure was for carriers not to partner other carriers, or for high-risk couples not to have children. In addition, there was a lack of community consultation and education, and a number of mandatory screening programmes were set up, which created bad feeling.

In summary, successful genetic screening programmes aimed at large populations have the following features: public education, community support, the consent of those screened, results given through genetic counsellors, confidentiality of results, assessment of the effectiveness of the programme in terms of disease reduction, and cost savings and benefits to society. Even if the programme achieves all these criteria, the ethical dilemmas remain. They become more acute when the prospect of extending genetic screening to an ever-widening range of conditions is considered.

9.6.5 Preventive screening

The area of medical genetics concerned with the interaction between environmental factors and different human genotypes is likely to become one of increasing importance. Many examples are now known of multifactorial diseases where individuals who inherit specific alleles of a gene have an increased risk of developing that disease when exposed to a particular environmental factor. An understanding of the link between particular genotypes and environmental agents in the development of many diseases opens up the possibility of a new strategy for health promotion — **preventive screening**.

● How could prevention of these diseases be promoted?

■ Population genetic screening could be used to detect people with particular genotypes and then counsel them about the environmental and other toxic agents they should avoid.

● Can you think of an example of this type of intervention?

■ The dietary restriction that helps to protect individuals with PKU. You may also have thought of the dietary advice given to people with a genetic predisposition to hypercholesterolaemia (high blood cholesterol) and greater risk of heart disease, for whom restriction of dietary cholesterol and fats is helpful.[12]

As part of the Human Genome Project, many hundreds of thousands of gene variants have been identified and, in the near future, we can expect to see many of them linked to susceptibility to disease in particular environments. For example, much of the variation in how people respond to pharmaceutical drugs is believed to be due to genetic variation. Up to 35 per cent of patients fail to respond to beta-blockers (used to control blood pressure) and as many as 50 per cent fail to respond to tricyclic antidepressants. In other cases, a sizeable number of patients over-respond or have dramatic side-effects to drugs used therapeutically.

Preventive screening for those individuals at high risk from genetic factors might enable them to modify their exposure to environmental hazards and thus lead a longer and healthier life. But as the techniques of genetic screening develop, should we extend it to include more subtle genetic effects, for example that might predispose people to common forms of lung cancer or heart disease if they smoke tobacco? Which is the preferable course: to live in ignorance of one's likely fate, or to have the chance to reduce the risk by never smoking?

Population genetic screening clearly demonstrates how modern-day 'high-tech' medicine has the potential to interact with modern culture and affect the frequency of genetic disorders and multifactorial diseases that have a genetic component. Is preventive medicine that relies on population screening medically sound? Would it make economic sense? Who and how many would benefit? Would it be seen as an invasion of privacy? Would individuals run the risk of possible stigmatisation or discrimination on the basis of having a genotype sensitive to particular environmental factors? These questions and others need careful consideration in the context of a preventive disease programme for the future.

---

[12] Coronary heart disease is the subject of a case study in *Dilemmas in UK Health Care* (Open University Press, 3rd edn 2001), Chapter 10.

9.7 Ethics of prenatal diagnosis and genetic screening

We have already touched on several ethical considerations arising from genetic screening and prenatal diagnosis, but there are many others. In 1993, the Nuffield Council on Bioethics published a report on genetic screening which highlighted these issues as they affect individuals and those with wider implications for society (see the list of Further sources at the end of this book).[13]

9.7.1 Termination of an affected fetus

At the personal level, the major ethical issue raised by prenatal diagnosis is that relating to abortion. Should a pregnant woman who agrees to prenatal diagnosis have made a *prior* commitment to terminate the pregnancy if she is carrying a fetus with a genetic (or other serious) disorder? What are the rights of the male partner in such a situation, and will health professionals bring undue pressure to bear on the parents' decision? Professor Robert Williamson, a medical geneticist, expresses this fear:

> While many professional geneticists regard the provision of information as important in its own right so as to facilitate choice, those concerned with the economics of health care may regard this as a frivolous luxury if the majority of those offered the information choose not to act upon it. (Williamson, 1993, p. 199)

Fewer than 5 per cent of fetuses examined by prenatal diagnostic techniques are, in fact, affected by the disease being screened for. Therefore, for the vast majority of prospective parents, prenatal diagnosis serves ultimately to reassure them that the unborn baby is *not* affected by the disease in question. However, there are anxieties inherent to screening; during the testing process, after notification of a positive result, and even before the first counselling session.

Many pregnancies end naturally in early miscarriage before the woman realises she is pregnant; this is often because the fetus has a genetic defect. By diagnosing abnormal genes before birth, medical science can shift the boundaries of the natural process of abortion to reduce the number of children born with genetic diseases. But a decision to go ahead with an abortion, or to continue the pregnancy, brings with it an often agonising personal decision and a degree of moral and social responsibility. If the disease detected by prenatal diagnosis is treatable, as in the case of PKU, then the question of abortion is quite different from what it would be if treatment were not available. Where a disease is life-threatening, with the child having little chance of reaching adulthood, then for some parents there may be little doubt as to what to do.

But what about diseases that in the main do not develop until adulthood, such as Huntington's disease? Here the affected people are destined to become incapacitated and generate a substantial cost to the state in terms of care and medical resource; yet before they become ill, they will contribute to society in many ways, including financially. Should prospective parents take into account this social interest when deciding whether to proceed with an affected pregnancy?

---

[13] These issues are illustrated in the audiotape 'Tinkering with nature', which OU students should listen to at around this point in the chapter. The notes in the *AV Media Guide* should be consulted beforehand.

● Can you suggest other dilemmas about whether to screen the population for Huntington's disease alleles?

■ The majority of individuals do not show any signs of the disease until *after* they have had children and hence have already passed on the mutant allele, so population screening could prevent this from happening. But prenatal screening of fetuses for alleles leading to Huntington's disease also inevitably reveals whether one or other *parent* has the mutation and is therefore destined to develop the disease themselves. This is something that the parent may prefer not to know.

9.7.2 Disclosure and discrimination

Disclosure of information accidentally revealed by genetic screening is another major concern. Should the parents be told that an unborn baby, although unaffected with the disease they agreed to be screened for, for example, the abnormal chromosome pattern associated with Down's syndrome, has another genetic disorder? Most genetic counsellors think that full disclosure should be given.

Disclosure and confidentiality are two aspects of population genetic screening that may have consequences not only for individuals and families, but also for society 'at large'. Genetic screening of the population would identify the carriers of certain inherited characteristics and so has the potential for creating and supporting social bias and subsequent hardship among those identified. This is especially worrying in diseases that occur more frequently in an ethnic group that already suffers discrimination, as in the case of sickle-cell disease in Blacks in the USA and Tay–Sachs disease in Jewish populations outside Israel.

It also raises questions about regulating the disclosure of genetic information about individuals who are likely to develop crippling and debilitating diseases while they are still part of the labour force? Will prospective employers and insurance companies begin to demand genetic screening of individuals *before* offering a job or agreeing to underwrite a policy?

Genetic screening tests are increasing in frequency. In Sweden, for example, thousands of newborn babies have already been screened for α_1-antitrypsin deficiency — a recessive genetic disorder caused by the lack of an enzyme, which leads to chronic lung and liver disease, particularly in smokers or in people exposed to smoke. Mass screening means that the medical condition of all those affected by this disorder in Sweden is already on record. The issues here are similar to those raised when insurance companies began asking life insurance applicants whether they had ever been *tested* for HIV (the virus that causes AIDS), even though the test had proved negative.

It is obviously uneconomical to screen everybody for everything, but since the number of genetic diseases or 'predispositions' that can be identified in carriers is rapidly increasing, these are questions of immediate concern to everyone. Concern has been voiced about the possible invasion of privacy, stigmatisation on the basis of an abnormal finding, the failure to obtain informed consent to screening, and the lack of confidentiality of results. Societies will increasingly have to debate and decide what will be permitted, what should be forbidden and what legislation should back it up.

Fears that genetic screening might damage individual freedoms emerged first in the USA, where most people depend on private insurance for health care and

Box 9.2 Guidelines for employment-based genetic testing

- Individuals should not be required to take a test and their 'right not to know' should be upheld;

- They should not be made to disclose the results of previous tests unless there is clear evidence that either they could not do the job safely or would be harmed by doing it;

- Employers should *offer* tests where known working conditions might harm people with known genetic variants;

- All test results must be accurate, with suitable information being communicated to the person concerned by trained professionals;

- All information derived from genetic testing is protected by Data Protection Principles. (based on HGAC, 1999)

9.8 Treating genetic disorders

Powerful DNA techniques currently being developed have the potential to make a dramatic impact on the treatment of genetic disorders but, despite their promise during the 1990s, these approaches have yet to have any major impact upon treatment. We begin with a brief overview of standard therapies in the treatment of genetic disorders, and then describe the strategy of gene therapy, its current stage of development and prospects for success.

Genetic disorders can often be treated by intervening at various stages in the complex pathway between the defective gene and the **clinical phenotype** of the individual (i.e. the 'signs and symptoms' of the disease, as diagnosed by a doctor). These levels of intervention are summarised in Table 9.2. But in many cases effective therapy is not available because insufficient is known about the pathology of the disease.

Earlier in this chapter, we discussed interventions at the level of the population and the family; here we briefly discuss techniques aimed at the lower levels in Table 9.2, before focusing extensively on the level of the mutant gene.

Table 9.2 Various levels at which intervention can occur in genetic disorders, with treatment strategies at each level. (The terms used are discussed further in the text below.)

Level of intervention	Treatment strategy
the population	population genetic screening and risk-factor counselling
the family	carrier testing; pre-conception testing; prenatal diagnosis; pre-symptomatic diagnostic testing; risk counselling; informed support; decisions about choice of partner, contraception or abortion
the individual clinical phenotype (signs and symptoms of the patient)	medical or surgical intervention for symptom control; informed support for behavioural coping strategies
the metabolic level (biochemical abnormalities in cells and tissues)	disease-specific treatments (e.g. drugs, implants, cell therapies, specialised diet)
the mutant protein	protein replacement, including with genetically engineered proteins
the mutant gene	modification of the genotype by gene therapy

9.8.1 Treating the phenotype

Intervention at the level of the clinical phenotype with surgery, medical treatment or education, are all forms of **phenotype modification**, so-called because the patient's clinical phenotype is altered by the treatment, but *without* affecting the underlying genotype. For example, surgical repair can successfully modify the clinical phenotype of some genetic disorders, including the commonest multifactorial conditions in newborn babies, such as cleft lip and palate, congenital heart defects and pyloric stenosis (constriction of the valve controlling emptying of the stomach).

Tissue and organ transplants were discussed in Section 9.2, but using transplants to treat genetic disorders is difficult. The mortality following transplants tends to be quite high; morbidity can also be high because of graft rejection, and there is a shortage of suitable organs and tissues. Nevertheless, there have been some good outcomes in the treatment of thalassaemia with bone marrow transplants. The prospect of fetal stem cell therapies or transplants from 'humanised' pigs and other genetically modified mammals in the future offers some hope for several other genetic disorders.

Intervention at the level of metabolic or biochemical abnormalities is another form of phenotype modification. To date, the genetic disorders that have been most successfully treated are those involving a metabolic abnormality, such as PKU and familial hypercholesterolaemia.

9.8.2 Genetically engineered proteins

Phenotype modification at the level of the mutant protein is routine treatment for only a few genetic disorders and involves **protein replacement therapy**. A prime example is infusion with the blood clotting protein Factor IX, to prevent internal bleeding in people with haemophilia, who cannot produce the normal protein themselves. The protein α_1-antitrypsin can be infused into people with α_1-antitrypsin-deficiency in doses large enough to maintain the correct protein concentration in the lungs. Both these proteins have been produced by genetic modification techniques (Figure 9.7).

●   Can you give another example where protein replacement therapy is the principal mode of treatment? (Think back to Chapter 7.)

■   Injecting insulin (a protein hormone) to treat diabetes mellitus.

Using laboratory techniques to isolate and manipulate 'normal' human genes, it is possible to produce large quantities of purified human proteins in laboratory cultures of bacteria and other micro-organisms. These **genetically engineered proteins** are rapidly replacing 'traditional' sources of replacement proteins used in therapy in the past, which were isolated directly from human donors or other mammals. For example, the majority of injectable insulin is still produced from the pancreas of cattle and pigs slaughtered for meat, but it is not identical in structure to human insulin and eventually elicits an immune response in the recipient against cow or pig epitopes in the hormone. However, genetically engineered human insulin has not always provided satisfactory regulation of blood glucose in at least some diabetic people.

●   The human blood clotting protein Factor IX has primarily been extracted from human blood donated by blood donors. What problem arose from this source and how might genetically engineered Factor IX overcome it?

The concept of gene therapy surfaced in the 1980s. Many trials are currently being undertaken around the world and the procedures and techniques in use are tightly regulated by various authorities (which we will not go into here). Despite the media hype attached to gene therapy, by the turn of the millennium, not a single patient had been cured of a genetic disorder and, indeed, there had been some fatalities amongst recipients. The expectation that gene therapy would be a panacea for human disease has been slowly tempered by the practical realities. Here we shall discuss the problems affecting this new technology, but note how some modest breakthroughs are being achieved.

It is very important to distinguish between gene therapy that alters the DNA in a person's 'body' cells (the *somatic* cells described in Chapter 3) or in their *gametes*. **Somatic gene therapy** aims to transfer a normal gene into the DNA of cells in the body *other than* the gametes, compensating for the defective allele which is the cause of the person's disease. It is currently (2000) being tried out in a few pilot studies and involves no new ethical concerns beyond those already raised in this chapter.

● Will somatic gene therapy prevent the treated person from passing on the disease allele to their children?

■ No, because the normal human gene transferred into the patient's DNA does *not* enter the DNA of their eggs (or sperm), so it cannot be transferred to the next generation.

Somatic gene therapy was originally envisaged as a potential treatment for adults or children, but recently the possibility of performing gene transfer to affected babies still in the uterus has been considered.

Germline gene therapy would (if it were allowed) result in the insertion of a normal human gene into the affected person's gametes, so that their offspring could inherit a normal allele. It carries a risk for future generations through the accidental introduction of new and harmful mutations, and is currently banned in humans in many countries. (However, it is legal to insert human genes into the germline of other species, as the case of Tracey illustrated.)

● There is an inherent dilemma in the decision to allow limited trials of somatic gene therapy, but to ban germline gene therapy. What is it?

■ Somatic gene therapy will enable people (who would otherwise have died young) to survive and have children, some of whom will inherit their affected parent's disease allele. Germline gene therapy could prevent these children from inheriting it at all.

Figure 9.8 overleaf outlines the simplest theoretical method of inserting genes into the patient's defective cells. Using either special viruses (which carry their DNA into a cell and insert their genetic material into the host's DNA), or liposomes (small fat-like structures which can carry DNA into a cell), human genes can be transferred into cells for gene therapy. Viruses, liposomes and other mechanisms used for this purpose are often referred to as **gene vectors**, a term that should remind you of Chapter 5 and the 'vectors' such as mosquitos that transport pathogens into new hosts.

Figure 9.8 *A technique for somatic gene therapy. A virus or liposomes are used to 'carry' the normal human gene into the patient's own cells in tissue culture, and insert the gene into the patient's DNA. The cells are then returned to the patient, where they colonise and repopulate the affected organs and tissues.*

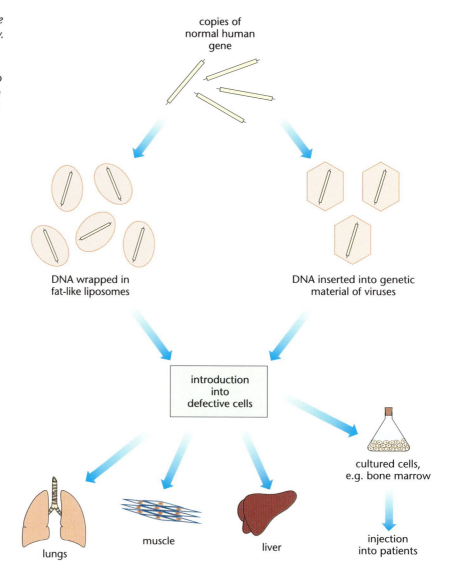

You will need to keep referring to Figure 9.8 as we discuss three of the major scientific hurdles that have to be overcome before the technique of somatic gene therapy can become more widely available.

9.8.4 Hurdles in the path of somatic gene therapy

The first difficulty is in getting the human gene into the patient's cells. Most ways of doing this are not very efficient, but the easiest is to use a virus. Normally such viruses reproduce extensively, killing the cell they have invaded. However, some viruses have been genetically engineered to contain the corrective human gene, but they are unable to reproduce and so do not kill their target cells. As in the example in Figure 9.8, adult bone marrow stem cells are one of the commonest targets for gene therapy because they are easily isolated, grown in tissue culture and re-implanted using existing medical techniques.

● What are the limitations of using adult bone marrow stem cells (Section 9.2.3)?

■ They replicate to produce red blood cells and lymphocytes, so this approach is only useful if the gene you want to deliver has a biological role in the blood — for example, treating sickle-cell disease or thalassaemia.

Delivery of a gene that has a biological role elsewhere, for example within the brain, would most likely have to occur within the target organ. In many cases, accessing the appropriate tissue and ensuring the gene can be delivered where it is needed, is a major problem — particularly if the gene is required in multiple tissues (e.g. muscles) all over the body. So the few host cells that 'accept' the transferred gene must survive within the recipient long enough to have a biological effect and must be capable of differentiating into many cell types.

● Given these criteria, which cells would have the highest chance of successfully recolonising the patient's many different tissues and organs?

■ Fetal stem cells fulfil all these criteria from a biological viewpoint, since they can differentiate into any cell type in the body; but ethical objections to the use of fetal cells may remain, even if they can be collected from umbilical cord blood.

The second hurdle is getting the inserted gene to become 'active' within the cell and lead to the production of the encoded protein. It is very important that the transferred genes express their proteins in the correct cell types, at levels that are appropriate to have an effect, and without interfering with or damaging existing normal genes.

Third, an immune response within the recipient can be a major problem.

● What might this immune response be directed against? (There are two potential targets and you will need to think back to Chapter 6 to work out what they are.)

■ The first is *viral* proteins present in the virus used as the gene vector; the immune system has adapted to be very efficient at detecting and attacking viruses, but in this case it would destroy the incoming therapeutic gene. The second target might be the patient's own cells carrying the inserted gene. If the patient has never previously expressed the *normal* protein, then the immune system will not have been programmed to ignore it as 'self'; as soon as the inserted gene is activated and the cells begin to make the protein for the first time, this may elicit an immune response.

The first recipient of gene therapy to die during treatment was killed by a 'whole body' inflammatory response against the new gene product, in much the same way as an allergic person may be affected by exposure to the allergen.

9.8.5 The story so far

A number of genetic disorders are potential candidates for correction by gene therapy, in particular blood conditions, such as thalassaemia and sickle-cell disease, and various forms of immunodeficiency diseases. In these conditions, the defective cells originate in the bone marrow — the tissue most suited for gene therapy. However, gene transfer into bone marrow cells may also be an effective treatment for diseases that do not affect bone marrow directly, such as PKU, familial hypercholesterolaemia and α_1-antitrypsin deficiency. The idea is that the treated bone marrow cells would produce the normal protein, which would then be transported in the bloodstream to wherever it was needed in the body.

The first candidate gene for somatic gene transfer in humans was the gene associated with *adenosine deaminase deficiency* (ADD). The gene codes for an enzyme (adenosine deaminase), which is normally present in high levels in white cells in the immune system; its absence causes severe immunodeficiency disease. The first transfers of the gene to correct the lack of the enzyme were successfully achieved in the early 1990s, but it was unclear whether the new genes were producing therapeutic quantities of the enzyme because the patients were maintained on standard pharmaceutical treatments. The only way to find out would be to stop all treatment and run the risk of a potentially fatal relapse.

Coupled with many other trials which gave either negative or inconclusive evidence for gene therapy, the National Institutes of Health (NIH; who fund most gene therapy trials within the USA) held an enquiry as to why the over-inflated promises made for gene therapy were not being reached. Among its conclusions was that the basic scientific understanding of the biology of the disease, the gene vectors being used and the host cells into which the genes were supposed to be transferred was inadequate.

At the beginning of 2000, over 300 trials of somatic gene therapy were in progress, three-quarters of these in the USA. Most were proceeding with a more realistic expectation that cures based on gene therapy for most genetic disorders are a long way in the future. Even these modest expectations have been tempered by the most serious incident involving a patient undergoing a trial gene therapy in which DNA was being carried into his cells using an *adenovirus*. Many people have been exposed to this virus in their normal lives, so they already have immune memory cells which recognise and attack it. Delivering human genes using adenovirus can, therefore, result in massive inflammation. In late 1999, one fatal case of just such a reaction lead to the regulatory authorities in the USA reviewing the efficacy and safety of the gene therapy trials it licensed.

9.8.6 A more realistic future

Cystic fibrosis is a candidate disease for gene therapy for which there is some reason to be fairly optimistic. A large number of young adults exist with cystic fibrosis whose informed consent for experimental gene therapy could be obtained. The lungs and gut of affected people are normal at birth, so the *early* insertion of a normal gene could correct the biochemical defect *before* damage is caused by the accumulation of mucus (a major feature of the disease). The lungs are very accessible sites, so gene transfer may be feasible without the need to remove the patients' cells to a laboratory culture. An aerosol containing viruses with the DNA sequence of the normal human gene can be sprayed at high pressure into the lungs.

The gut lining is also reasonably accessible to agents given 'by mouth', if a way can be found to deliver gene vectors that survive digestion (the problems should be evident from Chapter 7). Gene delivery systems are being tested in several inbred strains of mice, which carry mutations that give rise to a condition resembling cystic fibrosis in humans. Normal genes have been successfully transferred by direct application to the walls of arteries in their lungs. Animal tests have shown that if the normal gene can be transferred to only 5 per cent of cells in the lungs, this is sufficient to restore normal functioning.

We noted above that expression of the correct protein into the appropriate tissue is a major hurdle for gene therapy. For this reason, delivering genes to blood cells has obvious advantages, especially if only a small amount of the protein is required. Such is the case in haemophilia, where clinical trials are very promising for several reasons. (Open University students will have already encountered this example in the TV programme 'Bloodlines: A family legacy'.) First of all, haemophilia has been treated for many years with proteins isolated from either human blood, animals or through genetic manipulation of bacteria.

● Explain why this increases the chance of successful gene therapy.

■ It has allowed scientists to determine which patients will *not* initiate an immune response against the normal protein if gene therapy works.

Secondly, the proteins are required exactly where they would be generated — in the blood, transported around the body and forming part of the pathway by which blood clots. Thirdly, only very small amounts of these proteins are required, with a restoration to even 5 per cent of the usual levels being therapeutically successful. In addition, the body can tolerate as much as 150 per cent of normal levels with no ill effects.

Prospects for gene therapy in the first decade of the twenty-first century are more realistic than a decade earlier, as novel approaches are developed and successes accumulate. The routine use of this technique is predicted by geneticists within 10 to 20 years.

9.8.7 Weighing the risks

With any new therapy, there are concerns about risks versus benefits. The ethics of gene therapy do not pose any new issues as long as the germline is not involved. Some regard replacing a damaged gene as not much different from replacing a damaged organ such as a kidney, and as much less invasive than performing multiple transplants of the type which have been considered for patients with genetic disorders. However, some of the consequences may be far-reaching. Initial trials of somatic gene therapy are likely to involve disorders that are currently untreatable by other methods and have, until now, generally prevented the affected person from having children through illness or premature death.

● What are the likely consequences for the frequency of the disease allele in the population if somatic gene therapy successfully treats the disorder?

■ Recipients of gene therapy, although phenotypically normal, still carry the disease alleles in their germline DNA and could transmit them to their children. Somatic gene therapy could increase the frequencies of these alleles in the population because the treated person lives to reproduce.

Thus, somatic gene therapy has the potential to change the frequencies of disease alleles in the population. Note that this is true of *all* the treatment strategies listed earlier in Table 9.2, for the same reason. These examples illustrate how modern culture may affect human biological evolution in the future. However, other cultural forces are at work to counteract this tendency, making it unlikely that the frequency of genetic *disorders* will rise, even though the prevalence of disease *alleles* may increase. (This point is discussed further in the final chapter of this book.)

9.9   The 'new' genetics in context

The new millennium onwards may be viewed a few generations hence as the 'golden age of gene therapy', a time when diseases with a genetic predisposition could be overcome. Genetic medicine — screening, counselling and therapy — offers prospects that are both promising and disturbing. By tinkering with DNA we have the potential to influence our evolution and we need to consider the options carefully.

Some leading scientists, geneticists among them, have claimed that modern genetic techniques like gene therapy can only alter the course of human evolution 'in the most trivial way'?

● Can you explain this view?

■ If you think back to earlier chapters in this book — Chapter 5 in particular — you will see that compared to the worldwide burden of communicable disease, only a tiny fraction of the global population of 6 billion is affected by the 'single-gene' disorders that gene therapy may be able to cure. (Genetic disorders associated with a *single* gene account for only 2 per cent of total live births with any kind of disorder in the UK.)

Even in the developed world, the multifactorial diseases — such as coronary heart disease and other cardiovascular problems, cancers, diabetes, hypertension, arthritis, stroke, schizophrenia, depression and certain forms of obesity — affect and end the lives of a far greater number of people. These complex disease phenotypes depend on critical interactions between a large number of genes and environmental, social and cultural factors.

● Why is gene therapy an unrealistic option for multifactorial diseases?

■ A number of different genes are involved in these conditions and each gene has only a small effect, so multiple-gene therapy may be required; even if this were feasible, the effects of environmental factors on disease development could not be taken into account.

● What alternative approach to reducing the burden of multifactorial diseases is likely to be more productive than using new genetic technologies?

■ Tackling hostile environmental factors associated with the development of these diseases would help — using 'environment' in its widest possible sense to include factors such as poverty, housing and water quality, diet, employment and self-esteem.[15] We need to make the environment safe for our particular genotypes, rather than attempt to alter our genotypes to survive in unhealthy social conditions.

Detecting the genes associated with multifactorial diseases would enable individuals to make informed choices about their lives (for example, by weighing up a known personal risk from smoking or obesity), but think of the cost. If a nationwide programme of genetic screening was adopted as a form of preventive health care, what effect would its enormous cost have on the availability of other forms of

[15] The interaction of socio-economic, environmental and other factors in the causation of disease globally is discussed in detail in *World Health and Disease* (Open university Press, 2nd edn 1993; 3rd edn 2001).

health and social services? On a more positive note, discrimination (as envisaged by Benno Müller-Hill) could not be supported by genetic evidence if a genetic 'profile' of every citizen would be too costly to obtain.

Finally, we finish the story of tinkering with nature by turning to one of the 'founding fathers' of the genetic revolution we see today — James Watson, co-discoverer of the structure of DNA. In a short article 'Good gene, bad gene', he offers his personal viewpoint on genetic testing and the role of mutations in human evolution. His opinions, as an eminent scientist in the field of human genetics, provide a pragmatic approach to genetic disorders as a biological problem. He comes down firmly on the side of terminating affected fetuses as 'incomparably more compassionate than allowing an infant to come into the world tragically impaired'. Many will disagree with this view,[16] but he also sees genetic disease as 'the price we pay for the extraordinary evolutionary process that has given rise to the wonders of life on Earth.' (Open University students should read the article now; it is in *Health and Disease: A Reader*, Open University Press, 3rd edn 2001.)

The impact of genetics in medicine will be profound and many developments in gene technology are also on the horizon, which will raise other ethical and practical problems. For example, drugs that alter the activity of human genes are being actively researched; the pharmacist of the future may be able to reach into our DNA with a chemical 'spanner' and turn parts of the central mechanism of life on or off. One of the most active areas is cancer research, where methods for altering the expression of genes in tumour cells are already being tested in animals, with promising results. The practical problems are considerable but most biologists would agree they are not insuperable, given enough time and research resources. Ethical objections, however, may ultimately keep the spanner out of the works.

The *intentional* use of chemicals we call 'drugs' simply because they have been designed to alleviate or prevent disease is one way of tinkering with nature. As the next chapter shows, the *unintentional* use of chemicals we call 'pollutants' has been affecting the activity of human genes, cells and body fluids for over a century, with little concern being raised until recently about the consequences for the future health of the human species. We move on in Chapter 10 to examine human biology in the context of the chemical industrial environment.

OBJECTIVES FOR CHAPTER 9

When you have studied this chapter, you should be able to:

9.1 Define and use correctly, or recognise definitions and applications of, the terms printed in **bold** in this chapter.

9.2 Summarise the principal areas of public concern about the ethical aspects of organ transplants and cell therapies, and comment on the biological mechanisms that either support or undermine graft survival.

9.3 Discuss the biological, social and ethical implications of reproductive cloning.

[16] For example, the articles by Müller-Hill and by McGowan, referred to earlier in this chapter, raise concerns about the implications of routine genetic testing and termination of affected fetuses. Three other articles in *Health and Disease: A Reader* (Open University Press, 3rd edn 2001) also address this issue from different perspectives: Jenny Morris ('Pride against prejudice'), Peter Conrad ('Public eyes and private genes'), and Tom Shakespeare ('Brave New World II').

9.4 Discuss the practical and ethical issues raised by (a) genetic testing and prenatal diagnosis for individuals and families, (b) mass genetic screening at the level of populations. Identify the principal effects these techniques might have on human health and disease.

9.5 Distinguish between somatic and germline gene therapy and discuss the practical and ethical issues raised by these techniques. Evaluate their potential to affect human evolution in the future.

QUESTIONS FOR CHAPTER 9

1   (*Objective 9.2*)

A commentary in the leading scientific journal *Nature* by three American paediatricians who support the use of fetal tissue in research, argued for the following ethical framework:

> … the use of discarded fetal tissue for research and/or therapy should be to increase knowledge of human development and/or improvement of the human condition. Acknowledgement of the unique and non-trivial nature of the material should be mandatory. The review panels now assembling must ensure that human material is essential, and animal or substitute models should be used for preference when possible. (Bianchi *et al.*, 1993, p. 12)

(a) What criticisms could be made of this framework by opponents of the use of fetal tissue, and what safeguards does it refer to?

(b) What is the principal biological rationale for using fetal cells rather than their adult equivalents?

2   (*Objective 9.3*)

Explain why the creation of Dolly was a scientific breakthrough? Would it be technically feasible to undertake reproductive cloning using human cells? If so, which cells would be involved?

3   (*Objective 9.4*)

Imagine that you are addressing the Huntington's Disease Association. The disease, caused by a dominant mutation, is associated with degeneration of the nervous system and is usually first manifested in mid-life. A severely affected man, 40 years old, comments that he is not at risk of passing on the disorder because his parents are not affected with Huntington's disease and so his condition must be due to a new mutation. Evaluate this claim.

4   (*Objective 9.4*)

A new life-threatening disease called 'degeneration' is known to be inherited as a genetically recessive disease. It affects significant numbers of people living in small communities. Careful studies of DNA from normal and affected individuals identifies the gene associated with this disease. What factors should be considered before a programme of population screening for the defective allele is begun? (Give your answer in note form, as a list of numbered points.)

5   (*Objective 9.5*)

Describe the central aim of somatic gene therapy and explain how this example of modern culture might affect human evolution in the future.

CHAPTER 10

Living with the chemical industrial environment

Study notes for OU students

This chapter draws extensively on material in Chapters 3–8 of this book, so as well as being a 'case study' of a new and important topic, it also consolidates terms and concepts you have already been introduced to in other contexts. During Section 10.4 you will be asked to read an article called 'Climate and health' by Paul Epstein, which appears in *Health and Disease: A Reader* (Open University Press, third edition 2001). You may already have studied it during Chapter 11 of *World Health and Disease* (Open University Press, third edition 2001), where it was optional reading. The descriptions of the rise of industrialisation and its effects on health in Chapters 5, 6 and 8 of that book also provide background to the present chapter.

10.1   Effects of chemicals on the body

In Chapter 2 you saw something of how cultural evolution altered patterns of health and disease in early human settlements, over many thousands of years. But since the Industrial Revolution, which began in England in the middle of the eighteenth century and has since spread all over the world, human populations have undergone far more rapid changes. Industrialisation has affected all aspects of the environment we live in — physical, chemical, biological and social — with profound impacts on human health. It has brought with it enormous benefits in terms of increased wealth and employment, enabling nations in developing as well as developed countries to improve living standards, education, health care, transport and communication, among many other developments. But changes that occur at such speed, spanning only about ten generations of human lives, cannot be accommodated by evolutionary adaptation to *adverse* environmental circumstances arising as a consequence of industrialisation.

In this chapter, we focus on ways of evaluating the effects on health of changes in the chemical environment, caused by the production of synthetic chemicals for domestic, agricultural and industrial use, and by the linked production of waste. As you will see, it is extremely difficult to obtain reliable evidence about the long-term consequences for human health, even in the case of a well-documented chemical accident. This puts into context the far greater problems of estimating the impact of the industrial chemical environment on health at the global level.

We will start to examine the effects of chemical exposure on health by refreshing your memory about the body's capacity for defence against toxic chemicals, and its ability to repair damage; we also consider why some people may be affected by chemical exposure more than others. Then we examine direct toxicity, illustrated primarily through a case study of the health effects of the industrial chemical *dioxin*. We end by looking at some of the more indirect impacts on health of chemicals in our environment, mediated through local or global effects on the ecosystem, including global climate change.

10.1.1   Defence and repair

The study of evolution leads us to expect that the human body would have a wide range of defences against potentially harmful external influences, whether biological, physical or chemical. You have already learned a great deal about some of them in earlier chapters of this book. In Chapter 6 you saw how the body defends itself against harmful micro-organisms and larger parasites.

● Suggest some of the body's defence mechanisms against pathogenic organisms.

■ Defences range from simple barriers such as a relatively impermeable skin covering, to mucus protecting the respiratory lining, to the complex mechanisms of the innate and adaptive immune systems, including the actions of phagocytic cells and antibodies.

As Chapter 7 described, the liver contains a variety of enzymes that render toxic chemicals harmless by breaking them down — a process known as **detoxification**. However, sometimes these metabolic changes actually result in the conversion of a harmless chemical to a toxic form. The special role of the liver makes it particularly vulnerable to the action of many toxins, because such high concentrations are found there, and because the toxins may damage the liver before (or during) detoxification.

As well as defence mechanisms, there are repair mechanisms. If there is a lot of cell damage or death in a localised area, the body can often repair itself by cell division and the formation of scar tissue, made up from collagen fibres.

● From what you already know of collagen (Section 8.3.3), what do you predict will be its effect in scar tissue?

■ Collagen is a relatively inflexible protein, which accumulates in tissues as we age, making skin wrinkle and joints less mobile; in scar tissue, its strength holds the damaged tissue together.

Not all cells, however, retain the capacity to divide that they had during fetal life; nerve cells, for example, cannot divide after the fetal brain has formed and repair in the nervous system must then be carried out entirely by the deposition of collagen. By contrast, bone can heal almost entirely by the formation of new cells. Skin comes between these two extremes, with damage to the outer layer (the *epidermis*) being repaired perfectly by new cells growing up from the deeper layers (the *dermis*), which divide continuously throughout life. If the damage penetrates right through to the dermis then, although cells migrate in from the edges, collagen is laid down and, as a consequence, the repair leaves a scar.

● Why do you think older people with a poor circulation in the skin on their legs frequently have a diminished capacity to heal skin lesions such as leg ulcers?

■ The process of cellular repair depends on a good blood supply, because it needs energy and nutrients. (Note that it is implied therefore that the body is making an energy investment in repair.)

Maintenance and repair within cells involves a constant process of checking and eliminating mutations in the DNA and faulty proteins. Repair of DNA, either after spontaneous errors in replication or damage caused by radiation or chemicals, is a remarkable process, whereby mismatches in base pairs are identified and replaced, or more extensive damage is repaired by enzyme systems. If the damage is too extensive to repair, the cell may be triggered to undergo *programmed cell death* (or apoptosis, see Section 8.1.2). The natural turnover (breakdown and replacement) of proteins and lipids is another method by which damaged molecules can be disposed of, as you learned in Chapters 7 and 8.

So how do toxic and harmful chemicals get past this elaborate system of defence and repair? First, the system might quite simply be overwhelmed by an exposure that is so high or so prolonged that the body cannot compensate. Second, the body may be challenged by new toxins to which evolution has not had time to produce appropriate defences.

Third, the repair process itself can prevent *acute* (short-term) damage, but ultimately lead to *chronic* (long-term) disease. For example, the mucus in the respiratory tract produced after inhalation of harmful substances, eventually contributes to chronic bronchitis if it persists because of long-term exposure. Scar tissue is also a response to acute damage, but has disadvantages compared to normal tissue. Scar tissue in the brain can provoke neurological disorders. Scar tissue in the liver, characteristic of cirrhosis of the liver produced by excessive alcohol intake, is laid down following cell damage. Eventually, it compresses the liver cells and interferes with their function. Moreover, DNA repair itself, while protecting the integrity of the DNA molecule, can sometimes introduce new and harmful mutations.

● Suggest an evolutionary explanation for the fact that humans have not evolved defence and repair mechanisms that also protect against long-term damage.

■ The commitment of resources to maintenance and repair of the body has been balanced against investment in growth and reproduction (recall the discussion of energy 'trade-offs' in Section 5.3.3); in addition, the selection pressures favouring long-term protection from damage decline in importance after the reproductive phase of the life history, since characteristics developed in later life cannot be passed on to one's offspring (the evolution of ageing was discussed in Chapter 8).

So defence and repair mechanisms are inherently imperfect and natural selection cannot favour the evolution of a perfect self-repairing organism. As with all biological systems, where 'imperfection' exists there is an innate degree of variability between individuals as to the strength and efficiency of their defences.

10.1.2 Sensitivity and hypersensitivity

An important principle in the study of the relationship between the environment and health is the identification of sensitive or critical groups in the population. This is essential to achieve the aim of *equity* of access to a healthy environment. Equity means that each person has access to an environment that does not harm his or her health, and this varies from person to person, so it is important to identify those individuals who are most at risk in a given environment. The concept of a **critical group** is used here to refer to people who are most likely to be exposed to a chemical.

● Suggest some examples of critical groups.

■ There are many, but you may have thought of people in certain occupations, people with particular dietary habits, people who live in or near sites of high exposure, less affluent groups who have less financial or political power to avoid exposure, or particular age groups who might have a behaviour that makes them more likely to be exposed, for example children who eat soil.

Pollution from a chemical factory by the River Mersey, Widnes. People living nearby (and other life-forms in this location) are a 'critical group' at risk of exposure to accidental release of chemicals. (Photo: David Drain/Still Pictures)

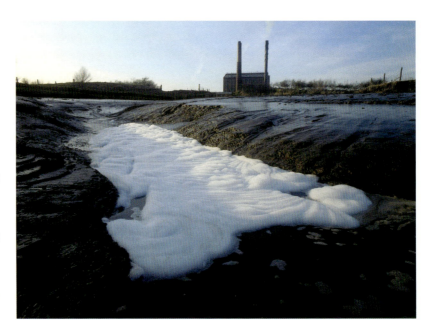

Sensitive groups

The concept of a **sensitive group** is used here to refer to people who *once exposed*, are more likely than others to develop adverse health effects. The newborn baby is one example: since it lacks or is deficient in several of the enzymes involved in the detoxification of chemicals, it eliminates drugs from the body more slowly, and has an inefficient **blood–brain barrier**. In adults, the walls of the blood vessels in the brain have a special structure that prevents many molecules getting from the bloodstream into the brain cells, but this is not fully developed in babies. Another example of a sensitive group is people who are genetically more predisposed to develop a particular disease, and react more strongly to environmental exposures.

- Can you think of examples from earlier chapters where genetic susceptibility affects the way people react to an environmental exposure?

- Chapter 9 referred to people with inherited α_1-antitrypsin deficiency, who are highly sensitive to tobacco smoke, which accelerates the progression of liver and lung disease. You may also have thought of the fact that white-skinned people are more susceptible than dark-skinned people to skin cancer caused by exposure to ultraviolet radiation (the lactose case study in Chapter 7).

Other examples of sensitive groups are people with *xeroderma pigmentosa*, a genetic defect that prevents the repair of ultraviolet radiation, who always develop skin cancer, and albino people, who have faulty melanin production (melanin is a protein that absorbs UV light and thereby protects other proteins in the skin), and also have a high incidence of skin cancers.

People with α_1-antitrypsin deficiency illustrate the interaction of environmental with genetic factors in the cause of disease. They have a genetic predisposition to *emphysema*, a serious lung condition, because they have a defect in a molecule that normally inactivates an enzyme released by white cells in response to inhaled bacterial or chemical irritants. If the enzyme is not inactivated in a short time, it speeds up the breakdown of protein in the lungs, particularly of elastin, the protein that gives elasticity to structures in the lung. The alveoli (tiny air-filled bags in the lungs where the exchange of oxygen and carbon dioxide takes place) become more rigid and breathing becomes extremely difficult. The environmental irritant means that the destructive enzyme is released and the inherited lack of the normal inactivator means that the destructive enzyme has widespread harmful effects on health.

Hypersensitivity reactions

A commonly encountered sensitive group in the population consists of individuals who are *hypersensitive*, or allergic, to particular industrial chemicals, certain metals, or organic material such as pollen and cat fur. **Hypersensitivity** is said to exist when the immune response to a harmless foreign substance produces harmful effects in the body. In other words, hypersensitivity is an example of the situation in which the body's defence itself leads to disease. Hypersensitivity reactions are of several types. We shall look at only two: one mediated by circulating antibodies and one by T lymphocytes (or T cells; the terms and mechanisms in the following account should already be familiar to you from Chapter 6).

A specific type of antibody circulating in the bloodstream is implicated in acute (rapid, short-term) hypersensitivity reactions, such as hay fever, some types of asthma, and hypersensitive reactions to wasp and bee stings (such reactions are commonly called *allergies*). When the *allergen*, the substance that triggers a hypersensitive reaction (for example, pollen, house dust mites, cat fur or insect venom), enters the body, it elicits the production of antibodies.

● Can you recall from Chapter 6 what happens if the allergen gets into the body again?

■ In any subsequent exposure to the allergen, it becomes bound to the mast cells by the antibodies, triggering the mast cells to release histamine and other irritant chemicals, which produce the hypersensitive reaction; blood vessels near the mast cells dilate and become 'leaky', so the area is flooded with fluid and white cells and becomes hot, swollen, red and sore.

This reaction is exactly the same as an acute inflammatory response to pathogens, except that it is triggered inappropriately by harmless proteins in organic sources such as pollen and bee venom. This type of reaction particularly affects mucous membranes (for example, in the nasal passages and inside the eyelids) and skin, where mast cells abound. In asthma, swelling of the mucous membranes and spasm of the muscles in the walls of the lungs causes narrowing of the airways and difficulty in breathing. The type of hypersensitivity found in asthma (often called *atopy*) and hay fever tends to run in families and there is some evidence that it has a genetic contribution.

The rates of reported asthma have continued to rise and the most recent prevalence data suggest that as we left the twentieth century the rates were as high as 1 in 7 children and 1 in 25 adults within the UK (National Asthma Campaign, 1999). Explanations as to why there is an apparent increase in the prevalence in asthma have ranged from a greater exposure to allergens like the house dust mite (possibly favoured by changes in housing such as central heating), to an increase in certain forms of air pollution (which may exacerbate sensitivity to a particular allergen or make asthmatic people more sensitive to other allergens). Alternative theories have referred to a change in the diagnostic category 'asthma', which may now be more generally applied to what was once labelled 'wheeziness'; better hygiene (it has been proposed that infections in early life protect against developing allergies); or dietary changes (methods of infant feeding and food additives).[1]

The second type of hypersensitivity is due to the action of T cells. The *cytotoxic* T cells normally attack the body's own cells only if they become infected with intracellular micro-organisms such as viruses. However, if certain chemicals come into prolonged contact with the skin they can combine with proteins to form allergens, which 'trigger' the cytotoxic T cells to attack otherwise healthy skin cells. The result is skin redness, blistering and weeping, known as contact dermatitis. Common allergens include rubber, tanning agents in leather, and nickel; some people react to components in the jewellery they wear. Initially, the reaction is localised in the region of the skin that has been in contact with the chemical, but later it may spread to other areas. Contact dermatitis is an important occupational health problem, but there is considerable uncertainty as to why some individuals are prone to it while most are not.

In the next section we move on to look at a specific industrial chemical — dioxin — which causes contact hypersensitivity reactions (among other health-damaging

[1] Childhood asthma and the evidence for these competing explanations for the rising incidence are discussed in a case study in *Experiencing and Explaining Disease* (Open University Press, 2nd edn 1996; colour-enhanced 2nd edn 2001), Chapter 5.

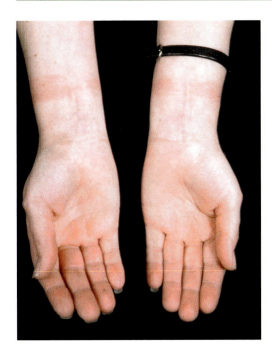
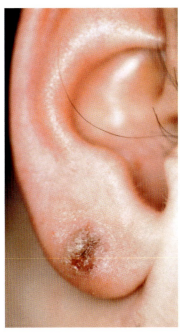

Contact dermatitis caused by a hypersensitive reaction to an environmental chemical that combines with proteins in the skin, forming a novel allergen. (left) Hypersensitivity to tanning agents in a leather watch strap, and (right) to nickel in earrings. (Photos: Dermatology Department, The Royal Hallamshire Hospital)

effects) in people who are exposed to sufficiently high doses. The case study also allows us to examine problems with collecting and interpreting evidence that a certain chemical is harmful to human health.

10.2   Chemical toxicity: the case of dioxin

A quick review of public, media and scientific concern in environmental health will reveal many currently unanswered questions about direct health effects from environmental exposure to electromagnetic radiation from power lines, microwave emissions from mobile phones and transmitters, radioactive waste contamination of ground and water supplies, and a concern that weakly oestrogenic (hormone-like) qualities of some chemicals, including PCBs (polychlorinated biphenyls), might lead to reproductive disorders such as falling sperm count. All these questions are the subject of active research. We are going to illustrate the subject of 'living with industrial chemicals' by looking at one called *dioxin*.

Why is there particular concern about dioxin, when people regularly come into contact with thousands of chemicals in, for example, household cleaning products, shampoo, makeup, deodorants and toothpaste? There are at least two scientific reasons for this, both of which are explored here. The first is its persistence in the environment and the *bioaccumulation* of this chemical (we explain this term below). Second, is the evidence from animal experiments of the strong toxicity of dioxin. In addition, the chemical has been associated in the public mind with well-publicised industrial disasters and warfare.

Dioxin is also an ideal example for a case study because of the long research history on the effects of this chemical, and the controversy that remains about its significance for human health at current exposure levels. There is also evidence that dioxin, as one of a class of persistent chlorine-containing chemicals, is becoming a global problem due to their spread in the atmosphere from the low to mid-latitudes where they originate, to polar regions, where they are a particular problem for traditional peoples consuming fish and mammals.

10.2.1 Dioxin exposures

On 10 July 1976, in Seveso, a quiet industrial town in the province of Milan in northern Italy, an explosion took place at a TCP (trichlorophenol) pesticide manufacturing plant. It released a large quantity of dioxin, a by-product in the manufacturing process, into the densely populated surrounding area. Many domestic and small animals grazing nearby died; there were over 400 cases of acute chemical burns affecting people, but there were no known human fatalities. However, acute toxicity in the form of *chloracne* (an acne-like skin disorder caused by exposure to certain chlorine-containing compounds) started to appear on the fourth day and was reported by nearly 200 residents and workers, some of whom also developed liver problems. Those living in the most contaminated area close to the plant were evacuated from their homes for several weeks.

The local effects of the explosion in a chemical factory in Seveso, Northern Italy, which took place on 10 July 1976, are illustrated in the face of four-year-old Alice Senno, photographed (left) on 18 June and (right) on 29 October that year. The sores are chloracne, caused by exposure to chlorine-containing compounds. (Photo: AP-Wirephoto)

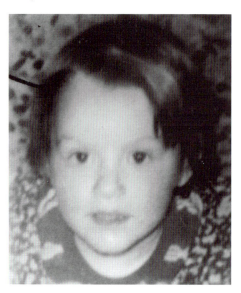
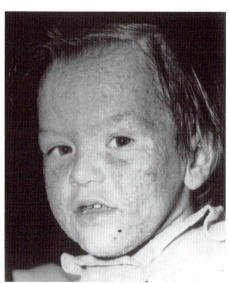

A much earlier and more extensive example of dioxin exposure was not publicised at the time, but evidence of its effects emerged over succeeding years. During the Vietnam war in the 1960s, Agent Orange, a herbicide, was sprayed from the air to defoliate jungles and destroy food crops. Agent Orange, like many herbicides and fungicides, is contaminated by dioxin. Vietnamese citizens and US veterans subsequently reported skin rashes, chronic depression, cancer and birth defects. Later in this chapter we discuss the difficulties in interpreting such reports.

In both these examples, the first effect of dioxin was chloracne. This is an example of **acute toxicity**, an immediate effect of a single exposure to a high dose. Industrial accidents are a typical situation in which acute toxicity occurs. Other situations in which acute toxicity is observed are when chemicals in common external use are accidentally consumed (for example, concentrated pesticides), or when food is contaminated by chemicals.

One notorious example of a food poisoning incident concerns a chemical closely related to dioxin, commonly known as PCB (polychlorinated biphenyl), which contaminated rice oil in Japan in 1968. Over 1 000 individuals were poisoned; they experienced chloracne, pigmentation of the skin, general weakness, numbness of the limbs, respiratory symptoms and impaired immune function.

There are, however, many sources of low-dose dioxin exposure where levels never reach the dose needed for an acute effect like chloracne. In Belgium in 1999, a large tank of fats was contaminated by PCBs and sold to animal feed manufacturers, who in turn sold their feed to farmers, mainly on chicken farms. Chickens showed signs of toxicity, including low fertility and deformed chicks. Exposure of humans to contaminated food was not high enough to result in chloracne, but poultry sales plummeted as public confidence in food safety took another blow.[2] The incident demonstrated the need for tighter control of food contamination, to prevent incidents such as this passing un-noticed. Concerns about a chemical such as dioxin stretch way beyond the immediate exposure, for reasons that will become more apparent shortly.

Apart from its presence as a contaminant in pesticides, dioxin is also produced by combustion (burning) processes in industry and in waste incineration; it is present in cigarette smoke; it occurs in some liquid industrial-waste effluents, and in products of paper and pulp manufacture which involve chlorine-bleaching. A Working Group set up by the Department of the Environment in the UK in the 1980s identified municipal incinerators, domestic coal fires, and vehicle exhausts (mainly from engines using leaded petrol) as the most important sources of dioxin in the UK. Their concerns, and EU directives imposed in 2000, have now led to much stricter controls being placed upon the siting and functioning of municipal incinerators.

A major concern is that long-term exposure to low or intermittent doses can also produce adverse effects on health, in other words the concern relates to **chronic toxicity**.

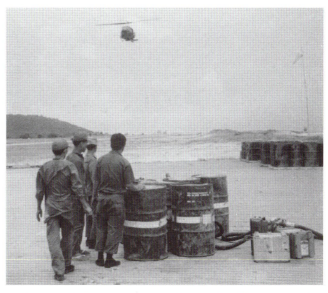

An American helicopter prepares to land and refill its tanks with pesticide at An-Thiot, after a defoliation mission to Phu Quoc island during the Vietnam war, 1968. (Photo: US Army Military History Institute)

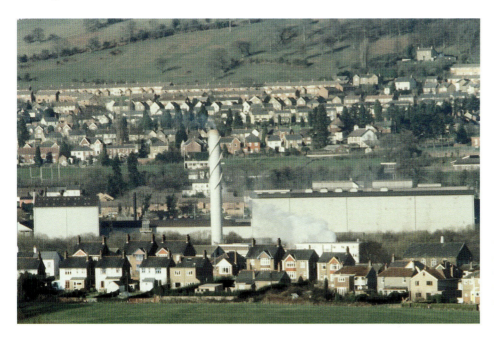

An industrial chemical incinerator disposes of toxic waste in the heart of a residential area in Pontypool, South Wales (Photo: Hoffman/ Greenpeace)

[2] The rise in food safety concerns and the effects on consumer confidence are discussed in *World Health and Disease* (Open University Press, 3rd edn 2001), Chapter 11.

10.2.2 Bioaccumulation and persistence of chemicals in the environment

Dioxin, and the related compounds PCBs, have special properties which cause them to build up in body tissue and in the environment. They are *lipophilic* (literally, 'liking fats'; in biological usage the term means 'readily dissolves in fats'); in practice, this means that they accumulate in body tissue where lipids are found, and are able to cross cell membranes and enter cells.

●   Why can dioxin cross cell membranes? (Refer back to Figure 3.7 if you need to remind yourself of membrane structure.)

■   Phospholipids (i.e. lipids with phosphate attached) form the basic framework of cell membranes, with proteins embedded or attached to them. Dioxin is lipophilic, so it is soluble in cell membranes and easily passes across.

Lipophilic compounds in general are not soluble in water, and thus dioxin tends to stick to soil or to sediment. Dioxin is also resistant to degradation, which means that it does not react easily with other chemicals or with air to form new compounds or breakdown products. Because of these properties, dioxin tends to accumulate in organisms as it passes up the *food web* (an example is shown in Figure 5.14). This phenomenon is known as **bioaccumulation**.

●   Can you think of some food webs that involve humans? How many 'levels' do your examples contain?

■   There are so many to choose from, but for example:
     human eats cow which eats grass (3 levels);
     human drinks milk from cow which eats grass (3 levels);
     human eats fish which eat smaller fish which eat plankton (4 levels);
     humans eat shellfish which eat plankton (3 levels);
     humans eat vegetables (2 levels).

Whatever we eat, we eventually excrete most of the material in one form or another, either in faeces, urine, perspiration or exhaled air (Chapter 7). Since dioxin (like many other lipophilic compunds) tends not to be excreted but remains in the fatty tissues, it accumulates in the body. When this happens at an early stage in the food web, and the animal (along with many others) is eaten by another animal, which is in turn eaten (again along with many others) by another animal, the chemical gets steadily more concentrated at each level of the food web.

●   Which of the food webs that end in humans would result in the highest dioxin exposure to humans?

■   Food webs with the most levels, since dioxin becomes more concentrated each time an animal eats another animal.

Food is the major source of exposure to dioxins and PCBs in humans; the highest levels are found in fatty foods, especially dairy products, eggs, meat and fish. However, there are also other exposure routes, such as inhalation of contaminated air, ingestion of contaminated water (remember that dioxin is not soluble in water but sticks to sediment), and absorption through the skin from soil or pesticide use, or handling other contaminated products. The main routes of exposure and level of exposure for different groups within the population depends on their dietary habits, contamination of their area of residence, and occupation. Thus, it is important to think of *critical groups* in the population, and not just *average* population exposure. This is particularly true of breast-fed babies.

● Why are breast-fed babies in contaminated areas likely to have a higher exposure to dioxins than bottle-fed babies?

■ Babies fed on breast milk receive a uniquely fat-rich milk in which accumulated dioxins and other compounds absorbed by the mother can be transferred to the baby.

A recent survey of breast milk in the UK found that it contained 10 to 40 times the normal levels of many chemical compounds, including dioxin (Lyons, 1999). Determining the exact health risks associated with these levels is extremely difficult due to the diversity of their effects and the difficulty in studying them in humans, as we shall discuss in the following sections. Despite this, the benefits of breast-feeding still outweigh the risks posed by dioxin contamination, for reasons discussed in Chapter 7.

It is estimated that once dioxin enters the body, its **biological half-life** is 6–10 years. 'Half-life' refers to the time it takes for a compound to reach half its original concentration or activity level. The term is most often used in relation to radiation; the half-life of a radioactive isotope gives a good idea of how long the radioactive exposure will persist in the environment. Radioactive iodine, for example, has a half-life of 8 days, whereas some forms of radioactive caesium have a half-life of 32 years. However, the *biological* half-life, or the half-life inside the body, refers not only to properties of the chemical itself, but also to how quickly the body transforms or excretes it. Thus, when the body is constantly absorbing it, the long half-life of dioxin leads to its accumulation in the body. Over a 40–50 year period the body can build up the equivalent of 5 000 times the acceptable daily dose. However, there are many difficulties in determining whether these levels of bioaccumulation are actually harmful to health. Even in accidents such as occurred at Seveso, where exposures were high, it is not straightforward to disentangle which of the long-term effects are related to the chemical — as the next section illustrates.

10.2.3 Evidence of toxicity from animal experiments

Depending on the exposure dose, dioxin has been found to be highly *carcinogenic* (cancer-causing) in rats and mice. Liver cancer is found in both these species, but other cancers seem to depend on species, sex, and the method of administration of the chemical. Dioxin is thought to belong to a small group of compounds that are carcinogenic but *not* **mutagenic** (i.e. dioxin does not cause mutations in the DNA of exposed cells); this finding is based on experiments upon both animals and isolated cells and tissues in laboratory cultures, which have failed to find a mutagenic effect.

The development of a cancer (carcinogenesis) is considered to be a multistage process requiring a number of different steps, as described in Section 8.6.1. These steps may include mutations, but also other events, called 'promoting' events, which lead to increased cell division and therefore the growth of the cancerous cells. Increased cell division may, in itself, promote mutation, since it is during cell division that the genetic material is most vulnerable to mutation. Thus, carcinogenic agents may either be mutagens, or non-mutagens that promote cell growth.

Dioxin has also been shown in animal experiments to be *immunotoxic*, i.e. it adversely affects the immune system, especially the developing (pre-adult) immune system. This could be expected to reduce resistance to infection.

10.2.4 Reproductive effects

Dioxin and the related compounds, PCBs, also cause *reproductive anomalies*, or 'adverse reproductive outcomes', in experimental animals: these include cleft palate, renal (kidney) anomalies, decreased fetal weight, increased fetal death rates, and adverse effects on sperm production in males, although the effects differ in different species. Dioxins belong to a varied group of chemicals which (among other functions) act as **endocrine disrupters**. This term is used to describe chemicals that can mimic the cellular effects of female sex hormones.

During early development, many embryos are extremely sensitive to minute changes in the levels of sex hormones (or molecules that can mimic them such as endocrine disrupters) and an imbalance can cause many problems including the loss of male genitalia. Many naturally occurring populations of animals (including fish, alligators and birds) have undergone such changes, with males showing a trend toward physical 'feminisation'. Increasing death of embryos and fetuses, as well as birth defects in wild populations have also been documented.

One particular compound, bisphenol, which is used widely in the plastics industry, is known to be a very powerful endocrine disrupter and its effects have been extensively studied (Lyons, 2000). As well as contaminating the environment in industrial waste, it may also have entered the human food web by contact with food stored in plastics. It has been hypothesised that the falling sperm count identified in human populations in industrialised countries over the last century is due to the action of such chemicals. However, inferring human health effects from animal experimentation or effects upon wild populations is very difficult, as the following section demonstrates.

10.3   Measuring and estimating toxicity

10.3.1 Extrapolating from animal experiments to human exposures

The effect of a chemical depends on how it is absorbed by the body, distributed in the body, broken down by the body (including detoxification in the liver), and excreted. Other animal species can be very different in these characteristics from humans.

For example, thalidomide, a drug prescribed around 1960 to alleviate morning sickness during pregnancy, proved to be highly *teratogenic*. A **teratogen** is an agent that causes congenital malformations (i.e. present at birth) if the fetus is exposed to it during pregnancy, usually during the first few months when the main formation of the organs takes place. In humans, thalidomide caused severe congenital limb malformations and other physical problems, but this effect is not seen in rats, one of the species used for safety-testing of drugs.

● Explain why an understanding of biological evolution suggests that the results of experiments on other animals are potentially applicable to humans, but that we should nevertheless expect differences from humans.

■   Humans and primates share a recent (in evolutionary terms) common ancestor, a more distant common ancestor with other mammals, and a yet more distant common ancestor with other vertebrates. The closer the evolutionary relationship between us and the animal species used as a substitute for humans in biomedical research, the more like ourselves biologically we can expect it to be, and the more reliably can the results of the research be applied to humans. However, no matter how close the relationship, an 'animal model' differs from humans in many aspects of its biology and behaviour, and this may crucially affect the outcome of the research, as the thalidomide tragedy illustrates.[3]

Each species of animal has, during the course of evolution, adapted to its habitual environment; this includes adaptation to the various chemicals it encounters in its diet and surroundings. Thus, different species have evolved biological responses to different chemicals, and the responses that have evolved even to the *same* chemicals may also differ between species.

It takes very intensive research on a particular chemical and how it is absorbed, distributed and metabolised in the bodies of different animals, to understand — at least to some extent — whether it is likely that human exposures will have similar effects. For example, dioxin concentrates particularly in the liver in rats, mice and hamsters, but in fat, muscle and skin in guinea pigs and rhesus monkeys. Not only is it difficult to predict the type of effect this will have, it is also not easy to estimate the human equivalent of the dose given to an animal.

Another aspect that needs consideration is *how* the animal has been exposed to dioxin. The same amount of dioxin administered in different ways is treated very differently by the body. Thus, if dioxin were injected straight into the bloodstream of animals, the relevance of the results to human exposures, which do not happen in this way, would be very uncertain. It is known that dioxin is better absorbed when administered in oil, but less well when it is stuck to soil or ash. Similarly, absorption through the skin depends on what the dioxin is mixed with. The general area of biological extrapolation from animal experiments to humans is the job of a *toxicologist*.

10.3.2   Interpreting the evidence for chronic toxicity in humans

What about evidence from exposed humans? In fact, evidence about chronic toxicity is generally difficult to obtain.

●   Why might it be easier to identify a source of *acute* toxicity than *chronic* toxicity?

■   Acute toxicity occurs very quickly after the exposure, and it is obviously easier to identify the source if the exposure and the disease are close together in time.

Other conditions that tend to apply to acute but not chronic toxicity, are if the disease is rare without such exposure, or if the disease almost always follows exposure.

Epidemiological studies of chronic toxicity tend to focus on high-exposure situations, where the health effects are either more frequent or more severe than low-dose exposures, and therefore easier to study. For dioxin, these include certain occupational groups who use herbicides or work in chemical plants, Vietnam veterans, and people living in a contaminated area like Seveso.

[3] The use of animals in biomedical research is discussed in *Studying Health and Disease* (Open University Press, 2nd edn 1994; colour-enhanced 2nd edn 2001), Chapter 9.

However, there are several problems for epidemiologists attempting to study chemical accidents or other high-exposure situations. After industrial accidents, it is common for the public-health response to be concentrated on practical measures to alleviate the immediate effects, but to neglect the gathering of information that might be useful to an epidemiologist for detailed study of health outcomes.

● It may also be difficult to distinguish between effects on health due to chemical toxicity and effects due to other consequences of the disaster. Can you suggest why?

■ After a disaster, people in the affected area are very likely to change many aspects of their normal behaviour (e.g. diet, sleeping patterns, use of stimulants such as alcohol, etc.) and they will probably experience high levels of anxiety and stress. Some of the adverse health effects after the disaster may be due to these changes rather than to the chemical exposure.

● What are the problems of relying on studies of high-exposure situations among certain occupations to predict environmental risks to the *general public* from low-dose chemical exposures?

■ It is often difficult to extrapolate reliably from the effects of high doses to the effects of low doses. Also, occupational studies tend to refer to men exposed during their working years, and it may be difficult to extrapolate to the effects on women, children, fetuses, newborns or elderly people, as well as sensitive groups in the population who are under-represented in the labour force.

Interpretation of epidemiological studies has to be very carefully conducted to determine whether a genuine association between an exposure and an outcome exists. Both false-negative and false-positive findings can occur (these terms were defined in Section 9.6). A long period of follow-up is needed after exposure in order to study cancer as a possible outcome, because it generally takes years to develop. Studies of small numbers of people cannot distinguish between real and chance effects. Large or multiple-site studies, which include many types of cancer, are likely to find one or two cancers increased in frequency by chance alone.

Another problem is that people are often exposed to a mixture of chemicals and it is difficult to know which chemical is the important one, or if the mixture itself is critical.

It may also be difficult to assess accurately the *extent* of the exposure to an individual, especially when it was in the past. This problem makes it particularly hard to estimate whether there is a **dose–response relationship** — a primary goal for public health regulation of industrial chemicals. For example, a dose–response relationship for a carcinogenic chemical means (broadly) that more highly exposed people have a higher incidence of cancer than less highly exposed people, and the less highly exposed have a higher incidence than the unexposed. It is clearly important to discover just how low a dose can be tolerated without causing an adverse response, and what outcomes can be expected for each extra increment of exposure. (We return to this point shortly.)

Another problem in estimating dose–response relationships is the potential for *bias* when the health status of an individual is ascertained by assessors who already know his or her exposure status, or conversely when exposure status is ascertained by assessors who already know the individual's state of health. After a major chemical accident, there may not be sufficient time or personnel to conduct assessments 'blind'.[4]

10.3.3 Outcomes of dioxin exposure in humans

The best evidence to date suggests that dioxin is not as strong a carcinogen in humans as would be expected from animal experiments. (The research evidence discussed below is reviewed by Bertazzi *et al.*, 1997, 1998 and 1999.) The 20-year follow-up study of the residents of Seveso examined cancer mortality across a range of exposures, from those with high levels to those with low levels, and found elevated rates for leukaemia and related cancers of the blood and lymphatic system, but not for the common cancers, e.g. of the breast, lung, stomach.

Human studies of teratogenic effects of dioxin have been very few. They include an epidemiological study of pregnant women at Seveso, which found no increase in congenital malformations. One theory is that dioxin is not teratogenic in humans because the doses that would be needed to produce a congenital malformation are also doses that would be clearly toxic to both mother and fetus. There is more evidence about the teratogenicity of the dioxin-related compounds, PCBs. After high-dose exposure, defects of skin, teeth, nails and hair have been reported, along with low birthweight and shorter duration of pregnancy. Currently, the research agenda for dioxin and PCBs is shifting to elucidating the effects of prenatal and early-life exposure on growth and development. This presents new challenges in the consistent measurement of subtle developmental effects.

10.3.4 Threshold effects in toxicity

Some long-term health effects of exposure to toxic chemicals or radiation do not show a smooth dose–response relationship, but instead demonstrate what is known as a **threshold effect**. Damage occurs only after the dose has exceeded a certain threshold level, and only beyond this threshold does the effect become more severe the greater the dose. For example, high exposure to certain kinds of radiation results in cataracts or sterility, but below a threshold level there seems to be no adverse effect.

● Toxic sources that display threshold effects tend to be those that cause destruction of tissues in the exposed organism. What biological mechanisms could underlie the threshold phenomenon? (Think back to the first section of this chapter.)

■ When a disease is a consequence of the destruction of tissue, it is reasonable to suppose that below a certain threshold the body's repair mechanisms are able to cope; but above the threshold, the amount of damage is more than the body is able to repair.

Many teratogenic effects, for example, are thought to need threshold doses before the fetus is no longer able to compensate, or repair the damage and develop normally; above the threshold, a dose–response relationship appears, in which the malformation may be more severe the higher the dose.

---

[4] The importance of assessors being 'blind' to the previous history of the subjects they are evaluating is discussed in the context of medical intervention trials in *Studying Health and Disease* (Open University Press, 2nd edn 1994; colour-enhanced 2nd edn 2001), Chapter 8.

By contrast, the development of cancers following a toxic exposure often does not show a threshold effect; the disease occurs with an increasing probability the higher the dose across a range of exposures, and there may be no relationship between the dose and the severity of the disease.

● Why aren't threshold effects generally seen in the development of most cancers after a toxic exposure?

■ Cancers develop as a result of a number of mainly genetic changes (mutations) within cells, which affect their growth relative to other cells (see Section 8.7). The lower the dose of exposure, the lower the probability that the mutation will occur (and the lower the probability that genetic repair mechanisms will miss the mutation). But although the probability becomes smaller and smaller, it is impossible to say *no* mutation will ever occur.

Dioxin belongs to the group of *non*-mutagenic carcinogens and, without knowing about its exact mechanism of action, it is difficult to know whether a 'no-threshold' model should apply to its adverse effects on human health. Knowledge of thresholds and the relationship between the dose and the probability or severity of disease is fundamental to the regulation of industrial chemicals, and is therefore the subject of much research.

10.4   Thinking about risks

To what extent should we attempt to minimise the exposure of human populations to the effects of the chemical industrial environment? At first sight this may seem obvious, but it is not a straightforward question. It is not easy to guage the extent to which minimising exposure is achieveable or even desirable.

The United Kingdom 1991 Environmental Protection Act introduced the *BATNEEC principle*: Best Available Technology Not Entailing Excessive Cost. Radiation protection operates on the *ALARA principle*: As Low As Is Reasonably Achievable. But what is 'excessive' or 'reasonable'?

One approach to answering this question is the *prioritisation of risks* to human health. Whilst the information provided by epidemiologists and toxicologists is a very important basis for prioritising the risks from environmental exposures, it does not in itself *constitute* prioritisation. When people are ranking environmental hazards, they are consciously or unconsciously taking account of many other variables, such as those illustrated by the questions in Box 10.1.

When thinking about risks, it can be useful to divide the subject into 'risk assessment' and 'risk management'. **Risk assessment** is mainly carried out by scientists who seek to characterise the potential adverse health effects of human exposures to environmental hazards. We have already discussed elements of this process, particularly the use of experimental data from animals and human data from accidental exposures, and the establishment of the relationship between dose and response. Another important part of risk assessment is finding out which parts of the population are exposed, by what route, and by how much. Risk assessments are generally very difficult, since they are almost always based on incomplete data and on assumptions. Finding ways to evaluate and include the 'uncertainty' in the risk assessment is essential for its use in risk management.

Box 10.1   Prioritising the risks from the chemical industrial environment

- Is the exposure voluntary or involuntary?

- Does the individual have any control over the extent of his/her exposure?

- Is it a predictable low-level exposure, or an unpredictable exposure with a possibility of disasters such as industrial accidents?

- Can we be confident that we know the possible health and environmental consequences?

- What would we lose in economic, social or personal terms from reduction of the exposure?

- Is everyone equally at risk or are there certain critical or sensitive groups?

- Is the distribution of risks and benefits in the population fair?

Risk management is the process of weighing policy alternatives and selecting the most appropriate regulatory action. It involves integrating the results of risk assessment with engineering data and with social, economic and political concerns in order to reach a decision about what actions to take. Risk management must weigh the health costs of the chemical (as revealed by risk assessment) and other costs, against its benefits. The example of dioxins in breast milk is a particularly complex example of weighing of costs and benefits.

There are sometimes question marks over the sustainability of the benefits we gain from some chemicals, for example many insect species are developing resistance to pesticides. Another increasingly important element in decision-making is that we cannot just look at risks to human health in terms of the *direct* toxicity of chemicals. We need to consider the *indirect* effects of chemicals at both local and, increasingly, global levels.

10.5   Effects of chemicals on the ecosystem

Since the 1980s awareness has increased about the *indirect* effects of industrialisation on human disturbance of the ecosystem and food sources. Locally, the indirect effects of chemical pollution of food sources are of particular concern in communities that depend on subsistence farming, fishing or hunting, or whose economy depends on the sale of these products. In newly industrialising countries, such as those of Asia and Latin America, the coexistence of small rural communities and industry, which is often inadequately subjected to pollution control, is a particularly difficult problem. For example, local communities can be devastated when chemical pollution depletes fish in rivers.

Chemicals can also exert effects on a global scale. You have already seen how dioxins and PCBs are distributed around the globe in the Earth's atmosphere and oceans and can exert effects at a distance from their source due to bioaccumulation. However, other chemicals from the burning of fossil fuels and from other industrial processes are also having major global effects upon our ecosystems.

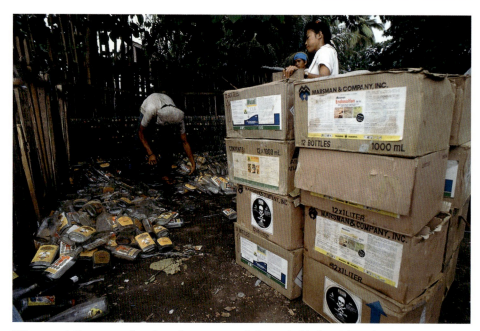

When regulations regarding the safe storage and disposal of industrial or pharmaceutical chemicals are broken, the impact on health locally and on food production can be devastating, particularly if fields and water sources become contaminated. Chemicals dumped at Cagayan on Mindanao Island, Philippines. (Photo: Julio Etchart)

10.5.1   Global warming

Chemicals can also impact on the ecosystem at a global level, with far-reaching consequences for health, not only of the human population but many other species. Of greatest concern is the contribution of the chemical industrial environment to global climate change. **Global warming** or the 'greenhouse effect' refers to the effects that the accumulation of carbon dioxide (produced in all combustion processes, whether industrial or in motor vehicles), and other gases such as methane and nitrous oxide, have on the temperature of the Earth's atmosphere.

The consequences of global warming were already evident at the start of the new millennium in an increase in the frequency of severe weather events around the world. It is too soon to say if this is the start of an accelerating trend. Hurricane winds, torrential rainfall and droughts cause massive destruction of property, livestock, farm land and human lives. But they may also leave in their wake another threat to health — infectious disease.

The association between 'Climate and health' is explored in an article under this title, written by Paul Epstein, a leading member of a scientific institution which is tracking the effects of global climate change. Figure 10.1 comes from Epstein's article and shows the geographical association between extreme weather events and subsequent major outbreaks of infectious disease among human populations in those areas. (The article appears in *Health and Disease: A Reader*, Open University Press, 3rd edn, 2001. Open University students should read it now.)

- According to Epstein, how do extreme weather events influence outbreaks of infectious disease?

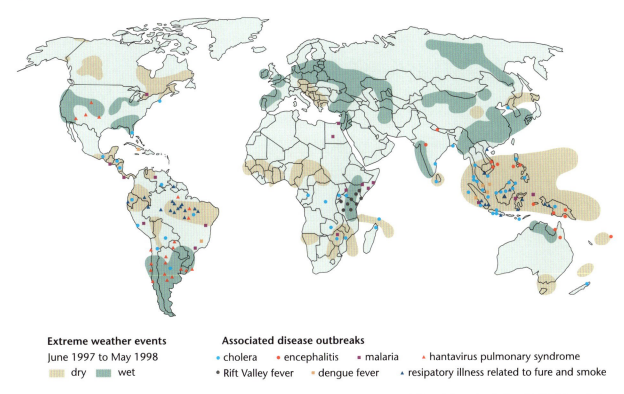

Extreme weather events
June 1997 to May 1998

▦ dry ▦ wet

Associated disease outbreaks

• cholera   • encephalitis   ▪ malaria   ▲ hantavirus pulmonary syndrome

• Rift Valley fever   ▪ dengue fever   ▲ resipatory illness related to fure and smoke

Figure 10.1 *Predicting disease outbreaks. The map shows regions of heavy rainfall and drought during 1997–98 and the associated clustering of outbreaks of emerging infectious disease. Extreme weather events have resulted in a surge in epidemics, particularly in tropical regions. Using climate data to predict the arrival of conditions that are likely to favour disease outbreaks can facilitate public-health interventions, such as vaccination and preparations at treatment facilities. (Source: Epstein, P. R. 1999, Climate and health, Science, 285(5 426), pp. 347–8)*

■ Precipitation and flooding lead to increased outbreaks of infectious diseases (e.g. cholera) through the spread of flood waters, or the generation of conditions more suited to the proliferation of insect vectors (e.g. mosquitoes) of diseases such as Rift Valley fever and malaria. Droughts can lead to predator–prey ratio changes, in turn leading to increases in the numbers of rodents carrying infectious agents (such as hantavirus), or they can lead to deforestation though fires, which then magnify subsequent flooding events. Environmental change might also see effects upon agriculture, including increases in pests and the spread of crop-related diseases.

Global warming has other predicted adverse effects on human populations, including population displacement and impoverishment through rising sea levels in low lying areas of the world; and changes in local economic activity and in land productivity (e.g. in agriculture and in the tourism industry); and the depletion of fresh water supplies.

10.5.2 Effects on the ozone layer

One of the major changes in the Earth's outer atmosphere, which underlies global warming, is a reduction in the concentration of *ozone* (an ozone molecule is formed from three oxygen atoms). Manufactured chemicals such as chlorofluorocarbons (CFCs) which, until the mid-1990s, were used extensively as refrigerants and propellants in aerosols, and nitrogen oxides (NO_x) which is generated from combustion engines, can react with ozone in the upper atmosphere and destroy it.

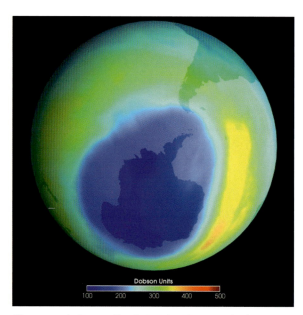

The ozone hole over the Antarctic, photographed on 6 September 2000 from the Total Ozone Mapping Spectrometer (TOMS) on board NASA's Nimbus 7 satellite. The size of the hole was far larger than scientists had predicted, covering the whole of Antarctica and extending almost to the tip of South America (visible at the top right-hand side). The colours represent a scale in Dobson Units which is a measure of the amount of ozone in a column of atmosphere, with blue indicating areas with low ozone (Photo: Courtesy of the TOMS Science Team/NASA)

Ozone acts as a natural ultraviolet (UV) block. It therefore reduces the intensity of the Sun's UV rays as they pass through the upper atmosphere, so **ozone depletion** will increase the risk of skin cancer and cataracts in humans, and could cause some degree of suppression of the immune system. Greater exposure to UV radiation could also destroy ocean-living phytoplankton, which are particularly vulnerable to UV damage.

● What might be the consequence of decreased numbers of phytoplankton? (You might want to look back to Figure 5.14.)

■ Phytoplankton form an important basis of food webs for all marine creatures and for land animals that take food from the sea. They are also a critical source of significant amounts of oxygen in the atmosphere. A reduction in phytoplankton will ultimately lead to global loss of animal and plant biodiversity.

In order to predict the impact of environmental pollution upon human health at a global level, the combination of future changes in pollution levels and the direct and indirect effects of pollution upon ecosystems and the climate, must all be put into the equation. While there are uncertainties in all these aspects, there is a general agreement within the scientific community that global changes are occurring.

10.6 Global solutions?

As we have just mentioned, much of the impetus for regulation of chemical production and waste emission now comes from the fear of adverse consequences for the *ecosystem*, and *indirect* effects on human health. These are even more difficult to measure or predict than the direct effects, since there is considerable uncertainty about how the ecosystem will be affected by changing industrial practices and patterns of industrial activity. International cooperation includes measures such as the Montreal protocol, an international agreement signed in 1987 aimed at tackling ozone depletion at a global level through the phasing-out of chemicals such as CFCs, and the Kyoto Treaty which aims at limiting the emission of carbon wastes such as carbon dioxide from industrialised countries. Despite being signed in 1997, this agreement had still to be implemented at the beginning of 2001. Other measures such as the Basel convention, signed in 1989, aim to reduce the export of toxic waste to developing countries with inadequate regulations protecting the environment and health. It is clear, therefore, that the world community needs to think carefully about how to live with the chemical products of industrialisation. In the next and final chapter in this book, we will take a broader view of modern industrial culture and its effects on health.

OBJECTIVES FOR CHAPTER 10

When you have studied this chapter, you should be able to:

10.1 Define and use, or recognise definitions and applications of, each of the terms printed in **bold** in the text.

10.2 Give examples of how the body can defend itself against, and repair damage from, environmental toxins and explain why disease sometimes results despite these mechanisms.

10.3 Distinguish between a critical group and a sensitive group (as defined in this chapter), and describe the mechanisms underlying hypersensitivity to certain chemicals.

10.4 Distinguish between acute and chronic toxicity and explain why knowledge of the chronic effects of environmental pollutants is very incomplete; refer to the difficulties of extrapolating from animal experiments to humans and the problems of risk assessment.

10.5 Summarise the various ways in which the chemical industrial environment can directly and indirectly affect human health, either through local exposures (as in the dioxin case study) or through changes in the global ecosystem.

QUESTIONS FOR CHAPTER 10

1 (*Objective 10.2*)

Explain how the process of cellular repair involving cell division might lead to disease. (You will also have to think back to Chapters 4 and 8 to answer this question fully.)

2 (*Objective 10.3*)

Distinguish between an acute inflammatory response to an infection in the respiratory tract and an acute hypersensitivity reaction to an inhaled allergen such as pollen. (You will also have to think back to Chapter 6 to answer this question fully.)

3 (*Objectives 10.3 and 10.4*)

   (a) Use the example of thalidomide exposure to illustrate the concept of a *sensitive group.*

   (b) What features of the thalidomide tragedy helped clinicians and epidemiologists to establish a *causal* relationship between the drug and limb malformations?

   (c) Suggest some reasons why toxicity testing of thalidomide in other species might fail to give an accurate assessment of the risk to human fetuses.

4 (*Objective 10.5*)

Based on your reading of Chapters 7, 8 and 10, how might the chemical industrial environment alter the level of ultraviolet (UV) radiation reaching the surface of the Earth, and what health effects might result?

CHAPTER 11

The impact of modern culture

Study notes for OU students

This short chapter brings together some key themes as it draws the book to a close and speculates about the future in terms of impacts on human health arising from the pace of cultural change. During Section 11.2.2 you will be asked to read an extract entitled 'The evolution of Utopia' by the geneticist Steve Jones, which appears in *Health and Disease: A Reader* (Open University Press, second edition 1995; third edition 2001).

11.1   Genetic and cultural evolution

In the earlier chapters of this book, we considered how genetic evolution, through natural selection, has made us what we are: multicelled, sexually reproducing, with long gestation, a complex brain and a complex immune system. We also considered why, despite our long evolutionary past, we are neither disease-free nor immortal.

Chapter 2 introduced the idea that cultural evolution also affects human health and disease, and other chapters have looked at the effects of modern cultural changes, including industrialisation, medical technologies, dietary changes, and the consequences of living longer. What are the essential differences between cultural evolution and genetic evolution? Now that you have almost completed this book, it is time to review the meanings of these terms.

11.1.1   Genetic evolution revisited

Genetic evolution, based on the theory of natural selection (as described in Chapters 2 to 4), begins with the four processes that create *genetic variability* between members of a population of organisms.

● What are the four processes? (All were described in Chapter 4.)

■ They are: crossing over of genetic material between chromosomes during meiosis when eggs and sperm are forming (Section 4.3.3 and Figure 4.8);

random assortment of chromosomes during meiosis (Figure 4.9);

the mixing of genes from both parents at fertilisation (Figure 4.9);

mutation (Section 4.10).

To summarise points made many times earlier in this book, sometimes a new genetic variant is beneficial, within a specific environment, in the sense that such an individual is more likely to survive and leave offspring in the next generation. In the 'shorthand' of evolutionary biology, this genetic variant will be *selected for*, that is, the frequency of this genetic variant will increase in the population over time. Conversely, natural selection will *act against* genetic variants that reduce reproductive success, and these will tend to decrease in the population over time.

● Can you think of examples of this process discussed earlier in this book?

■ The genes for sickle-cell disease and thalassaemia are believed to have increased in the population because they confer some protection against malaria to individuals who inherit a single copy of the disease allele; this advantage more than offsets the genes 'lost' from the population due to the reduced reproductive success of people who inherit two copies of the mutant gene.

There are three important features of evolution by natural selection that are worth emphasising before we move on.

First, the classical theory of genetic evolution is based strictly on the reproductive success of the *individual*. You might even think of it as based on the 'reproductive success' of particular genes, because natural selection *cannot* favour the persistence of a gene that codes for a characteristic that is *not* good for the individual or their closest kin (who have genes in common). Natural selection could not favour such a gene *even* if it happened to be good for the wider group or community, because it is individuals (not groups) who live long enough to reproduce or who die early.

Natural selection can only favour the 'survival of the fittest' *individuals*. However, you may have come across a rival theory called 'group selection', which is incompatible with the classical theory of natural selection. Advocates of this idea claim that 'altruistic' genes may have evolved which code for behaviours that benefit the group as a whole, even if they are disadvantageous to some individuals.

Second, the classical theory of natural selection also predicts that characteristics that produce benefits for the individual *only* during the post-reproductive years cannot be selected for *unless* they produce benefits for close kin (if you are unclear about why this is so, look back at the discussion in Chapter 8 on the evolution of ageing).

● Can you think of an example of a post-reproductive characteristic that may have evolved by natural selection?

■ The extended period of post-reproductive longevity among female primates, including humans, is believed to have been favoured by natural selection because it maximises the time available for parental care, and thus increases the survival chances of a female's own offspring and those of her closest relatives.

However, there is a question mark over the prediction that natural selection cannot favour late-acting characteristics. During the twentieth century, the mortality rate among older people in many high-income countries began to slow down — a phenomenon known as enhanced old-age survival. It is not clear whether this is simply due to the most robust members of a population surviving to become a cadre of the 'healthiest old', or if there is some evolutionary selection process at work that reduces one's chances of dying after you reach a certain age.[1]

The third feature of genetic evolution by natural selection is lack of foresight or strategy. A gene cannot increase (or decrease) in frequency in *readiness* for a future change in the environment, but only in *response* to a change that has already occurred. There is no disagreement among biologists on this point!

11.1.2 Cultural evolution revisited

Cultural evolution can be distinguished from genetic evolution by three features that are the antithesis of the classical theory of natural selection. First, human societies can choose to change their cultural practices so that they will benefit the whole community, not just the individual (this is the equivalent of group selection).

Second, we can and do introduce cultural practices that will favour the survival of people in their post-reproductive years — for example, state pensions, winter fuel payments, or residential care.

Third, we can look ahead to the consequences of our actions in future generations and decide to forsake some of our temporary well-being for the sake of those who come after us. For example, any attempt to reduce the pace of global warming must include a reduction in our use of fossil fuels such as petrol, which may reduce living standards in the gas-guzzling Western world, or at least constrain travel opportunities. People may nevertheless make this choice, which cannot benefit them in their own lifetimes.

---

[1] Enhanced old-age survival has also been observed in a wide range of invertebrates, which increases the possibility that the phenomenon may be a more general feature of genetic evolution. An article by Vaupel *et al.* (1999) discusses this possibility; it can be found in *Health and Disease: A Reader* (Open University Press, 3rd edn 2001).

● Can you see a way in which cultural evolution might itself be an expression of genetic evolution?

■ If certain forms of human behaviour are influenced by genes and these behaviours have been selected for (e.g. by increased reproductive success or avoidance of death!) then such genes might themselves influence cultural evolution. It has been controversially argued by some scientists that behaviours as wide ranging as fear, excitement-seeking (such as hang-gliding), sexual-philandering and criminal activities can be at least partially explained by the genes we inherit. Human behaviour is vastly complex and claims that our social behaviour are genetically determined are highly controversial.

Human health, as defined by the World Health Organisation in its frequently quoted constitution of 1958, is 'a state of complete physical, mental and social wellbeing and not merely the absence of disease and infirmity'. In this sense, much of human endeavour and culture can be seen as an effort to improve health. However, it is not always clear *whose* health. By improving the health of one subgroup of the population, does this damage the health of others, or of future generations? Does society do enough to assess the impact of cultural change on health, and who is included in this impact assessment?

Cultural evolution, itself perhaps inexpertly aimed at promoting health, causes problems to the environment and to human biology, which require further cultural adaptation to combat, not only for the survival of the human species but also for the survival of the global ecosystem. However, the capacity of both humans and other species to adapt to environmental change, whether through genetic or cultural adaptation, depends not only on the *nature* of the change, but also on its *speed*. It has been the speed of change in industrialised societies that has caused particular concern in recent years.

11.1.3 The pace of change

Genetic adaptation is a very slow process because it cannot begin until new mutations or genetic variants appear that are better adapted to the current environment, and then these have to spread through the population from generation to generation. Probably a sequence of genetic variations, each building on the last, will be necessary before any lasting adaptation occurs. However, maintenance of a high degree of genetic diversity in a population, whether human or otherwise, can speed up this evolutionary 'response time'.

● Can you explain why?

■ It increases the chance of a favourable combination of genes or gene variants (alleles) occurring, which can be passed on to subsequent generations.

Cultural adaptation means that human societies must recognise what the problem is, devise a solution, and change the behaviour of the population in order to implement that solution. This might happen extremely quickly (as in the introduction of car seat-belt legislation), or it might take many generations (as in the slow decline of cigarette-smoking among men in the UK). An important concern is that the speed of cultural change in the second half of the twentieth century may *in itself* have been psychologically damaging and thus have had a direct adverse effect on health, which is likely to accelerate in the new millennium.

11.2   Impacts of modern culture on human genetic evolution

Although cultural evolution is now a predominant force in explaining changes in human health and disease, we can still expect genetic changes to occur. Framed in terms of genetic evolution, a disease could be thought of as a state that lowers individual *fitness* (Chapter 3). However, many 'diseases' no longer affect fitness. For example, infertility treatments have changed the reproductive prospects of infertile couples, and some children born with severe genetic birth defects now survive to reproductive age following treatment of their conditions (Chapters 4 and 9).

Other genetic characteristics may have less influence *now* on explaining differences in reproductive success between individuals than was the case in the past. For example, people who are more genetically susceptible to infection may now be protected from pathogens by antibiotics, effective sanitation and vaccination (Chapter 6). People with visual impairments can have their sight corrected with glasses, or can adopt a lifestyle that prevents their visual impairment from being a major handicap. In future, screening for genetic susceptibility to disease may allow early interventions, whether directed at the genes or the environment of the susceptible person, which will reduce the risk of developing the screened disease (Chapter 9).

●   What is the likely effect of the health interventions described above on the frequency of disease alleles in the population?

■   Many cultural developments are leading to a relaxation of the *power* of natural selection to act against (reduce the frequency of) formerly disadvantageous genetic characteristics in the population. This relaxation of natural selection will inevitably lead to *increases* in the frequency of certain disease alleles.

On the other hand, we also have the potential to impose stronger selective pressures against those alleles, for example by prenatal screening and selective abortion, or if we engage in the future in forms of gene therapy that result in heritable changes to the genetic material (we return to this point below). As explained in Chapter 9, gene therapy involving germline changes to the DNA was not sanctioned in the UK or in other industrial democracies, at the time of writing (2000). Society is becoming increasingly conscious of the need to clarify and regulate the ways in which we are interfering with our genetic inheritance. Cultural change may also create strong selection pressures that alter our genetic make-up, as the following example illustrates.

11.2.1   The 'thrifty genotype' hypothesis

Scientists have long been speculating about the genetic evolutionary basis of an epidemic of *non-insulin-dependent diabetes* in the Pacific island of Nauru. This form of diabetes is not caused by insulin deficiency (in contrast to insulin-dependent diabetes mellitus, as discussed in Chapter 7). Over a short time period, the economy of the island was transformed from one of subsistence farming and fishing, to phosphate mining. The Nauruans quickly became wealthy, and this manifested itself in high calorie intake, obesity and low physical activity: well-known risk factors for this form of diabetes. Diabetes subsequently rose to epidemic proportions in young adults after 1950.

One hypothesis to explain the rise of diabetes in Nauru is known as Neel's **thrifty genotype hypothesis** after the American geneticist who formulated it in 1962. According to Neel's hypothesis, the reason why the genotype associated with non-insulin-dependent diabetes was so frequent before the Nauruans adopted a Western lifestyle is because it (thriftily) favoured fat deposition during periods of plentiful food. This genotype would be advantageous in situations where food sources are unpredictable; the fat stored during 'good times' would be used up quite quickly when food became scarce again and, as a consequence, diabetes did not develop. However, when the Nauruans' lifestyle changed suddenly to one of permanent plenty, they remained obese and became prone to diabetes.

● Since 1975, diabetes among Nauruans has been found to decline markedly in prevalence and incidence. Can you suggest a hypothetical explanation for this decline, even though their calorie intake, levels of obesity and inactivity remained as high as before?

■ The decline may be due to natural selection, in that people with diabetes-prone genotypes with a high-calorie, low-activity lifestyle might have *fewer* children than other Nauruans who don't have this genotype. In such a situation, the 'thrifty' genotype would gradually decline in frequency in the population, and so would the incidence of diabetes.

In Western populations, the 'thrifty' genotype may have decreased in frequency over a much longer period of stable food supply, when it was no longer advantageous.

There is little hard evidence to support this hypothetical evolutionary explanation of events on Nauru, but we can identify two important general points in this example: the *interdependence* of cultural and genetic evolution, and the potential *speed* of genetic evolution under strong selection pressure from sudden cultural change.

11.2.2 Future trends in gene frequency

Speculating about the future evolution of human genes is a risky venture, but Steve Jones, a leading British geneticist, has attempted to do this in his book *The Language of the Genes* (1993, 2nd edn 2001). An extract from the final chapter, entitled 'The evolution of Utopia', appears in *Health and Disease: A Reader* (Open University Press, 2nd edn 1995; 3rd edn 2001). (Open University students should read it now and then answer the following questions.)

● What effect on the frequency of serious human genetic diseases, such as cystic fibrosis, does Steve Jones predict will occur when medical treatments enable children with previously fatal disease alleles to survive and reproduce, thereby passing on their genes?

■ He thinks it will have little effect for three reasons. First, most serious genetic diseases are caused by *recessive* alleles and disease results only if *two* copies of the disease allele are inherited; most of the copies of these alleles in the population occur in unaffected 'carriers', so increasing the total number of disease survivors in the population will produce little increase in the total number of disease alleles. Second, the increase in the number of disease alleles passed on to the next generation by affected people (who survive to reproduce as a consequence of medical treatment) is likely to be offset by a decrease in the birth of affected babies, as more genetic advice is available to potential parents, who then decide against having affected children. Third, increased population movements and intermarriage between people from different parts of the world greatly *decreases* the chance of two carriers of a disease allele having a child.

● What cultural change does Jones predict *will* have a significant effect on the frequency of human genetic diseases arising by new mutations?

■ The falling age at which people now *complete* their families will reduce the mutation rate. (Even though the age at which parents have their *first* child is tending to increase, the age at which they have their *last* child has fallen sharply.) The gametes of younger parents are less likely to carry mutations and hence new disease alleles will arise less often.

Jones thinks that the pace of human evolution is slowing down, for three reasons. First, remember that natural selection acts on genetic variations which are partly determined by the rate of new mutations. Jones thinks that industrial sources of radiation and chemicals have a much smaller effect on the mutation rate than do natural sources (such as radon gas leaking from granite), so — even as industrialisation spreads — the effect on mutation rate will be insignificant. At the same time, falling parental age (mentioned above) will also tend to reduce the mutation rate. Lower mutation rate means less genetic variability for natural selection to act on and hence the pace of human evolution will slow down.

Second, important genetic differences between individuals in terms of evolution are those affecting their fertility and the survival rates of their offspring. Jones points out that, as people have *fewer* children, *most of whom survive*, these evolutionarily significant differences are tending to decrease. Greater longevity and the decline of infectious diseases in many parts of the world mean that genetic differences between individuals will, in future, tend to affect susceptibility to the degenerative diseases of the *post-reproductive* years, when natural selection cannot act directly.

Third, he argues that random genetic change will also be less likely as genetically isolated small population groups disappear and intermarriage becomes commonplace (a point also made at the end of Chapter 4 of this book).

11.3 The impact of modern culture on human health

Since the Industrial Revolution, average life expectancy has increased very significantly through the combined effects of improved diet (in quality, quantity and predictability), sanitation and protection from pathogens, protection from physical environmental extremes (e.g. by improved housing), and medical innovation and access to health services. For example, in China, life expectancy at birth soon after the end of World War II (1946–49) was 39 years; by 1981 it had risen to 68 years — an increase of almost 30 years of life expectancy in a period of just over three decades.[2]

Much of the disease burden in modern culture now occurs in old age. Ageing is associated with the degeneration of many different biological processes and systems, as Chapter 8 described. There is currently much research and debate over the extent to which age-associated disease, as well as its progression to disability, is potentially preventable (or postponable) by social and medical interventions or lifestyle changes during youth, as well as during old age. The evolutionary heritage

[2] These data are quoted in an article in *Health and Disease: A Reader* (Open University Press, 3rd edn 2001), entitled 'Health sector reform: lessons from China' by Gerald Bloom and Gu Xingyuan. Global trends in longevity and the underlying causes are discussed extensively in another book in this series, *World Health and Disease* (Open University Press, 3rd edn 2001).

of 'post-reproductive degeneration' need not be seen as inevitable; as with all biological processes, genes and environment have a complex interaction and we can alter the expression of our genes by changing our environment.

We can consider changes to the 'environment' in three categories: the physical and chemical (usually abbreviated to physico-chemical) environment, the biological environment, and the psycho-social environment.

11.3.1   Cultural change and the physico-chemical environment

Industrialisation has been characterised by a rapid use of resources beyond their capacity for self-renewal, the production of a range of synthetic chemicals, and the production of wastes at a rate too great for their absorption in the environment. The negative impact of these processes on human health via changes in the *physico-chemical environment* (including both the direct and indirect health effects discussed in Chapter 10), depends on society's ability or will to regulate industrial processes.

Complex economic and political forces have restricted the regulation of industry and its waste emissions. In the poorer newly industrialising countries, the situation is particularly serious, since these communities have the least power to ensure that the negative effects of industrialisation are reduced to a sustainable level.

Unfortunately, we are also limited by our lack of knowledge of the health effects of many environmental contaminants, and this lack of knowledge further limits the ability of citizens to ensure that costs and benefits of industrial activities and processes are properly balanced. Threats such as global warming and ozone depletion are beset with difficulties, not just in understanding the relationship between environmental change and health, but in predicting just what that environmental change will be.

The impact of industrialisation on the physical, chemical and biological environment — particularly in newly industrialising countries — is encapsulated in this scene of men unloading sulphur for the chemical industry; Cochin port, Kerala, India, 1980. (Photo: E & P Ragazzini/ Corbis Images)

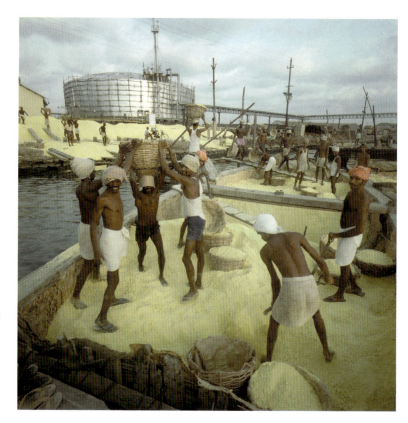

11.3.2 Cultural change and the biological environment

Human health depends on the *biological environment* for food, for oxygen (produced by plants and by phytoplankton in oceans and lakes), for shelter from the elements, and for recreation. The vast range of pathogens in the biological world also presents some of the greatest challenges to human health.

The biological environment is being affected by changes in the physical and chemical environment: for example, in the use of pesticides to increase crop yields, by the effects of chemical pollution on plants and animals and, on a larger scale, by the possible effects of global warming on the distribution and survival of pathogenic organisms and food sources. It is also subject to direct destruction or manipulation. Agricultural practices, such as the chopping down of rainforests for farming (e.g. in Brazil), may result in direct environmental degradation, as can population pressure and sprawling urbanisation on fragile or marginally fertile areas. Problems of sanitation, particularly in urban areas in developing countries, far outweigh the health effects of local industrial pollution.

The exploitation of genetic variability in other species has been at the basis of agriculture and innovations in drug development (e.g. penicillin, derived from a fungus). The reduction of biological diversity (biodiversity) is therefore of great concern, not only for its own sake, but for its implications for human well-being. As you saw in Chapter 5, coevolution with pathogens is a driving force in evolutionary change, and may even be the basis of the evolution of sexual reproduction itself.

Humans are interfering with this coevolution by introducing very strong and uniform selective pressures on pathogens. One example is the use of antibiotics, which was discussed in Chapter 5.

● How do bacteria become resistant to antibiotics?

■ Within each population of bacteria, there is a range of resistance to antibiotics. Bacteria have very short generation times, so unless all are destroyed by the drug, the most resistant survivors will rapidly increase in subsequent generations. In addition, in each generation there is an opportunity for a new mutation to arise, which gives the mutant bacterium greater or even total resistance to the antibiotic, greatly increasing its reproductive success and the survival of its genes.

The simplest part for humans to play in the 'coevolutionary race' is to keep changing the antibiotic and so keep one step ahead of the bacteria, but this is very difficult and expensive. There is a real possibility that certain strains of bacteria (such as some that cause tuberculosis, or infect wounds and burns in hospitals) are becoming resistant to all our antibiotics — the so called *multi-drug resistant strains* (Section 5.7.1).

Several strategies are in operation to combat the threat of **antibiotic resistance**.

● What is the most important strategy? (Chapter 5)

■ Of greatest importance is to use antibiotics less often and only when absolutely necessary, so that bacteria are less likely to encounter them and become resistant; and when antibiotics *are* used, to complete the dosing regimen even if symptoms are resolved before all the prescribed doses have been taken.

Other strategies are to give several different antibiotics at once, so that any bacterium has to have more than one mutation to overcome the effect and survive; and to improve hygiene conditions, especially in hospitals, so that bacteria become less of a disease threat, irrespective of the use of antibiotics.

Pharmaceutical companies are also extracting potential new antibiotics from other species, exploiting the ability of organisms as diverse as alligators, moths, frogs and sharks to defend themselves against their own pathogens. These new drugs have never been used against human pathogens, which cannot therefore have evolved resistance to them — but our resort to plundering the world's biodiversity to protect ourselves from 'superbugs' should remind us of the interconnected web of life in the biological environment.

Two further examples of humans interfering with the biological environment are evident in the countryside of developed economies: agricultural *monoculture* — the continuous growing of one type of crop over a large area, which wipes out biodiversity — and the indiscriminate use of pesticides and herbicides, often to maintain those monocultures.

Human ability to devise new methods of affecting the biological environment may be close at hand with the development of genetic technologies to modify crop species and domestic livestock. Whether the outcomes are generally beneficial or have unwanted consequences, we must take care not to deplete the reserves of genetic variability in nature. The preservation of biodiversity may be in our own interest, as well as a 'moral good'.

11.3.3   Cultural change and the psycho-social environment

One of the more complex areas of human biology is that of the biological basis of stress and psychological adaptation, or the interaction of mind and body. This is part of what is often termed the *psycho-social environment.* Modern culture is characterised by speed — not only the speed of our communication networks which require constant response, but also the speed of change in the form of technological developments and the structure of society and social support. How this can influence human health via psychological effects is beyond the scope of this book, but is as important a part of human biology as the other factors we have discussed.[3]

We should also mention a specific area of social interaction, that of human conflict. While conflict in the rest of the animal kingdom is limited to direct predator–prey interactions, or competition between animals for mates or breeding sites (which rarely end in fatal injuries), human conflict is distinguished by the sophisticated use of 'tools' of warfare. Modern culture has produced the escalation of armaments to weapons of potential mass destruction. The health effects are not only those that directly result from the use of such weapons, but also from the massive diversion of resources from welfare-related productivity to the arms industry, and the destruction of people's homes and livelihoods. In addition, war can wreak destruction on the physico-chemical and biological environments.

[3] The psychological dimensions of human health and illness are discussed extensively in *Birth to Old Age: Health in Transition* (Open University Press, 2nd edn 1995; colour-enhanced 2nd edn 2001); there is also a case study on schizophrenia in *Experiencing and Explaining Disease* (Open University Press, 2nd edn 1996; colour-enhanced 2nd edn 2001), Chapter 6.

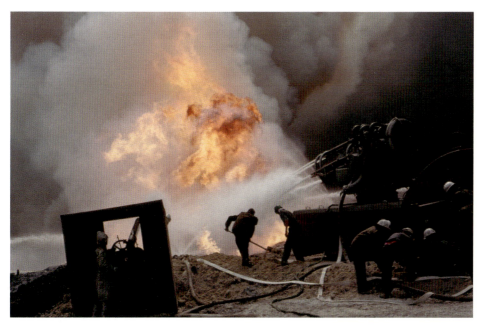

As the army of Iraq retreated from Kuwait at the end of the Gulf War in 1990, more than 500 oil wells were set ablaze, sending millions of tons of burning oil into the atmosphere. It took over a year for all the wells to be capped (this scene was photographed in October 1991), causing incalculable environmental damage, in addition to the direct and indirect health effects of the pollution and of the war itself. (Photo: Robert van der Hilst/Corbis Images)

War, however, is not the only means by which one group of humans can cause the destruction of another. The massive reduction in the populations of Native Americans and Aborigines in Australia, for example, has resulted not only from genocide, but from the results of exposure to new diseases (as you read in Chapter 5), economic impoverishment, and the health problems that result from disintegration of cultural identity. Modern Western culture also poses a continuing threat to the health of many populations in the developing world, since its 'success' is currently underpinned by the unequal distribution of resources.

Some of the limitations of human biology can be overcome by cultural developments, but it is notable how inequitable the effects can be for different population groups within and between societies. We can also see how inadequate is our knowledge of the complexities of human ecology for predicting the consequences of our actions. The future of human life on Earth need not be determined by blind natural selection, but there are many challenges in developing an informed and ethical structure for human cultural evolution, which will lead to an overall improvement of human health in its broadest sense, while preserving biological diversity. Using what you have learnt in this and other books in this series, you may like to reflect on whether 'nature knows best'.

OBJECTIVES FOR CHAPTER 11

When you have studied this chapter, you should be able to:

11.1 Define and use, or recognise definitions and applications of, each of the terms printed in **bold** in the text.

11.2 Distinguish between genetic and cultural evolution and give examples of ways in which they interact with each other and with the environment in affecting human health and disease; comment on ways in which modern culture may have an impact on human evolution in the future.

QUESTION FOR CHAPTER 11

1 (*Objective 11.2*)

In times of persistent plenty, Nauruans with the diabetes-prone 'thrifty' genotype may be at a reproductive disadvantage compared with others in the population who lack it. Yet in the research article in which J. V. Neel first proposed the thrifty genotype hypothesis to explain the epidemic of diabetes on Nauru, he stated that:

> … efforts to preserve the diabetes genotype through this transient period of plenty are in the interests of mankind. (Neel, 1962)

(a) Justify this statement and use the Nauruan example to illustrate the interaction between genotype, phenotype and environment.

(b) Explain why, in times of persistent plenty, the thrifty genotype cannot be preserved through natural selection. How then might it be preserved?

References and further sources

References

Alberts, B. and Klug, Sir A. (2000) The Human Genome must be freely available to all humankind, *Nature*, **404**, p. 325.

Beardsley, T. (1997) The start of something big? Dolly has become a new icon for science, *Scientific American*, **276**, pp. 15–16.

Begon, M., Harper, J. L. and Townsend, C. R. (1990) *Ecology: Individuals, Populations and Communities*, 2nd edn (1st edn, 1986), Blackwell Scientific Publications, Oxford.

Bertazzi, P. A., Bernucci, I., Brambilla, G., Consonni, D. and Pesatori, A. C. (1998) The Seveso studies on early and long term effects of dioxin exposure, *Environmental Health Perspectives*, **106**, Supplement 2, pp. 625–33.

Bertazzi, P. A., Pesatori, A. C., Bernucci, I., Landi, M. T. and Consonni, D. (1999) Dioxin exposure and human leukemia and lymphomas: lessons from the Seveso accident and studies on industrial workers, *Leukemia*, **13**, Supplement 1, pp. 572–4.

Bertazzi, P. A., Zocchetti, C., Guercilena, S., Consonni, D., Tironi, A., Landi, M. T. and Pesatori, A. C. (1997) Dioxin exposure and cancer risk: a 15 year mortality study after the 'Saveso accident', *Epidemiology*, **8**, pp. 646–52.

Bianchi, D. W., Bernfield, M. and Nathan, D. G. (1993) A revived opportunity for fetal research, *Nature*, **363**, 6 May, p. 12.

Bloom, G. and Xingyuan, G. (1997) Health sector reform: lessons from China, *Social Science and Medicine*, **45**(3), pp. 351–60; an edited extract also appears in Davey, B., Gray, A. and Seale, C. (eds) (2001) *Health and Disease: A Reader*, 3rd edn, Open University Press, Buckingham.

Bogin, B. (1993) Why must I be a teenager at all? *New Scientist*, 6 March, pp. 34–8; reprinted in Davey, B., Gray, A. and Seale, C. (eds) *Health and Disease: A Reader*, (1995) 2nd edn and (2001) 3rd edn, Open University Press, Buckingham.

Brines, R., Hoffman-Goetz, L. and Pedersen, B. K. (1996) Can you exercise to make your immune system fitter?, *Immunology Today*, **17**, pp. 252–4.

Brundtland, G. H. *et al.* (1980) Height, weight and menarcheal age of Oslo school children during the past 60 years, *Annals of Human Biology*, **7**, pp. 307–22.

Campbell, N. A. (ed.) (1993) *Biology*, 3rd edn, The Benjamin/Cummings Publishing Company, Inc., Redwood City, California and Wokingham, Surrey.

Council of Europe (1996) *Convention for the Protection of Human Rights and the Dignity of the Human Being with regard to the Application of Biology and Medicine*, Council of Europe, Strasburg, France.

Cuatrecasas, P., Lockwood, D. H. and Caldwell, J. R. (1965) Lactase deficiency in the adult, *Lancet*, **7375**, pp. 14–18.

Daintith, J. and Isaacs, A. (eds) (1989) *Medical Quotations*, Collins Reference Dictionary, Collins, London and Glasgow.

Davies, C. T. M. and Young, K. (1983) Effect of temperature on the contractile properties and muscle power of *triceps surae* in humans, *Journal of Applied Physiology*, **55**, pp. 191–5.

Dawkins, R. (1976) *The Selfish Gene*, Oxford University Press, Oxford.

Department of the Environment (1989) *Dioxins in the Environment: Report of an Interdepartmental Working Group on PCDDs and PCDFs*, Pollution Paper No. 27, HMSO, London.

Diamond, J. (1992) *The Rise and Fall of the Third Chimpanzee*, Vintage Books, London; an edited extract appears in Davey, B., Gray, A. and Seale, C. (eds) *Health and Disease: A Reader*, (2001) 3rd edn, Open University Press, Buckingham.

Dobson, A. (1992) People and disease, Chapter 10.4 in Jones, S., Martin, R., Pilbeam, D. and Bunney, S. (eds), *The Cambridge Encyclopedia of Human Evolution*, Cambridge University Press, Cambridge.

Durham, W. H. (1991) *Coevolution, Genes, Culture and Human Diversity*, Stanford University Press, Stanford, California.

Epstein, P. R. (1999) Climate and health, *Science*, **285**(5 426), pp. 347–8; also reproduced in Davey, B., Gray, A. and Seale, C. (eds) *Health and Disease: A Reader*, (2001) 3rd edn, Open University Press, Buckingham.

Ewald, P. W. (1993) The evolution of virulence, *Scientific American*, **268**, pp. 86–93.

Fiennes, R. N. T. W. (1978) *Zoonoses and the Origins and Ecology of Human Disease*, Academic Press, London.

Følling, A. (1934) Über Ausscheidung von Phenylbrenztraubensaüre in den Harn als Stoffwechselanomalie in Verbidung mit Imbezillität, *Hoppe-Seyler's Z. Physiol. Chem.*, **227**, pp. 169–76.

Gabriel, S. E., Brigman, K. N., Koller, B. H., Boucher, R. C. and Stutts, M. J. (1994) Cystic fibrosis heterozygote resistance to cholera toxin in the cystic fibrosis mouse model, *Science*, **266**, pp. 107–9.

Hamilton, W. D. and Zuk, M. (1982) Heritable true fitness and bright birds: a role for parasites, *Science*, **218**, pp. 384–7.

Health Technology Assessment (1997) *Neonatal Screening for inborn errors of metabolism: costs, yield and outcome*, **1**, number 7, Department of Health. Available from http://www.hta.nhsweb.nhs.uk/ [accessed March 2001].

Hebb, D. O. (1953) Heredity and environment in mammalian behaviour, *British Journal of Animal Behaviour*, **1**, pp. 43–7.

Herzog, V., Sies, H. and Miller, F. (1976) Exocytosis in secretory cells of rat lacrimal gland, *Journal of Cell Biology*, **70**, pp. 692–706.

Human Fertilisation and Embryology Authority (1994) *Donated Ovarian Tissue in Embryo Research and Assisted Conception*, Human Fertilisation and Embryology Authority, London.

Human Genetics Advisory Commission (1997) *Implications of genetic testing for Insurance*, Office of Science and Technology. Available from http://www.dti.gov.uk/hgac/papers/paperb1.htm [accessed March 2001].

Human Genetics Advisory Commission (1999) *Implications of Genetic Testing for Employment*, Office of Science and Technology. Available from http://www.dti.gov.uk/hgac/papers/paperg1.htm [accessed March 2001].

Jones, S. (1993) *The Language of the Genes*, HarperCollins, London (hardback) and (1994) Flamingo, London (paperback); extracts from Chapter 16 'The evolution of Utopia', reprinted in Davey, B., Gray, A. and Seale, C. (eds) *Health and Disease: A Reader*, (1995) 2nd edn and (2001) 3rd edn, Open University Press, Buckingham.

Jones, S., Martin R., Pilbeam, D. and Bunney, S. (eds) (1992) *The Cambridge Encyclopedia of Human Evolution*, Cambridge University Press, Cambridge.

Kirkwood, T. G. L. (1992) Biological origins of ageing, Chapter 2.1 in Evans, J. G. and Williams, T. F. (eds) *Oxford Textbook of Geriatric Medicine*, Oxford University Press, Oxford.

Lerner, I. M. and Libby, W. J. (1976) *Heredity, Evolution and Society*, 2nd edn, W. H. Freeman, San Francisco.

Lin, Y. J., Seroude, L. and Benzer, S. (1998) Extended life-span and stress resistance in the Drosophila mutant methuselah, *Science*, **282**, pp. 943–6.

Lindgren, G. (1976) Height, weight and menarche in Swedish urban school children in relation to socio-economic and regional factors, *Annals of Human Biology*, **3**, pp. 501–28.

Lyons, G. (1999) *Chemical Trespass: A Toxic legacy*, World Wildlife Fund, Washington DC, USA.

Lyons, G. (2000) *Bisphenol: A known Endocrine Disrupter*, World Wildlife Fund, Washington DC, USA. Available from http://www.worldwildlife.org/toxics/pubres/ [accessed March 2001].

Mackinnon, T. L. (2000) Overtraining effects on immunity and performance in athletes, *Immunology and Cell Biology*, **78**, pp. 502–9.

Maes, M., Song, C., Lin, A. H. *et al.* (1998) The effects of psychological stress on humans: increased production of pro-inflammatory cytokines and Th1-like response in stress-induced anxiety, *Cytokine*, **10**, pp. 313–18.

Marshall, G. D., Agarwal, S. K., Lloyd, C. *et al.* (1998) Cytokine dysregulation associated with exam stress in healthy medical students, *Brain, Behaviour and Immunity*, **12**, pp. 297–307.

Martin, R. D. (1992) Primate locomotion and posture, Chapter 2.8 in Jones, S., Martin, R., Pilbeam, D. and Bunney, S. (eds) *The Cambridge Encyclopedia of Human Evolution*, Cambridge University Press, Cambridge.

May, R. M. (1992) How many species inhabit the Earth?, *Scientific American*, **267**, pp. 42–8.

McGowan, R. (1999) Beyond the disorder: one parent's reflection on genetic counselling, *Journal of Medical Ethics*, **25**, pp. 195–9; reprinted in Davey, B., Gray, A. and Seale, C. (eds) *Health and Disease: A Reader*, (2001) 3rd edn, Open University Press, Buckingham.

Meltzer, D. J. (1992) How Columbus sickened the New World, *New Scientist*, **136**, pp. 38–41.

Migliaccio, E., Giorgio, M., Mele, S., Pelicci, G., Reboldi, P., Pandolfi, P. P., Lanfrancone, L. and Pelicci, P. G. (1999) The p66shc adaptor protein controls oxidative stress response and life span in mammals, *Nature*, **402**, pp. 309–13.

Modell, B. (1983) Screening for carriers of recessive disease, in Carter, C. O. (ed.) *Developments in Human Reproduction and their Eugenic, Ethical Implications*, Academic Press, London.

Modell, B., Kuliev, A. M. and Wagner, M. (1991) *Community Genetics Services in Europe*, WHO Regional Publications, European series no. 38, WHO Regional Office for Europe, Copenhagen.

Modell, B., Petrou, M., Layton, M., Varnavides, L., Slater, C., Ward, R. H., Rodeck, C., Nicolaides, K., Gibbons, S., Fitches, A. and Old, J. (1997) Audit of prenatal diagnosis for haemoglobin disorders in the United Kingdom: the first 20 years, *British Medical Journal*, **315**, pp. 779–84.

Modell, M., Wonke, B., Anionwu, E., Khan, M., Tai, S. S., Lloyd, M. and Modell, B. (1998) A multidisciplinary approach for improving services in primary care: randomised controlled trial of screening for haemoglobin disorders, *British Medical Journal*, **317**, pp. 788–91.

Müller-Hill, B. (1993) The shadow of genetic injustice, *Nature*, **362**, pp. 491–2; reprinted in Davey, B., Gray, A. and Seale, C. (eds) *Health and Disease: A Reader*, (1995) 2nd edn and (2001) 3rd edn, Open University Press, Buckingham.

National Audit Office (2000) *The Management and Control of Hospital acquired infection in Acute NHS Trusts in England*, NAO, London.

National Asthma Campaign (London) (1999) *National Asthma Audit 1999/2000*.

A summary can be seen at http://www.asthma.org.uk/newspr08.html [accessed March 2001].

Neel, J. V. (1962) Diabetes mellitus: a thrifty genotype rendered detrimental by 'progress'?, *American Journal of Human Genetics*, **14**, pp. 353–62.

Nieman, D. C. (2000) Exercise effects on systemic immunity, *Immunology and Cell Biology*, **78**, pp. 496–501.

Nuffield Council on Bioethics (1993) *Genetic Screening: Ethical Issues*, Nuffield Council on Bioethics, London.

O'Brien, P. M, Wheeler, T. and Barker, D. J. (1999) Fetal programming: influences on development and diseases in later life, *Proceedings of the 36th Royal College of Obstetricians and Gynaecologists Study Group*, RCOG, London.

Passmore, R. and Robson, J. S. (1980) *A Companion to Medical Studies, Volume 2, Pharmacology, Microbiology, General Pathology and Related Subjects*, 2nd edn, Blackwells Scientific Publications, Oxford.

Penrose, L. S. and Smith, G. F. (1966) *Down's Anomaly*, 1st edn, Churchill Livingstone, Edinburgh (2nd edn, 1976).

Perry, M. M. and Gilbert, A. B. (1979) Yolk transport in the ovarian follicle of the hen *(Gallus domesticus)*: lipoprotein-like particles at the periphery of the oocyte in the rapid growth phase, *Journal of Cell Science*, **39**, pp. 257–72.

Simoons, F. J. (1978) The geographic hypothesis and lactose malabsorption: a weighting of the evidence, *American Journal of Digestive Diseases*, **23**, pp. 963–80.

Stern, C. (1973) *Principles of Human Genetics*, 3rd edn, W. H. Freeman, San Francisco.

Strassburg, M. A. (1982) The global eradication of smallpox, *American Journal of Infection Control*, **19**, pp. 53–9; reprinted in Black, N. *et al.*, (eds) *Health and Disease: A Reader*, 1st edn, and in Davey, B., Gray, A. and Seale, C. (eds) *Health and Disease: A Reader*, (1995) 2nd edn and (2001) 3rd edn, Open University Press, Buckingham.

Strehler, B. L., Mark, D. D., Mildvan, A. S. and Gee, M. V. (1959) Rate and magnitude of age pigment accumulation in the human myocardium, *Journal of Gerontology*, **14**, pp. 430–9.

Strickberger, M. W. (1990) *Evolution*, Jones and Bartlett, Boston, Massachusetts.

Suzuki, D. T., Griffiths, A. J. F. and Lewontin, R. C. (1981) *An Introduction to Genetic Analysis*, 2nd edn, W. H. Freeman, San Francisco.

Tanner, J. M. (1992) Human growth and development, Chapter 2.13 in Jones, S., Martin, R., Pilbeam, D. and Bunney, S. (eds), *The Cambridge Encyclopedia of Human Evolution*, Cambridge University Press, Cambridge.

Thornton, R. (1987) *American Indian Holocaust and Survival: A Population History since 1492*, University of Oklahoma Press, Norman, Oklahoma and London.

UNESCO (1997) *Declaration on the Human Genome and Human Rights*, Article 6. Available from http://www.unesco.org/human_rights/hrbc.htm [accessed March 2001].

Vaupel, J. W., Carey, J. R., Christensen, K. *et al.* (1998) Biodemographic trajectories of longevity, *Science*, **280**, pp. 855–60; an edited extract appears in Davey, B., Gray, A. and Seale, C. (eds) *Health and Disease: A Reader*, (2001) 3rd edn, Open University Press, Buckingham.

Voltaire, F. M. A. de, (1759) *Candide*, translated by Lowell Bair (1959 edn), Bantam Books, New York.

Walker, D. W., McColl, G., Jenkins, N. L. *et al.* (2000) Evolution of lifespan in *C. elegans*, *Nature*, **405**, pp. 296–7.

Ward, E. (1997) Attitudes to Xenotransplantation, *Lancet*, **349**, p. 1 775.

Watson, J. D. (2000) *A Passion for DNA: Genes, Genomes and Society*, Cold Spring Harbour Laboratory Press/Oxford University Press, Oxford; the chapter appears in Davey, B., Gray, A. and Seale, C. (eds) *Health and Disease: A Reader*, (2001) 3rd edn, Open University Press, Buckingham.

Watson, J. D. and Crick, F. H. C. (1953) Molecular structure of nucleic acids: a structure for deoxyribose nucleic acid, *Nature*, **171**, 25 April, pp. 737–8.

Weiner, D. B. and Kennedy, R. C. (1999) Genetic vaccines, *Scientific American*, **281**, pp. 50–7.

Williamson, R. (1993) Universal community carrier screening for cystic fibrosis?, *Nature Genetics*, **3**, pp. 195–201.

World Health Organisation (1958) *Constitution of the World Health Organisation*, Annex 1, WHO, Geneva.

World Health Organisation (1999) *Infectious Diseases Report*, WHO, Geneva

World Health Organisation (2000a) *Tuberculosis*, WHO Fact Sheet No. 104, revised April 2000, WHO, Geneva. Available from http://www.who.int/inf-fs/en/fact104.html [accessed February 2001].

World Health Organisation (2000b) *The World Health Report 2000 — Health Systems: Improving Performance*, WHO, Geneva.

Wyllie, F. S., Jones, C. J., Skinner, J. W., Haughton, M. F., Wallis, C., Wynford-Thomas, D., Faragher, R. G. and Kipling, D. (2000) Telomerase prevents the accelerated cell ageing of Werner syndrome fibroblasts, *Nature Genetics*, **24**, pp. 16–17.

Yorke, J. A. and London, W. P. (1973) Recurrent outbreaks of measles, chickenpox and mumps: II, Systematic differences in contact rates and stochastic effects, *American Journal of Epidemiology*, **98**, pp. 469–82.

Further sources

General

The following books and articles are highly recommended to anyone who wishes to read very broadly about human evolutionary biology and the interaction with human culture; they are relevant to many of the chapters in *Human Biology and Health: An Evolutionary Approach*. They are followed by further reading of a more specialist nature, linked to specific chapters.

Boyden, S. (1987; reprinted 1992) *Western Civilization in Biological Perspective*, Clarendon Press, Oxford. An exploration of the interplay between biological and cultural processes in human affairs, from the early evolution of *Homo sapiens* to the present day.

Campbell, N. A. (ed.) (1998) *Biology*, 5th edn, Addison-Wesley Longman Publishing Co (paperback). Hardback 5th edn (1999) published by Benjamin Cummings Publishing Company Inc., California, includes a CD-ROM. A wonderfully illustrated and produced general textbook of biology, at an astonishingly low price for such a weighty hardback. Each main section (for example, on the cell, the gene, animal and plant form and function, and on evolutionary history) is written by leading biologists and takes an evolutionary perspective throughout.

Cohen, M. N. (1991) *Health and the Rise of Civilization*, Yale University Press, New Haven and London. A historian's view of human health through the ages, and of attempts to avoid, eradicate or cure disease.

Diamond, J. (1992) *The Rise and Fall of the Third Chimpanzee*, Vintage, London (paperback). A wide-ranging, popular vision of human evolution with an overview of history and speculation about the future of our species, written by a distinguished physiologist and ornithologist.

Haviland, W. (2000) *Human Evolution and Prehistory* (5th edn) Harcourt Publishers Ltd College Publishers, Fort Worth and London. This text offers a comprehensive and balanced presentation on the views of human evolution and prehistory. If focuses on selected aspects of physical anthropology and prehistoric archaeology as they related to the origin of culture and the development of human biological and cultural diversity.

Jones, S. (2000) *The Language of the Genes*, Flamingo, London. Based on the highly acclaimed BBC Reith Lectures, broadcast by Steve Jones in 1991, this is a revised edition of the book first published in 1993. It is a readable and fascinating book covering the scope of modern genetics from the fine details of individual genes to the broad sweep of human evolution and its interaction with human culture. It is readily accessible to non-biologists and contains a wealth of illuminating examples, anecdotes from history, references to literature and much else besides, written in the author's direct and amusing style which reveals his penetrating insight into human society as well as human biology.

Jones, S., Martin, R., Pilbeam, D. and Bunney, S. and Dawkins R. (eds) (1994) *The Cambridge Encyclopedia of Human Evolution*, Cambridge University Press, Cambridge. A wide-ranging introduction to the human species that places modern humans in an evolutionary perspective. This definitive text on human evolution, although enormous, is broken down into sections by theme, each subdivided into short and accessible chapters on specific topics contributed by experts in (among others) genetics, functional anatomy, palaeontology, anthropology, archaeology, medicine and agriculture.

McKeown, T. (1991) *The Origins of Human Disease*, Blackwell Publishers, Oxford. A physician's account of the many causes of disease in humans from primeval to modern society, and of habits and policies that reduce or perpetuate disease.

McMichael, A. J. (1995) *Planetary Overload: Global Environmental Change and the Health of the Human Species*, Cambridge University Press, Cambridge. A discussion of global environmental problems and their consequences for health within an ecological framework.

McNeill, W. H. (1976) *Plagues and Peoples*, Basil Blackwell Ltd, Oxford (paperback). A historian's account of the incidence of disease from prehistory to the beginning of the twentieth century, and its military and political consequences.

Meltzer, D. J. (1992) How Columbus sickened the New World, *New Scientist*, October, pp. 38–41. A readily obtainable article that discusses why early European settlers in the USA passed serious infectious diseases to Native Americans, and why this was a largely one-way process. Most central libraries have this journal in their reference section.

Chapter 2

Much of the information in Chapter 2 is derived from sources already listed in the above: Cohen (1991), Diamond (1992), Jones *et al.* (1994), McKeown (1991), and McNeill (1976), and from the sources listed below, which provide far more detail and assume much more background knowledge, than the Open University's *Health and Disease* course requires.

Clutton–Brock, J. (1999) *A Natural History of Domesticated Mammals*, Cambridge University Press, Cambridge. The 2nd edition of this popular, profusely illustrated account of the origin and modern biology of domesticated animals. This book describes the origins of domestication and its spread, both biologically and culturally, across the world.

Fiennes, R. N. T. W. (1978) *Zoonoses and the Origins and Ecology of Human Disease*, Academic Press, London. The definitive study of how and when diseases transfer between people and animals, based upon a lifetime's experience of veterinary medicine in zoo and wild animals.

Heiser, C. B. (1990) *Seeds to Civilization: The Story of Food*, Harvard University Press, Cambridge, Massachusetts. A botanist's popular account of the wild origins, domestication and modern cultivation of major food crops.

Lewin, R. (1998) *Human Evolution: An Illustrated Introduction*, 4th edn, Blackwell Science (USA). The biological mechanisms and palaeontological record of human evolution, as told by an anthropologist.

Chapter 3

Campbell (1998), already listed above, is an excellent general textbook of biology.

James D. Watson (1956) *The Double Helix*, Penguin Books, London. A perosnal account of the discovery of the structure of DNA written by one of the co-discoverers and this book is still an addictive read.

Jones, S. (2000) *Almost Like a Whale: the Origin of Species Updated,* Anchor Books, London. New edition of Steve Jones' work (first published in 1999) updating the theories of Darwin's 'The Origin of the Species'. It highlights the relationships of the living world using twentieth century science to breathe life into Darwin's nineteenth century theory.

Sayre, A. and Kevles, D. J. (Introduction) (2000) *Rosalind Franklin and DNA,* W. W. Norton, London. This recently re-issued book details the story of Rosalind Franklin, whose research into the structure of DNA played a crucial role in the breakthrough of Watson and Crick.

Chapter 4

The most relevant texts are listed in the general section above: Diamond (1992), Jones (2000), and Jones *et al.* (1994). In addition, we recommend:

Mueller, R., Young, I. and Emery, A. (1998) *Emery's Elements of Medical Genetics,* Churchill Livingstone, London. This is an excellent textbook of medical genetics covering both the scientific basis and clinical practice of medical genetics.

Chapter 5

See Meltzer (1992), listed in the general section above, together with the following:

Brown, P. (1992) The return of the big killer, *New Scientist,* October, pp. 30–7. A readily obtainable article that discusses the reasons why tuberculosis is once again becoming a major problem in developed countries, such as the United States, from which it was previously largely eradicated. Most central libraries have this leading journal in their reference section.

Ewald, P. W. (1993) The evolution of virulence, *Scientific American,* April, pp. 56–62. A readily obtainable article that reviews the evidence that pathogenic organisms may become either more or less virulent in response to selection pressures imposed by their environment. Most central libraries have this leading journal in their reference section.

Hamilton, W. D. and Zuk, M. (1982) Heritable true fitness and bright birds: a role for parasites, *Science,* **218,** pp. 384–7. A very significant paper in evolutionary theory, which sets out the theoretical argument that bright plumage in male birds indicates to females that they carry low infestations of parasites. Most central libraries have this leading journal in their reference section.

Hudson, P. J., Dobson, A. P. and Newborn, D. (1992) Do parasites make prey vulnerable to predation? Red grouse and parasites, *Journal of Animal Ecology,* **61,** pp. 681–92. A paper reporting a field study of how parasites affect the behaviour of red grouse in northern England and, in consequence, influence the risk of the grouse being taken by predators; the authors raise general issues about the relationship of parasites to predation.

Lively, C. M. (1987) Evidence from a New Zealand snail for the maintenance of sex by parasitism, *Nature,* **328,** pp. 519–21. The hypothesis that sexual reproduction is an adaptation against the harmful effects of parasites is clearly difficult to investigate, but supportive evidence is reported in this study of New Zealand snails, which use sexual reproduction where parasites are abundant and asexual reproduction where parasites are rare. Most central libraries have this leading journal in their reference section.

Chapter 6

Cohen, S. and Williamson, G. M. (1991) Stress and infectious disease in humans, *Psychological Bulletin,* **109,** pp. 5–24. A comprehensive review of experiments to determine whether or not stress leads to an increase in the incidence of infection. The authors explain the difficulties of investigating this question scientifically, and make clear the all-important distinction between, on the one hand, demonstrating (as many have done) that the immune system changes under stress and, on the other hand, showing that this has any consequences for human health.

Roitt, I., Brostoff, J. and Male, D. K. (eds) (2001) *Immunology* (6th edn) Harcourt Publishers Ltd., London. This lavishly illustrated paperback is aimed at biology undergraduates, nurses, medical students and anyone who requires a general introduction to the theory and practice of immunology. The same authors have also produced a CD-ROM — *Immunology Interactive*, version 2.1, by Male, D. K., Gray, A., Brostoff, J. and Roitt, I. (1998) Harcourt Publishers Ltd., London.

Roitt, I. (2001) *Essential Immunology*, 10th edn, Blackwell Science, Oxford. One of the most popular and influential textbooks of basic immunology. The subject is taught to first degree (and in places to postgraduate) level and yet will be accessible to anyone with a basic grounding in biology; its accessibility rests on a clearly and often amusingly written text, supported by excellent diagrams and photographs. The author regularly updates this highly recommended textbook, so check if a more recent edition has been published.

Weiner, D. B. and Kennedy, R. C. (1999) Genetic vaccines, *Scientific American,* **281**, pp. 50–7.

Chapter 7

Vander, A. J., Sherman, J. H. and Luciano, D. S. (2000) *Human Physiology: the Mechanisms of Body Function*, 8th edn, William C. Brown, Publications. One of the best modern textbooks of human physiology, written primarily for nurses and other medical workers.

Domingo, J. L. (2000) Health risks of GM foods: many opinions but few data, *Science* **288**, pp. 1 748–9.

Chapter 8

Dice, J. F. (1993) Cellular and molecular mechanisms of ageing, *Physiological Reviews*, **73**(1), pp. 149–59. A review article that gives more detail of biological mechanisms than was possible in Chapter 8. It will be of particular interest to those with some prior knowledge of biology.

Kirkwood, T. (2000) *Time of Our Lives*, Phoenix House, London. An excellently written and easily readable book by a leader in the ageing field and speaker in the BBC 2001 Reith Lectures. The book examines the subject of why we age from a wide variety of perspectives.

Martin, G. M. (1992) Biological mechanisms of ageing, Chapter 2.2 in Evans, J. G. and Williams, T. G. (eds) *Oxford Textbook of Geriatric Medicine*, Oxford University Press, Oxford. This review will be most relevant to anyone working in geriatric medicine, with a reasonable knowledge of biochemistry.

Olshansky, S. J., Carnes, B. A. and Cassel, C. K. (1993) The ageing of the human species, *Scientific American*, April, pp. 18–24. This is a clear account of demographic trends and evolutionary theories of ageing. This readily obtainable article also considers the social and ethical implications of an ageing human population.

Young, S. (1993) Against ageing, in 'Mind and Body', *New Scientist* supplement, 17 April, pp. 10–12. This article is written for non-biologists and is enjoyable and informative; most central libraries stock this journal.

Chapter 9

Certain of the texts already listed in the general section are also relevant here: Jones (2000), Jones *et al.* (1994). Also Mueller *et al.* (1998) in the list for Chapter 4 is of interest.

Department of Health Report on Human Cloning (1998) This report is the government response to the report by the Human Genetics Advisory Commission and the Human Fertilisation and Embryology Authority on cloning issues in reproduction, science and medicine Department of Health. Available from http://www.doh.gov.uk/cloning.htm [accessed March 2001].

Harper, P. S. (1998) *Practical Genetic Counselling*, 5th edn, Arnold, London. The author outlines the main steps in the process of genetic counselling and, though fairly technical, it is one of the few definitive texts in this area.

Nuffield Council on Bioethics (1993) *Genetic Screening: Ethical Issues*, Nuffield Council on Bioethics, London. A summary of the conclusions of this report can be seen at http://www.nuffieldfoundation.org/bioethics/publication/geneticscreening/rep0000000062.html [accessed April 2001].

Trent, R. (1997) *Molecular Medicine*, Churchill Livingstone, London. An easily understandable book covering all the applications of modern genetics and DNA techniques in diagnosis and therapy.

Wilmut, I. (1998) Cloning for medicine, *Scientific American*, **279**, pp. 58–63. A personal account of the cloning of Dolly and an exploration of some of the possible applications.

Chapter 10

We recommend McMichael (1995), listed in the general section, together with the following:

McLachlan, J. and Arnold, F. (1996) Environmental Estrogens, *American Scientist*, September–October 1996. Available from http://www.sigmaxi.org/amsci/articles/96articles/mclachla%2D1.html [accessed March 2001]. A comprehensive guide to chemicals which are believed to be 'feminisers' in the environment and their effects on the ecosystem.

Ott, W. R. and Roberts, J. W. (1998) Everyday exposure to toxic pollutants, *Scientific American*, **278**, pp. 86–91. A clear and easily accessible review of exposures to chemicals in the environment.

Power, H., Elsom, D. M. and Longhurst, J. W. S. (eds) (2000) *Air Quality Management*, WIT Press, Southampton. This book provides details of on-going research projects in the field of air quality management.

Rodericks, J. V. (1993) *Calculated Risks*, Cambridge University Press, Cambridge. An exploration of the scientific basis of public concerns about environmental pollution and chemicals.

Timbrell, J. A. (1999) *Principles of Biochemical Toxicology*, 3rd edn, Taylor & Francis, London. A comprehensive textbook on all aspects of toxicology, clearly laid out and designed for self-study.

Chapter 11

See Boyden (1987, reprinted 1992), listed in the general section.

Rose, H. and Rose, S. (2000) *Alas Poor Darwin*, Jonathan Cape, London. In this collection of essays, various evolutionary biologists challenge the claims of evolutionary psychology.

Internet database (ROUTES)

A large amount of valuable information is available via the Internet. To help OU students and other readers of books in the *Health and Disease* series to access good quality sites without having to search for hours, the OU has developed a collection of Internet resources on a searchable database called ROUTES. All websites included in the database are selected by academic staff or subject-specialist librarians. The content of each website is evaluated to ensure that it is accurate, well presented and regularly updated. A description is included for each of the resources.

The URL for ROUTES is: http://routes.open.ac.uk/

Entering the OU course code U205 in the search box will retrieve all the resources that have been recommended for *Health and Disease*. Alternatively if you want to search for any resources on a particular subject, type in the words which best describe the subject you are interested in.

Answers to questions

Chapter 2

1 (a) Most non-human primates, including nearly all monkeys, are active by day and live in tall trees where they locate their food. This is often coloured fruit or flowers which are visible from some distance. They jump across gaps between trees, where scent trails would be useless but good vision is essential. Many species also live in social groups and communicate with each other by means of visual signals such as facial expressions and gestures, as well as by sounds.

   (b) The typical primate diet consists of soft, easily digested, fresh food, such as fruit, flowers, leaves and small animals which does not require massive teeth.

   (c) Primates move by climbing and leaping, using their opposable fingers and toes to grasp branches, while they swing from their arms or tail. Fingernails and toenails are not used in climbing, but may facilitate delicate handling of small objects.

2 The upper part of the human pelvis became shorter and wider while the lower part became narrower than the pelvis of non-human primates (see Figure 2.1). The spinal column became more curved, particularly at its lower end, and the sacrum broader. The ilium curved forwards around the contents of the abdomen, supporting larger muscles that stabilise the hip and thigh (Figure 2.1c). These changes permitted humans to take longer, more powerful strides than is possible in apes.

However, the more compact human pelvis is less efficient for birth, particularly that of babies with enlarged heads; limited observational evidence suggests that birth complications are much more common in humans than in apes (Section 2.3.2). The aperture of the human pelvis in females does not reach full size until several years after fertile eggs are first produced, so difficulties in giving birth are commonest among very young mothers.

There are major sex differences in the shape of the human pelvis: that of females is wider relative to the size of the body as a whole, and more rounded, forming a pelvic canal that is more satisfactory for birth than the narrower pelvis of males; as a consequence, most women cannot run as fast as most men of a similar age.

3 (a) Living in caves and shelters over many generations permitted the evolution of a species of flea and a species of louse that breed only in association with humans; these ectoparasites trouble us with their irritating bites and lice can transmit the bacteria that cause typhus. The occupation of caves and shelters may have brought humans into contact with the fleas of wild mammals such as rats, badgers and bats, which 'shared' the same shelters and whose fleas can transmit life-threatening or disabling infectious diseases, including plague and rabies (Section 2.6.3). The later use of fire to protect and heat living areas greatly increased the incidence of burns and damage from the inhalation of smoke.

   (b) Humans who settle permanently in one place, in the absence of modern public health measures, remain in close association with their own debris and excrement, thereby promoting the spread of many infectious diseases and parasites. Permanent settlements enabled the development of agriculture and animal husbandry, but the latter practice brought people into close, continual contact with domestic livestock, from which they acquired parasites, many of which were pathogenic. Agricultural crops and domestic livestock form a less diverse diet than wild food, which often led to poorer nutrition. Living permanently in one place also fostered the concept of land ownership, which promoted internecine warfare and diminished the status of women, both of which increased human morbidity and mortality (Section 2.6.6).

4   (a) Blood-sucking insects act as diseases vectors by transmitting pathogenic micro-organisms (e.g. those that cause sleeping sickness, malaria, yellow fever) and multicellular parasites (e.g. the nematodes that cause river blindness and elephantiasis), from other species of mammal to humans, and between infected and uninfected people. Examples of such insect vectors include ectoparasites such as lice and fleas, and mosquitoes (e.g. *Anopheles*) and blackflies (*Simulium*) which suck the blood of many different kinds of mammals as well as humans.

     (b) Several species of freshwater snails and shrimp-like animals are essential secondary hosts for *Schistosoma* and guinea worm; most mosquitoes, including those that carry the pathogens that cause malaria and yellow fever, breed in fresh water. When fish became an important food many thousands of years ago, people would spend more time standing or swimming in fresh water (and defaecating in or near it) than would have been necessary when they hunted land mammals. More recently, artificial irrigation systems created additional habitats for the snails that serve as the secondary host for *Schistosoma*.

     (c) People can contract *Toxocara*, a nematode worm that is normally a parasite of dogs, cats and their rodent prey; the larvae can cause abdominal pain and (rarely) blindness. Measles virus may have arisen from canine distemper virus, and dogs have long been a major route of infection for the virus that causes rabies.

Chapter 3

1   The three mechanisms are: *passive diffusion*, by which small molecules such as oxygen, carbon dioxide and water pass freely through a membrane without expenditure of energy, in response to a concentration gradient across the membrane; *active transport*, in which transport proteins in the membrane bind to molecules outside the cell by lock-and-key interactions, and then carry them through the membrane, using up energy in the process; and the processes of *endocytosis* and *exocytosis*, by which large molecules are carried through the membrane, packaged in bags of membrane called vesicles (see Section 3.3.4 and Figures 3.8 and 3.9). Lock-and-key mechanisms (Section 3.3.5 and Figure 3.10) are involved in the processes of *endocytosis* and *exocytosis*.

2   The bases (A, T, C or G) in adjacent nucleotides along a length of DNA are arranged in a series of three nucleotides termed codons, such as CAG or TTA. A 'meaningful' sequence of these codons is one way of describing a gene. Each triplet in a gene uniquely specifies a particular amino acid. The complete message, encoded in the series of many hundreds of codons in the gene, is transcribed into an messenger RNA molecule and the code is translated. The

order of the codons corresponds to the order of amino acids, which are joined together in a unique sequence to give a unique protein molecule (see Section 3.6.2 and Figures 3.15 and 3.16).

3   Both cells have virtually identical DNA, because they were both derived by cell division from a single fertilised egg, so they have exactly the same genes. This set of genes forms the unique genotype of the individual whose body contains these cells. However, there are differences in which of these genes are 'switched on' and which are 'switched off' in the two cells. For example, the gene that carries the instructions for making the protein insulin (the gene product) is active in the cell from the pancreas, but switched off in the skin cell. Conversely, the gene that encodes the structure of the pigment protein is active in the skin cell, but inactive in the pancreatic cell. The differences between which genes are on and off is the mechanism by which the wide variety of structures and cell functions is achieved within the human body (see Section 3.6.1).

4   Within individual cells, homeostasis is maintained primarily by the cell membrane, which selectively takes in or expels substances when their levels fall below or rise above some optimum level (see Sections 3.8.2, 3.9.4 and Figure 3.18). For example, cells must maintain a certain optimum level of glucose which provides enough energy to fuel chemical reactions, but not so much that it damages the cell. Similarly, the body must maintain a constant temperature for the optimal performance of cellular functions. In addition to the sum total of these cellular homeostatic processes being carried out in all the billions of cells in the body, large multicellular animals also regulate their internal environment by adjusting internal bodily mechanisms, under the control of the nervous system (Figure 3.22) and hormonal system, which alter the animal's temperature, respiration, digestion, immune defences, blood supply (Figure 3.21), etc., within certain limits. Homeostasis can also be assisted by actions, such as moving to another location; in the case of humans, some actions may be consciously willed, e.g. the blood sugar homeostasis can be affected by eating a sugar-rich snack or fasting or even administering an insulin injection.

5   Figure 3.23 gives the correct sketch. As you can see, if the body temperature rises, a feedback system alerts the body sensors which in turn lead to a response mechanism (such as sweating) which leads to body cooling. The reverse occurs for the cold body, the response being to warm up the body (such as shivering, putting on more clothes).

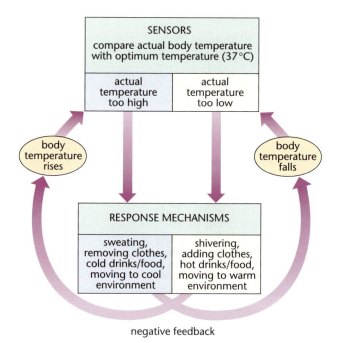

negative feedback

Figure 3.23 *Schematic diagram of a negative feedback circuit to maintain human body temperature by homeostasis.*

best explained as being due to chance or random processes preserving the disease allele in an 'isolated' population. A description of these types of occurrences can be found in Section 4.11.3.

(b) The evidence suggests that the allele involved in thalassaemia is maintained by natural selection in certain regions of the world, particularly those in which malaria is, or was, rife. Thalassaemia seems to work in a similar way to sickle-cell disease, conferring an advantage on carriers (who have only one copy of the disease allele and are not anaemic), in that it gives some resistance to malaria. For OU students, this is explained further in the TV programme 'Bloodlines: A family legacy'. The process of natural selection preserves the thalassaemia gene in populations exposed to malaria because carriers have a reproductive advantage over non-carriers. This is similar to another case you have studied, sickle-cell disease, in Section 4.11.4.

(c) The occurrence of neurofibromatosis, a dominant disorder, in families with no previous history, suggests that affected individuals have inherited a new mutation. (In fact the mutation rate for this disease is as high as 1 per 1 000 gametes, but the reason for this is unknown.)

Chapter 5

1   Parasites are described in detail in Section 5.3. A microparasite is a very small organism, typically visible only with the aid of powerful microscopes. Examples include all viruses, bacteria, protoctists and some fungi. Most microparasites are endoparasitic, living within the bodies, often within the cells, of their hosts. The microparasite derives some benefit from this relationship, at a cost to the host. This may simply be by diverting small amounts of food from the host, but some microparasites are *pathogenic*, that is, they cause disease.

A vector is an organism that carries a pathogen from one host individual to another. For example, mosquitoes are the vector of malaria.

Virulence is a measure of how severely a pathogen affects its host. It is expressed as the percentage of infected host individuals that die from an infection.

2   You might have thought of the following from this chapter or from Chapter 2.
    1   Cholera, TB, measles virus.
    2   Thrush (*Candida*), hepatitis, *Chlamydia*, gonorrhoea and syphilis.
    3   Tetanus bacteria in the soil.
    4   Malaria (mosquito), plague (rat fleas), yellow fever (mosquito), *Trypanosoma* (tsetse flies).

3   Coevolution refers to intimate relationships between species, such as pathogens and hosts, over extremely long periods of time, in which an adaptation in one species leads to an appropriate adaptation in the other (Section 5.6). For example, the evolution of increased virulence in a pathogen leads to the evolution of greater resistance to that pathogen in the host. An example is that of myxomatosis in rabbits.

4   Three important adaptations which are defences against pathogens are:
    (i)   Possession of an effective and flexible immune system, which can protect the host from significant harm, including reduction of reproductive success, and counter any new strains that emerge as a result of mutation within a species of pathogen.

(ii) The evolution in a host species of widespread resistance to those pathogenic organisms that are commonly found in that environment. Resistance is determined by genes that enable the host's immune system to make an effective and flexible response to those pathogens.

(iii) Sexual reproduction may have evolved, at least in part, as an adaptation against pathogens, because it increases genetic diversity among a host's offspring and thus reduces the susceptibility of those offspring to pathogens that infected the parent.

5   Four important factors in destabilising host–pathogen relationships are:

(i)   Mutation, which may give rise to more-virulent or less-virulent varieties of pathogen and to more-resistant or less-resistant hosts.

(ii) Changes in the proportion of susceptibles and immunes in a host population: new susceptibles are added to the population, by birth and immigration, and susceptibles and immunes are removed through death (from any cause) and emigration. Immunes increase sharply after an epidemic from which most infected people recover and vaccination can dramatically increase the proportion of immunes in a very short time.

(iii) Pathogens that have been associated with one particular host species may start to infect a new species (zoonotic diseases); typically, the pathogen is much more virulent in the new host species, which has not yet been able to evolve greater resistance.

(iv) Cultural factors in the history of a host population, which affect its long-term exposure to pathogens, can influence the stability of host–pathogen relationships. For example, the history of exposure to zoonotic diseases derived from domesticated animals was quite different for people in Europe up to the end of the fourteenth century, compared with Native Americans.

6   Micro-organisms such as bacteria and plankton make up the largest proportion of the total biomass of life on Earth. They are 'producers' (along with plants), at the base of all food webs. Phytoplankton are also major contributors to atmospheric oxygen, required for respiration by most other organisms (Section 5.9).

Chapter 6

1   The evolution of human biology and human culture are continuously interacting. The enormous repertoire of non-self epitopes that the human immune system can recognise has been selected for as a consequence of, and/or has facilitated the evolution of: the longevity of humans and the unusually prolonged juvenile phase before reproduction takes place; the wide range of habitats that humans have colonised; the wide range of foodstuffs that humans can safely eat; the communal living habits of most human populations; and the close proximity of humans with many domesticated species.

2   Each time a person is infected with a particular rhinovirus, a primary *adaptive* immune response results which leaves the person less susceptible to that virus on subsequent encounters. Young children have not developed immunity to any of these viruses from previous encounters, so they are susceptible to all of them and suffer repeated colds, each time with a different rhinovirus. As time passes, fewer and fewer rhinoviruses remain which have not been encountered before and by old age a person may have developed immunity to all but the rarest rhinoviruses as a result of previous encounters.

3   Three aspects of the biology of HIV contribute to its resistance to destruction by the immune system of the host:

(i)   Like all viruses, it replicates inside the host's own cells, where it derives some protection from the immune system's essential self-tolerance.

(ii)   The genes that code for epitopes on the surface of the virus particle are highly liable to mutate, thereby changing the shape of the epitopes; this 'antigenic drift' prevents an effective *secondary* immune response from developing.

(iii)   Most important of all, the cells that HIV colonises and destroys are the helper T cells, which are essential for the activation and effectiveness of all the other kinds of white cell involved in both innate and adaptive immunity.

4   Having the complete DNA sequence of HIV allows the identification of every gene within the virus and hence the order of each amino acid within its proteins. This knowledge can be harnessed to help create vaccines through genetic engineering by producing HIV proteins in bacteria which can be used to illicit a protective immune response in humans. Having the complete genome sequence also allows the potential development of DNA vaccines which have the advantage that they stimulate both antibodies and cytotoxic T cell production and can be made to target many epitopes in a single injection (Section 6.9).

Chapter 7

1   These are described in Sections 7.2 and 7.5.3.

(a)   The stomach muscles contribute to digestion by churning the food, breaking it into fragments and mixing it with acid and a few enzymes secreted by cells in the lining of the stomach. A few molecules (e.g. alcohol) dissolve in the membranes of the cells lining the stomach, but no active absorption takes place there. Sensors in the stomach monitor its contents and thereby regulate the secretion of hormones and neural signals that activate and coordinate the rest of the gut, so it has an indirect role in the digestion and absorption of nutrients into the bloodstream further down the gut.

(b)   The pancreas secretes several different digestive enzymes into the duodenum (first portion of the small intestine). Other cells in this gland are sensitive to the concentration of glucose and other fuels in the blood and synthesise and secrete the hormones insulin and glucagon; these hormones stimulate a variety of metabolic changes in the liver, muscles and adipose tissue, which regulate the concentration of fuels in the blood. The pancreas is not involved in the absorption of nutrients.

(c)   The liver secretes bile into the duodenum, which breaks down fats and oils into small droplets, exposing a greater surface area to the action of digestive enzymes. The blood supply from the gut passes directly to the liver, which removes from the bloodstream excess nutrients absorbed from the gut (e.g. glucose, amino acids and fats) and stores them until required; it also takes up a variety of non-nutritive molecules such as flavouring substances and toxins, some of which are broken down and made harmless.

(d)   Cells in the lining of the small intestine secrete many different digestive enzymes. The small intestine is the major absorption site in the gut: its lining contains transporters for glucose (and other carbohydrates) and amino acids, and fats pass freely across the lining into the bloodstream and lymphatic system. Muscles in its walls produce peristaltic movements that mix up the food and move it along the intestine.

(e) In humans, symbiotic bacteria are normally present only in and near the large intestine, where they digest many of the materials, particularly carbohydrates, that the human digestive processes did not break down. They also facilitate the uptake of vitamins and may themselves be taken up by endocytosis into cells lining the large intestine, where they are digested.

2   Food selection and appetite are determined by many complex mechanisms including the smell and taste of food and sensations arising from the stomach (Section 7.5). Vomiting and diarrhoea prevent the absorption of toxins or parasites by expelling potentially harmful food before digestion is complete, or by accelerating its passage through the small and large intestines. Anorexia (loss of appetite) reduces food intake and so conserves energy normally expended in digestion and absorption of nutrients from the gut, and conserves the large quantities of protein, salts and water in digestive secretions. The body switches from using nutrients absorbed from the gut to using reserves of fuel and protein.

3   (a) Blood glucose is increased by eating a meal rich in glucose or digestible carbohydrate, or by a rise in the level of the hormone glucagon in the bloodstream together with a fall in the level of insulin, which together cause stored fuels (principally glycogen) to be converted into glucose and released into the bloodstream.

     (b) Blood glucose falls following strenuous exercise (which breaks down glucose at a high rate to yield energy), and in starvation, or if there is a rise in insulin levels, which promotes its uptake by muscles and the liver for conversion into stored fuels.

     The balance between these two processes is shown in Figure 7.3 and discussed in Section 7.6.

4   (a) All suckling mammals can digest lactose, the major carbohydrate of milk, but most human populations and all other mammals lose this ability after weaning, when fresh milk disappears from or becomes a minor component of the diet. Retention after weaning of the capacity to secrete lactase, the enzyme that digests lactose, evolved among humans for whom milk obtained from domesticated animals was (and still is) a major food. Dairy farmers, among whom the ability to absorb lactose was rare or absent usually convert milk into cheese or yoghurt, which renders it digestible.

     (b) Skin de-pigmentation probably evolved in people who migrated to cooler, cloudier regions where protection from strong sunlight was less necessary than for ancestor populations living closer to the Equator. Essential precursors of vitamin D are synthesised in the skin during exposure to UV-B radiation. Less pigment in the skin reduces the shading of the molecules involved in this mechanism, making it more efficient at producing vitamin D at low intensities of UV-B radiation. Wearing clothes would further promote natural selection favouring individuals who could maintain efficient synthesis of vitamin D in areas of skin that remain exposed.

     This is discussed in Section 7.8.

5   The potential benefits include the potential for 'golden rice' to be used as a dietary source of beta-carotene and so help reduce vitamin A deficiency, a major cause of blindness (see *World Health and Disease*, Section 11.5). The risks include the possibility of potentially harmful chemicals which might be generated in the rice and which are not tested for as the food is considered

'substantially equivalent' to non-GM rice. An additional risk is the possible spread of the inserted daffodil gene to other plants in the environment by pollen dispersal, with unknown ecological consequences (see Section 7.9.1).

Chapter 8

1   This argument is not based on the theory of natural selection, which can only operate on individuals. It assumes (incorrectly) that since prevention of overcrowding will benefit the *species*, this will be favoured by natural selection. However, there is no advantage to the individual in ageing and dying, so natural selection cannot favour this process. This is outlined in Section 8.2. (You may be interested to know that data for organisms in natural communities suggest that mortality, through predation and disease, is typically so high that overcrowding is a problem only for a few species at certain times, and so cannot provide a general explanation for ageing.)

2   Joints become stiffer and movement more restricted, the lens of the eye becomes less flexible and focusing is more difficult, skin becomes wrinkled (which may be depressing in a youth-oriented culture), and arteries can become hardened, which leads to a rise in blood pressure and an increased risk of stroke or coronary heart disease. All these changes are due in part to the loss of elasticity in collagen as the cells that produce it age and the fact that the rate of breakdown of 'old' rigid collagen and the synthesis of new flexible collagen slows with age.

3   Genetic evidence from fruit-flies (*Methuselah*) and mice (*p66rhc*) suggests that the presence of free radicals in cells is a factor in ageing; damage is caused by the oxidation of various molecules within the cell eventually leading to cell death. Chromosomal damage through the shortening of telomeres with age might also play a role, as the loss of, or damage to, genes would be detrimental to the cell and result in its death. DNA damage, if not repaired, can lead to a cell undergoing programmed cell death or apoptosis.

4   As outlined in Section 8.6, in order to progress from a normal cell to a cancerous one, three things must occur: (a) positive growth signals activating the cell must increase through the mutation of oncogenes, (b) negative growth controls imposed upon it by the proteins which are synthesised from tumour suppressor genes must decrease, and (c) the process of programmed cell death or apoptosis must be prevented from occurring. This is a multistage process where the changes in cell behaviour occur sequentially (as shown in Figure 8.6) and, at each stage, cells with the new mutations proliferate faster than the earlier cell mass in a process similar to natural selection. Inheritance of a faulty gene in the process shown in Figure 8.6 would increase the risk of that person developing a cancer in their lifetime and may result in cancer at an earlier time of life. This is due to the fact that cells would only have to undergo two mutations in total to become cancerous (that is they would go straight from green to orange). This occurs in several forms of inherited human cancers.

Chapter 9

1   An outline of the properties of fetal cells and their uses for cell therapy can be found in Section 9.2.

   (a) All research on fetal tissue could be claimed to 'increase knowledge of human development' or have the potential to 'improve the human condition', so nothing is ruled out as unethical by this framework. Neither does it suggest how the unique nature of fetal tissue would be 'acknowledged'. However, the 'review panels' mentioned are intended to assess the potential value and ethical implications of research using fetal tissue and bring consistency to decisions about what is sanctioned and what is banned.

(b) The major attraction of fetal implants from the biological viewpoint is that relatively few fetal stem cells can multiply in the implant recipient to replace a missing cell population. These cells are totipotent, and are capable of forming many different cell types without being attacked by the recipient's immune system.

2   Dolly was created from a somatic cell, as described in Section 9.3.2. It had always been thought that these cells had undergone so many changes (such as DNA mutations), which are associated with differentiation into adult cells, that they would not be capable of generating a complete new animal. Reproductive cloning could be used with human cells as early human fetal cells are totipotent and many of the techniques for handling human embryos are already in place in IVF clinics. Any somatic cell could (in theory) be used as a source of the genetic material.

3   The man's disease is probably due to a new mutation, since neither of his parents were affected. The inheritance of Huntington's disease is discussed in Section 9.4.2 and the pattern of inheritance is shown in Figure 9.5. Further details of the genetic inheritance pattern for the disease and the mutation process can be found in Sections 4.7.3 and 4.10. The man is mistaken about not passing the Huntington's gene to his children; there is a one in two risk of passing on the new mutation.

4   The following important factors should be considered:

(i)   Is the disease treatable? If so, population screening of newborn babies could be undertaken, as in the case of PKU. If not, prenatal diagnosis combined with selective abortion might be considered, but this has ethical implications (see point (v) below).

(ii) Could the at-risk communities be educated effectively about the risks of carrying the gene and the benefits of screening? Are the communities in favour of a programme of population screening, or are there religious, cultural or other objections?

(iii) How reliable is the screening test? What would be the frequency of false negatives, i.e. individuals who were incorrectly reassured that they or their unborn child did not carry the gene? (False positives are not generated by screening tests that directly detect the presence of a faulty allele in the DNA.)

(iv) Would genetic counselling be available, so that an individual or couple could learn about and discuss the options available in a supportive and impartial situation?

(v)   What are the ethical consequences of such a screening test being available? For example, would screening be optional or enforced? If prenatal screening detected an affected fetus, would the parents be pressured to accept an abortion? Would the results of the test be kept confidential, and would employers, insurers or other family members try to obtain the information?

5   The central aim of gene therapy is to insert normal alleles of the affected gene into the appropriate tissues of an individual with a genetic disease and thus permanently correct the disorder (as discussed for cystic fibrosis). Practical problems include delivering the DNA to the appropriate cells within the body, ensuring the gene is 'active', and is producing a protein product which is at the appropriate concentration, and ensuring that a rejection response from the recipient's own immune system is avoided (Section 9.8). A consequence of somatic gene therapy might be that the frequencies of defective alleles may increase in the population because the normal gene inserted by gene therapy does not enter the germline and the treated person lives to reproduce and pass the defective allele on to succeeding generations. In germline therapy, any inserted DNA would be inherited in subsequent generations.

Chapter 10

1   Cell division always involves the risk of mutations caused by errors in assembling new strands of DNA alongside the template of the original strands (Section 4.10). Although most such mutations are detected and repaired by special enzymes, some persist and may damage either the cell or, indirectly, the whole organism; for example, a mutation may activate oncogenes and lead to the normal cell transforming into a cancerous one (Section 8.6).

2   The mechanisms involved in an acute inflammatory response to a respiratory-tract infection and an acute hypersensitivity reaction to an inhaled allergen such as pollen are exactly the same: antibodies produced in response to the infection or the allergen bind to mast cells in the mucus membranes of the respiratory tract and trigger the release of irritant chemicals, including histamine. The difference is that the inflammatory response is an appropriate, short-term defensive reaction against a pathogen, whereas the hypersensitivity reaction is an inappropriate, prolonged and damaging response to harmless material such as pollen.

3   (a) The drug thalidomide was not toxic to the pregnant women who were prescribed it to relieve morning sickness, but it was highly *teratogenic* to the fetuses, particularly in the first few months of pregnancy. In this example, the young fetuses are a *sensitive group*.

     (b) The exposure and the fetal malformation occurred quite close together in time (although not close enough to be considered an example of acute toxicity; the malformation was usually only discovered several months after the drug had been taken). Limb malformations of the type seen in the babies of women who had taken thalidomide are extremely rare in the absence of exposure to the drug, and (you may recall from news reports at the time) a very high proportion of exposures resulted in malformations. Note that teratogenicity is a special case of chronic toxicity, because the toxic agent has its effect only during a short sensitive period during fetal development.

     (c) The risk to the fetuses of experimental animals may have been much less than it was to human fetuses for two reasons:

          (i) Humans and other mammals may differ in their ability to resist or repair damage from certain chemicals because their different evolutionary history has resulted in adaptation to chemicals to which they have been persistently exposed in their natural environment; for example, the drug did not affect rats, so perhaps they have already adapted to a chemical that resembles thalidomide, whereas humans have no prior exposure to it.

(ii) The experimental animals may have been affected if they had been given a different dose of the drug, or were given it at a different stage of pregnancy, or via another route. (You may be interested to know that the reasons why different species differ in their response to thalidomide during fetal development is still an active area of research; for example, they could differ in whether or to what extent the drug crosses the placenta from the mother to the baby, whether it is broken down in the liver, the speed at which it is excreted, and its effects on cell metabolism.)

4   The chemical industrial environment might lead to an increased level of UV radiation through effects upon the Earth's atmosphere, particularly to ozone (Section 10.5). Industrial gases such as CFCs and combustion products such as nitrogen oxides can react with ozone in the upper atmosphere and destroy the gas. Ozone acts to absorb UV radiation and as its levels fall the amount of UV reaching the Earth increases. UV radiation can directly affect both the ecosystem and human health. Phytoplankton (which are at the base of many food webs) are sensitive to UV radiation and a reduction in their numbers impacts both upon the organisms which are within the same food web but also upon the level of oxygen they release into the Earth's atmosphere. UV radiation is also a cause of DNA mutations and exposure can lead to the formation of cancers in humans.

Chapter 11

1   The thrifty genotype is discussed in Section 11.2.

(a) A high degree of genetic diversity in a species should, in theory, enable it to adapt more rapidly and more effectively to sudden environmental change. If the future food supply of human populations becomes unpredictable, and periods of plenty are interspersed with scarcity, then the 'thrifty' genotype will again become advantageous. Individuals with that genotype are likely to leave more offspring than those without it. The Nauruan example illustrates that the same genotype can be expressed in either an adaptive (fat-storing) or deleterious (obese diabetic) phenotype, depending on environmental conditions.

(b) In times of persistent plenty, the thrifty genotype results in diabetes, which is damaging to the individual and to their reproductive success. It cannot be preserved in the population by natural selection, because characteristics are only favoured (selected for) if they give the individual or their closest kin (who have some of the same genes) a reproductive advantage. Natural selection cannot favour a characteristic that damages the individual, even if it would be 'in the interests of mankind' as a whole. Neither is natural selection capable of 'foresight'; a characteristic cannot be selected for in the expectation that it will become advantageous in the future (e.g. the thrifty genotype cannot be preserved by natural selection 'foreseeing' that food supplies might suddenly change). The only way to preserve it is by medical treatment and dietary counselling of the diabetic Nauruans, so that they have as many children as non-diabetic Nauruans.

Acknowledgements

Grateful acknowledgement is made to the following sources for permission to reproduce material in this book:

Figures

Figure 1.1 (bottom left-hand image) Camera Press; *Figure 1.1 (other images)* Marion Hall, Mike Levers, Caroline Pond, Jonathan Silvertown, Tina Wardhaugh, Mike Wibberley; *Figures 2.1, 2.2, 4.21, 4.22* Jones, S., Martin, R., Pilbeam, D. and Bunney, S. (eds) (1992) *The Cambridge Encyclopedia of Human Evolution*, Cambridge University Press; *Figures 3.4b (left and right) 3.5b, 3.6* Heather Davies/The Open University; *Figure 3.9a* photos from Perry, M. M. and Gilbert, A. B. (1979) *Journal of Cell Science*, **39**, p. 266, The Company of Biologists Ltd; *Figure 3.9b* photo from Herzog, V., Sies, H. and Miller, F. (1976) *Journal of Cell Biology*, **70**, p. 698, reproduced by copyright permission of the Rockefeller University Press; *Figure 3.12* Dr Gopal Murti/Science Photo Library; *Figures 3.17a, 3.17b* Eye of Science/Science Photo Library; *Figures 3.19a, 3.19b, 3.20b* S101 course material/The Open University; *Figures 4.1a, 4.11b* Mike Levers/Open University; *Figure 4.2* Dr Yorgos Nikas/Science Photo Library; *Figures 4.3a* Department of Cancer Studies, The Medical School, University of Birmingham; *Figures 4.3b, 4.20* L. Willatt, East Anglian Genetics Service/Science Photo Library; *Figures 4.4, 7.2b* CNRI/Science Photo Library; *Figure 4.10* redrawn from Suzuki, P. T., Griffiths, A. J. F. and Lewontin, R. C. (1981) *An Introduction to Genetic Analysis*, W. H. Freeman, San Francisco; *Figure 4.22* Strickberger, M. W. (1990) *Evolution*, Jones and Bartlett; *Figure 5.5* adapted from Bradley, D. J. (1977) *Origins of Pest, Parasite, Disease and Weed Problems*, Cherrett, J. M. and Sagar, G. P. (eds), Blackwell Science Ltd; *Figure 5.9* Adapted from Yorke, J. A. and London, W. P (1973) 'Recurrent outbreaks of measles, chickenpox and mumps, II systematic differences in contact rates and stochastic effects', *American Journal of Epidemiology*, **98**, pp. 469–82, by permission of Oxford University Press; *Figure 6.2a* Juergen Bergen, Max Planck Institute/Science Photo Library; *Figure 6.2b* Professor S. H. E. Kaufmann and Dr J. R. Golecki/Science Photo Library; *Figure 6.3* Courtesy of Professor Robert Dourmashkin, St Bartholomew's and The Royal London School of Medicine and Dentistry, London; *Figures 7.4, 7.5* Durham, W. H. (1991) *Coevolution, Genes, Culture and Human Diversity*, Stanford University Press; *Figure 8.2* Reprinted with permission from *Geriatrics*, **12**(40) 1957. Copyright © Advanstar Communications Inc. Advanstar Communications Inc. retains all rights to this material; *Figure 8.5a* Hemel Hempstead General Hospital, Radiography Department; *Figure 8.5b* Milton Keynes General Hospital, Radiography Department; *Figure 9.6* Modell, B., Kuliev, A. M. and Wagner, M. (1991) *Community Genetics Services in Europe*, WHO, Regional Office for Europe, Copenhagen; *Figure 10.1* The New York Times.

Tables

Table 4.1 Newman, H. H., Freeman, F. N. and Holzinger, K. J. (1937) *Twins: a Study of Heredity and Environment*, University of Chicago Press; *Tables 5.2, 5.3* World Health Organisation; *Table 7.1* Adapted from Durham, W. H. (1991) *Coevolution, Genes, Culture and Human Diversity*, Stanford University Press.

Un-numbered photographs/illustrations

pp. 19, 40 Caroline Pond; *p. 20* Karl Amman/BBC Natural History Unit Picture Library; *p. 23* Dr Franz B. M. de Waal, Living Links Center, Emory University; *p. 25* Yvonne Ashmore; *pp. 28, 136* John Birdsall Photography; *pp. 30, 43* Mike Wibberley; *p. 39* John Paul Kay, Peter Arnold Inc./Science Photo Library; *p. 41* London Aerial Photo Library; *p. 45* Jeremy Hartley/Panos Pictures; *p. 47* Hulton Getty Picture Collection, *p. 73* A. Barrington-Brown; *p. 97* The Grabowski family; *p. 128 (left)* Reuters/Popperfoto; *p. 128 (right)* Ali Jarekji/Reuters/Popperfoto; *p. 139* Muriel Nicolotti/Still Pictures; *p. 141* David Turnley/Corbis Images; *p. 143* Wellcome Trust Photo Library; *p. 162* EM Unit, VLA/Science Photo Library; *p. 167* Courtesy of the Multiple

Index

Entries and page numbers in orange type refer to key words which are printed in bold in the text. Indexed information on pages indicated by *italics* is carried mainly or wholly in a figure or a table.